LUNG FUNCTION TESTS:
PHYSIOLOGICAL PRINCIPLES
AND CLINICAL APPLICATIONS

Commissioning Editor: Maria Khan
Project Editor: Rachel Robson
Project Supervisor: Mark Sanderson
Typeset by Saxon Graphics Ltd
Printed in China

LUNG FUNCTION TESTS: PHYSIOLOGICAL PRINCIPLES AND CLINICAL APPLICATIONS

Edited by

Professor J M B Hughes

and

Professor N B Pride

Division of Respiratory Medicine
Imperial College School of Medicine,
Hammersmith Hospital,
London W12 0NN

W.B. SAUNDERS
London • Edinburgh • New York • Philadelphia • Sydney • Toronto

W.B. SAUNDERS
An imprint of Harcourt Publishers Limited

© Harcourt Brace and Company 1999. All rights reserved.
© Harcourt Publishers Limited 2000. All rights reserved.

 is a registered trademark of Harcourt Publishers Limited

No part of this publication may be reproduced, stored in a retrieval system, or transmitted in any form by any means, electronic, mechanical, photocopying, recording or otherwise, without the prior permission of the publishers (Harcourt Publishers Limited, Robert Stevenson House, 1-3 Baxter's Place, Leith Walk, Edinburgh EH1 3AF), or a licence permitting restricted copying in the United Kingdom issued by the Copyright Licensing Agency, 90 Tottenham Court Road, London W1P 0LP.

ISBN 0-7020-2350-7

First published 1999
  Reprinted 2000
  Reprinted 2001

British Library Cataloguing in Publication Data
A catalogue record for this book is available from the British Library

Library of Congress Cataloging in Publication Data
A catalog record for this book is available from the Library of Congress

Medical knowledge is constantly changing. As new information becomes available, changes in treatment, procedures, equipment and the use of drugs become necessary. The authors and publishers have, as far as it is possible, taken care to ensure that the information given in this text is accurate and up to date. However, readers are strongly advised to confirm that the information, especially with regard to drug usage, complies with latest legislation and standards of practice.

The publisher's policy is to use paper manufactured from sustainable forests

Printed in China by RDC Group Limited
C/03

Contents

Foreword P T Macklem		ix
Preface J M B Hughes, N B Pride		xi
Acknowledgements		xii

Section I SPIROMETRY AND MECHANICS

1.	Tests of forced expiration and inspiration N B Pride	3
2.	Airflow resistance N B Pride	27
3.	Lung volumes and elasticity G J Gibson	45
4.	Respiratory muscles J Moxham	57

Section II GAS EXCHANGE, CONTROL OF BREATHING, EXERCISE

5.	Pulmonary gas exchange J M B Hughes	75
6.	Diffusing capacity (transfer factor) for carbon monoxide J M B Hughes	93
7.	Control of breathing P M A Calverley	107
8.	Measurement of breathlessness P W Jones	121
9.	Exercise testing M D L Morgan	133

Section III APPLICATIONS OUTSIDE THE ROUTINE LABORATORY

10.	Sleep-disordered breathing J R Stradling	151
11.	Pediatric pulmonary function M Silverman, J Stocks	163
12.	Pulmonary function in the intensive care unit P D Macnaughton, T W Evans	185
13.	Domiciliary oxygenation and assisted ventilation A K Simonds	201

Section IV APPLICATIONS WITHIN THE ROUTINE LABORATORY

14.	Assessment of airway responses and the cough reflex *P W Ind, N B Pride*	219
15.	Pre-operative evaluation for thoracic surgery *P A Corris*	233
16.	Pulmonary vascular disease *J M B Hughes*	245
17.	Interpretation of the diffusing capacity (transfer factor) with special reference to interstitial lung disease *J M B Hughes*	259
18.	Examples of pulmonary function in different conditions *J M B Hughes*	273
19.	Presentation of pulmonary function test results to the clinician *J M B Hughes*	287
	Glossary of Abbreviations	297
	Index	303

Contributors

Professor PMA Calverley,
Aintree Chest Centre,
University Hospital,
Aintree, Liverpool L9 7AL

Dr PA Corris,
Department of Respiratory Medicine,
Freeman Hospital,
High Heaton,
Newcastle upon Tyne NE7 7DN

Professor TW Evans,
Intensive Care Medicine,
Imperial College School of Medicine,
Royal Brompton and Harefield NHS Trust,
London SW3 6NP

Professor GJ Gibson,
Department of Respiratory Medicine,
Freeman Hospital,
High Heaton,
Newcastle upon Tyne NE7 7DN

Professor JMB Hughes,
Division of Respiratory Medicine,
Imperial College School of Medicine,
Hammersmith Hospital,
London W12 0NN

Dr PW Ind,
Division of Respiratory Medicine,
Imperial College School of Medicine,
Hammersmith Hospital,
London W12 0NN

Professor PW Jones,
Division of Physiological Medicine,
St. George's Hospital Medical School,
London SW17 0RE

Dr PD Macnaughton,
Director of Intensive Care,
Derriford Hospital,
Plymouth PL6 8DH

Dr MDL Morgan,
Department of Respiratory Medicine &
Thoracic Surgery,
Glenfield Hospital,
Leicester LE3 9QP

Professor J Moxham,
Department of Respiratory Medicine,
King's College School of Medicine & Dentistry,
London SE5 9PJ

Professor NB Pride,
Division of Respiratory Medicine,
Imperial College School of Medicine,
Hammersmith Hospital,
London W12 0NN

Professor M Silverman,
Department of Child Health,
University of Leicester,
Robert Kilpatrick Clinical Sciences Building,
Leicester Royal Infirmary,
Leicester LE2 7LX

Dr AK Simonds,
Royal Brompton Hospital,
Royal Brompton & Harefield NHS Trust,
London SW3 6NP

Dr J Stocks,
Reader in Respiratory Physiology,
Portex Unit,
Institute of Child Health,
Great Ormond Street Hospital for Children,
London WC1N 1EH

Dr JR Stradling,
Osler Chest Unit,
Churchill Hospital,
Headington, Oxford OX3 7LJ

Foreword

How appropriate it is that this book has been written. When I was asked to undertake the pleasant task of writing a foreword I quickly accepted, not only because it is an honour to do so, but also because in North America, at least, respiratory physiology is at risk of becoming a lost art, a 'paleoscience'. Knowledge of respiratory function, nonetheless, is absolutely crucial to the understanding, diagnosis and management of chest disease.

Today, molecular biology, which has given us such a wealth of exciting new knowledge, is also undermining the foundations upon which good medicine is based. Medicine has become so fascinated by molecules that it is in danger of ignoring important features that can neither be predicted nor understood by studying the parts of a system in isolation. Asthma, for example, is a disease characterized by the potential for almost unlimited airway narrowing in response to the trigger of an attack. Normal people usually do not respond to these triggers, but if they do, they are protected by a mechanism that constrains the degree to which airways can narrow to safe limits. The excessive response of the asthmatic and the limited response of healthy people are integrated phenomena. The understanding of functional integration is health and disease is fundamental to physiology and medicine. This is what this book is all about and that is why it is so welcome.

Respiratory function tests, represent the most powerful tools we have available for the diagnosis of many respiratory diseases. Just as one cannot make a diagnosis of hypertension without measuring blood pressure, so one cannot diagnose COPD, asthma, restrictive disorders, respiratory muscle weakness and many other chest diseases without function tests. To understand the natural history of many lung diseases and to determine how they respond to therapy also requires function tests. Sadly, this seems to have been forgotten in recent years.

I congratulate the editors and authors of this volume for producing a book which emphasizes the practical aspects of respiratory function testing. Hopefully, this will bring about a renaissance of the science of respiratory pathophysiology and restore it to its rightful pre-eminence in respiratory medicine.

Peter T. Macklem
Professor of Medicine
McGill University

Montreal Chest Institute
3650 St Urbain Street
Montreal, Quebec
Canada H2X 2P4

Preface

This book arose from the Hammersmith Hospital Course on Clinical Applications of Pulmonary Function which took place every 1–2 years between 1980 and 1995. The external speakers on the course have kindly agreed to expand their lectures into chapters for the book.

Attendance on the Course in the early years mainly comprised doctors in training who expected to be running a Pulmonary Function Laboratory as one of their clinical responsibilities. Latterly, non-medically qualified laboratory staff (those who actually make the measurements) tended to outnumber the doctors. In the planning, writing and editing of this book, we have tried to cater for both groups. Lung Function Tests are performed to help clinicians in their management of patients' illness. Many of these tests require considerable co-operation from the subjects; indeed, one of the main attractions (and, occasionally, frustrations) of working in a Lung Function Laboratory is the one-to-one contact with the patient. Laboratory staff need a good knowledge of the underlying physiology and clinical indications for these tests, perhaps more now than before with the development of automated techniques which remove much of the repetitive drudgery, but carry the risk of accepting each test as a 'black box'. If staff have a good understanding of the reasons for performing the tests, they will be better equipped to obtain the necessary confidence and co-operation of their patients and to answer the questions they inevitably pose in the pauses between repeating the measurements.

The horizons of pulmonary function are continually widening. A good grasp of physiological principles is still required, as outlined in Sections I and II. Section III of the book deals with measurements of pulmonary function not normally associated with a routine lung function laboratory, and demonstrates the expanding scope of the subject. The last section returns to the routine laboratory, and reminds the reader of the many referrals to the lung function laboratory which come from non-respiratory teams. The theory behind the commonly used pulmonary function tests is explained, not as a lesson in pure physiology, but in the context of clinical application. This is not a technical manual; the focus is "why you do it and what it means", not "how you do it".

There is still no sign of agreement between North America and Europe over the question of units (we have tended to give both SI and traditional) although we have the impression that the *système internationale* (SI) is gaining ground. As with many other specialised areas of medical science, many terms and abbreviations which are not in common use have been introduced over the years. Becoming familiar with these represents a considerable first hurdle for newcomers to the field. Attempts to develop these systematically have had only limited success – as is inevitable if the area is not completely static – and synonyms abound. In this book we have had to make our own choice of terms and abbreviations, but have included a Glossary which attempts to help the reader through this tiresome area. The spelling is American, i.e. as English used to be! Overall, in our choices, we hope we have not offended both sides of the Atlantic.

JMB HUGHES
NB PRIDE

Acknowledgements

We wish to thank our colleagues who have contributed chapters, to the clinical laboratory staff in pulmonary function at Hammersmith Hospital over the last decade or so, especially Ann Watson, Carin Mordin, Caroline Dixon, Matthew Higham, Richard Magee, Jo Spring and Joanne Curtis, to Evelyn Fuggle for research assistance, to Jan Marshall for secretarial help, to Doig Simmonds for help with the artwork and to our clinical registrars and research fellows who are too numerous to mention individually.

Section I: SPIROMETRY AND MECHANICS

1 Tests of Forced Expiration and Inspiration

N B Pride

- **SPIROMETRY**
  Forced expiratory volume in one second (FEV_1)
    Applications
  Differences between slow (relaxed) and forced vital capacity
  Other spirometric measurements
  Maximum voluntary ventilation
  Flow-volume analysis

- **PHYSIOLOGICAL BASIS**
  Maximum expiratory flow
  Maximum inspiratory flow

- **TECHNICAL ASPECTS**
  Performance of the forced expiratory vital capacity maneuver
    Dependence on effort
    Quality control using MEFV curves
  Instruments
  Selection of 'best' tests and repeatability
  Variation in the normal population and reference values
  Performance of the forced inspiratory vital capacity maneuver

- **MAXIMUM EFFORT FLOW-VOLUME CURVES**
  Standard techniques
    Intrathoracic airways obstruction
    Extrathoracic airways obstruction
    Respiratory muscle weakness
    Restrictive lung disease
  Special techniques
    Role of lung recoil in reducing maximum expiratory flow
    Localization of site of airflow obstruction
    Maximum effort flow-volume curves via the nose
    Maximum effort flow-volume curves during cough
  Tidal flow-volume curves
    Changes between rest and exercise
    Detection of expiratory flow limitation
    Detection of inspiratory flow limitation

- **PEAK EXPIRATORY FLOW**
  Physiological basis
  Technical aspects
  Applications
  Intrathoracic airway obstruction
  Extrathoracic airway obstruction
  Restrictive lung disease
  Nasal peak inspiratory and expiratory flow

SPIROMETRY

Forced expiratory volume in one second (FEV_1)

Analysis of the volume versus time curve during a maximum effort forced expiratory vital capacity maneuver started from total lung capacity (TLC) is by far the most performed test of respiratory mechanics, having spread from the laboratory to the wards and outpatient clinics and gradually into the offices of general practitioners. In particular, FEV_1 is the best characterized test of respiratory function; information on changes with age, gender, ethnic group, growth, and disease is more developed than for any other test, repeatability is good, and it provides useful information across the whole range from normal to advanced disease. Extensive recommendations on the performance and standardization of spirometry are published by the American Thoracic Society[1] and European Respiratory Society[2] and should be known to all those undertaking spirometry; the most important technical points are dealt with later in this chapter, after factors determining maximum expiratory flow have been discussed.

Applications

Reductions in FEV_1 reflect the total effects of reduction in total lung capacity, obstruction of the airways, loss of lung recoil and, relatively uncommonly, gross weakness of respiratory muscles. The FEV_1 is mainly used to assess intrathoracic airways obstruction, either in clinical practice or in epidemiological surveys. In chronic obstructive pulmonary disease (COPD), the level of FEV_1 is used to grade the severity of obstruction, and FEV_1 is linked better to prognosis than any other single test of lung function. FEV_1 is not particularly sensitive in detecting mild changes, however, and once obstruction is severe, there is not a close relationship between FEV_1 and dyspnea. A major application of FEV_1 is the assessment of bronchodilator and bronchoconstrictor responses; this is discussed in Chapter 14.

Reductions in FEV_1 may also reflect reduction in TLC (restrictive disease of the lungs), such as occurs with widespread fibrosis of the lungs or removal of a lung. Whereas obstruction is associated with slower lung emptying, reduction in TLC is associated with normal or even accelerated lung emptying. This distinction is simply assessed by measuring the ratio of FEV_1 to the total volume expired in the forced expiration (forced vital capacity, FVC) or to a separately obtained slow vital capacity (VC). Normally the FEV_1/VC ratio is greater than 70–75% although it does fall slowly with increasing age.

For initial assessment, it is useful to measure the FEV_1/VC ratio but because VC is less repeatable than FEV_1 in airflow obstruction, the variability of the FEV_1/VC ratio is greater than for FEV_1. For follow-up of mild airways obstruction the change in FEV_1 usually provides more reliable information.

Differences between slow (relaxed) and forced vital capacity

In the United Kingdom and North America, vital capacity is usually measured during a slow expiration from TLC, with increasing effort used below functional residual capacity (FRC) to expire to residual volume (RV). In normal subjects a full VC may be expired in 3 s, and a slow VC equals FVC.

Figure 1.1 Measurements from the spirogram

(a) Forced expiratory and forced inspiratory vital capacity maneuvers

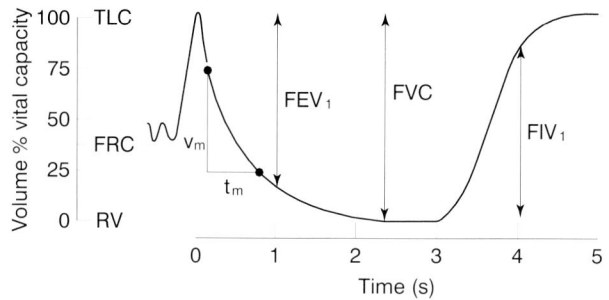

Maximum mid-expired flow (MMEF) is calculated by measuring the time to expire the middle 50% of the FVC. MMEF = $\dot{V}m(L)/tm(s)$. This gives an average expiratory flow between 75 and 25% FVC.

Other time intervals (0.5, 0.75 and 3 s) have been tried for FEV but are rarely used.

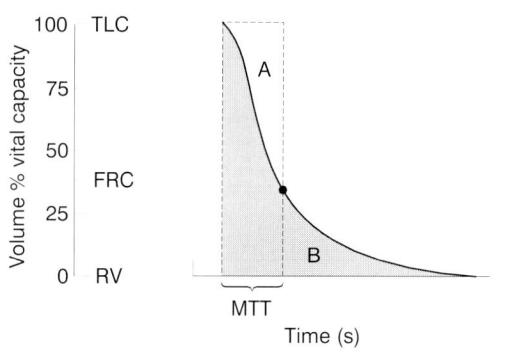

Mean transit time (MTT) The area under the normalized forced expired spirogram (diagonal shaded area) is measured. MTT is the point on the time axis where area A = area B. The distribution of transit times is calculated by dividing the spirogram into 20 ml volume decrements and calculating time from onset of expiration to the mid point of each volume decrement.

(b) Maximum voluntary ventilation (MVV) is measured as the sum of the tidal expired volumes during 12 or 15 s of rapid breathing with maximal inspiratory and expiratory efforts and expressed as $L.min^{-1}$.

(c) Vital capacity (VC)

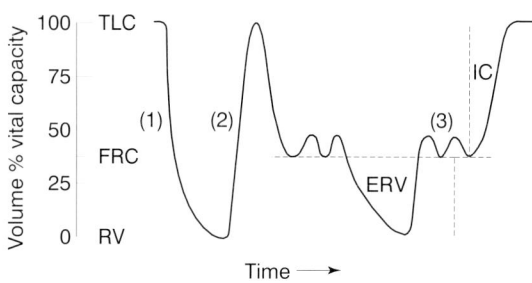

Vital capacity can be measured as (1) the volume expired from TLC to RV during a forced expiration (FVC) or a slow (relaxed) maneuver, (2) as the volume inspired from RV to TLC, (3) as the sums of inspiratory capacity (volume inspired from FRC to TLC) and expiratory reserve volume (volume expired from FRC to RV). In healthy subjects all these methods give similar results, but FVC is lower than other methods in patients with intrathoracic airflow obstruction.

In other European countries the standard technique has been first to expire to RV and then to measure an inspiratory VC up to TLC. Again there is no systematic difference between an inspiratory and expiratory VC in normal subjects.

The value of VC is much more dependent on the technique used when there is airways obstruction. In general, inspiratory VC gives the largest values, while slow expiratory VC started from TLC is consistently larger than the FVC. VC is sometimes obtained by measuring inspiratory capacity (IC) and expiratory reserve volume (ERV) separately, and with airway disease this two-part maneuver also usually gives larger values than FVC from forced expiration. The reasons for expiration being terminated at a larger volume during a forced maneuver than in one using less expiratory effort are poorly understood.

Other spirometric measurements

FEV_1 is a rather insensitive method for detecting changes in mild intrathoracic airways obstruction, and so other analyses of the forced expiratory spirogram have been used. The longest established is the maximum mid-expiratory flow (MMEF) which gives an average flow over the mid-portion of the spirogram. Several other measurements to assess the curvilinearity of the spirogram have been proposed but none has been established as useful.

When airway disease is distributed unevenly between parallel pathways, the most obstructed pathways take longer to empty during forced expiration than normal pathways. This inequality of lung emptying can be assessed by measuring the mean transit time and the distribution of transit times of the forced expiratory spirogram. The analysis may be useful for detecting minor abnormalities because it is biased towards the terminal part of the spirogram which changes most with normal aging and in the early stages of airway disease.

Occasional use has been made of spirometry during a forced inspiratory vital capacity maneuver to assess obstruction to inspiratory airflow. Usually the forced inspiratory volume in one second (FIV_1) has been measured but this is reduced only when inspiratory obstruction is severe; FIV_1 in normal subjects is usually about 95% of inspiratory FVC.

Maximum voluntary ventilation

Before the introduction of the FEV_1, the major dynamic spirometric test was maximum voluntary ventilation (MVV), in which the subject was asked to breathe in and out of a spirometer as fast and as deeply as possible for 12–15 s; the results were expressed as $L.min^{-1}$. This could be exhausting and depended on coaching the subject; repeated testing was required to ensure a maximum result which was obtained, usually with a small tidal volume at an elevated lung volume and a high frequency of breathing (a pattern of breathing similar to that used in strenuous exercise by patients with COPD but not by normal subjects). In patients it was recognized that reductions in MVV were usually associated with expiratory slowing. After the introduction of the FEV_1, MVV was measured much less often; instead $FEV_1 \times 35$ or 40 was used to predict an 'indirect' maximum breathing capacity. While these estimates were adopted for normal subjects, they have proved less successful in predicting whether patients with COPD and other respiratory diseases reach ventilatory limits on strenuous exercise (or during CO_2 rebreathing). In general, maximum ventilation on exercise in COPD patients with severely reduced FEV_1 is greater than 40 times FEV_1. This problem is alluded to in Chapters 7 and 9.

One obvious problem is that a 15 s MVV could not be expected to predict the maximum ventilation which could be sustained over several minutes of exercise; a more relevant test is measurement of the MVV that can be sustained over 4 minutes. The level of end-tidal PCO_2 has to be maintained at a constant level by adding CO_2 to the circuit and the test is rarely performed. Whereas normal subjects can only sustain about 60% of their 15 s MVV for 4 minutes, patients with COPD and a reduced 15 s MVV are able to sustain this level of ventilation for 4 minutes.

Various attempts have been made to improve prediction of maximum exercise ventilation in COPD from measurements made at rest, using either FEV_1 alone or FEV_1 and maximum inspiratory flow or maximum inspiratory pressure (PImax) or, more directly, from complete maximum flow-volume curves. None of these predictions has yet become established for clinical use. Direct measurements of MVV should be informative also in respiratory muscle weakness where single measurements at rest probably exaggerate the ability to sustain ventilation on exercise.

- FEV$_1$ is the measurement of choice for diagnosing intrathoracic airflow obstruction and for assessing its progression, and for epidemiological studies of airway function.
- Forced vital capacity is similar to slow inspiratory or expiratory vital capacity in healthy subjects, but smaller in patients with COPD: when reporting FEV$_1$/VC ratio, it should be stated if FVC or VC has been used.
- Maximum voluntary ventilation can be measured directly or estimated as 35 (or 40) × FEV$_1$; the latter may underestimate maximum exercise ventilation in patients with COPD.
- Other measurements from the forced expiratory spirogram may be useful for detecting mild intrathoracic airflow obstruction.

Flow-volume analysis

The most informative alternative to spirometry for analyzing maximum effort vital capacity maneuvers is the maximum flow-volume curve. The flow-volume analysis has been particularly informative in understanding the factors underlying the generation of maximum flow, but its use is often qualitative; only peak expiratory flow (PEF) has been adopted as a stand-alone test for clinical use.

PHYSIOLOGICAL BASIS

Maximum expiratory flow

Tests of forced expiration were introduced on an empirical basis by clinicians; however, extensive subsequent research showed that these tests reflect the mechanical properties of the lungs, providing a sound physiological basis for their use. The factors determining maximum expiratory flow are best explained by considering pressure and flows at one lung volume.

During breath-holding with open glottis, the pressure in the alveoli (Palv) and all airways is atmospheric; pleural pressure (Ppl) is negative (Figure 1.3a) and exactly balances the positive lung recoil pressure (PL) which is the difference between Palv and Ppl. Increases in pleural pressure at this volume result in a positive Palv and expiratory flow (Figure 1.3b). The positive pleural pressure however also compresses the airways, especially the central intrathoracic airways, increasing their resistance. Airway closure does not occur because the driving pressure for expiratory flow (Palv) is also increased by increases in Ppl. Above a certain minimum expiratory pressure, the increased driving pressure precisely counterbalances the increased resistance so that, at any given lung volume, expiratory flow via the mouth reaches a maximum plateau value which remains constant with further increases in pressure (Figure 1.4). The compressed central airways act as flow-limiting segments (FLS; also known as 'choke points') and the plateau value of maximum expiratory flow provides the basis for the relative independence from the precise expiratory pressure applied.* The factors determining maximum expiratory flow at each lung volume are the lung recoil pressure, the dynamic resistance of the airways up to the site(s) of FLS, and the mechanical properties of the airways at FLS, so flow during

Figure 1.2 Forced expiratory maneuver shown as expired volume versus time (spirogram) and expiratory flow versus expired volume (maximum expiratory flow-volume – MEFV – curve) in a normal subject

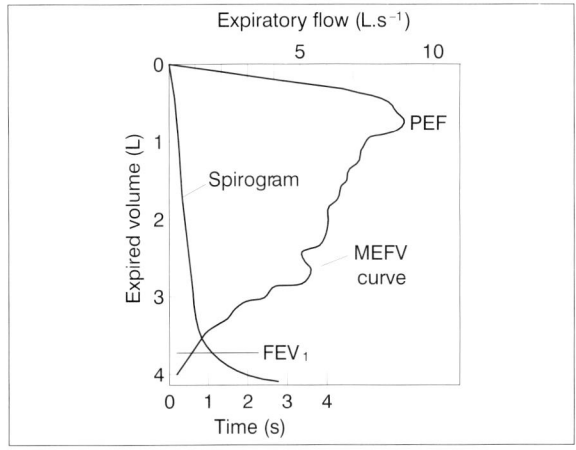

* The actual mechanism limiting maximum expiratory flow is the achieving of a critical 'wave speed' in some part(s) of the tracheobronchial tree (usually either the trachea or in several parallel lobar or segmental bronchi).[3]

Figure 1.3 Pressures during breath-holding and breathing

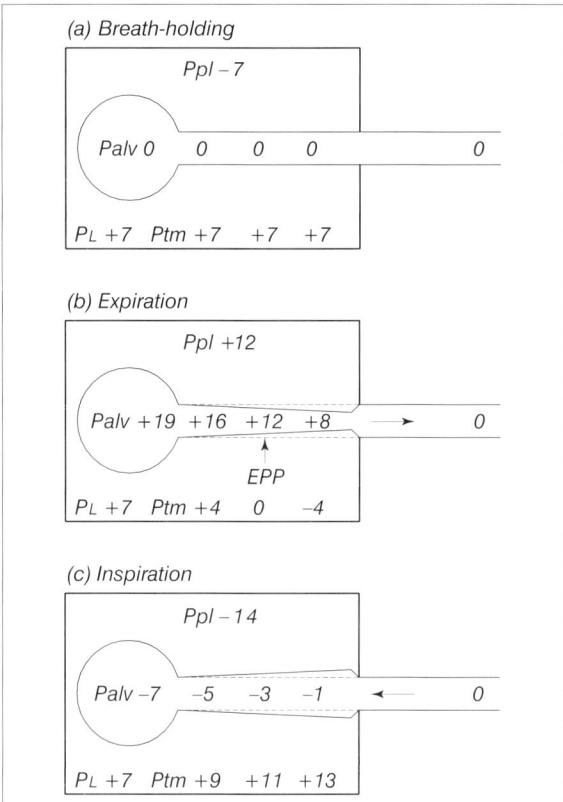

The three panels schematically show pressures (cmH$_2$O) at the same lung volume, where lung recoil pressure (P$_L$) is +7 cmH$_2$O.

Ppl = pleural pressure, Palv = alveolar pressure, P$_L$ = static transpulmonary pressure (Palv–Ppl), Ptm = transmural pressure of airway.

Ptm of all the airways are positive (distending the airways) during breath-holding and inspiration, but may be negative (compressing the airways) during forced expiration. The point in the airway where airway pressure = Ppl and Ptm = 0 has been termed the equal pressure point (EPP).

Figure 1.4 Isovolume pressure-flow curve at mid vital capacity

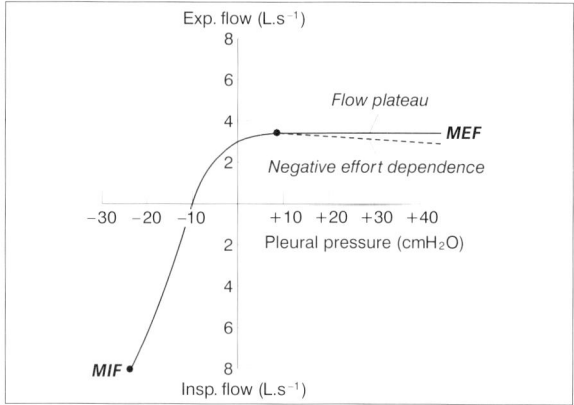

Schematic relation between pleural pressure (Ppl) and flow at one lung volume (mid-vital capacity). This relation is obtained by performing many expirations and inspirations with varying effort.

On expiration, flow reaches a maximum (MEF) at a Ppl of about 9 cmH$_2$O; further increases in Ppl usually generate unchanged values of MEF, which is then described as independent of effort. In a few subjects there may be a small fall in expiratory flow as Ppl is increased (negative effort dependence).

On inspiration, flow increases as Ppl is reduced and maximum inspiratory flow (MIF) is determined by the most negative dynamic Ppl and is therefore effort dependent.

forced expiration reflects the important mechanical properties of the lungs. At large lung volume, driving pressures in excess of those required to achieve maximum expiratory flow cannot be achieved in normal subjects. While peak expiratory flow (PEF) may be associated with achieving flow limitation in the trachea, the value of flow depends on the rapidity with which expiratory pressure is increased; the more rapidly this is generated, the larger the lung volume at which peak flow is achieved, and the higher the value of peak flow. In normal subjects, while FLS are probably in the trachea or central extrathoracic airways at volumes greater than functional residual capacity, over the last 25% of the vital capacity they move towards the alveoli.

When there is intrathoracic airway obstruction with slowing of lung emptying, dynamic expiratory alveolar pressures are *larger* than in normal subjects while pressures required to achieve maximum flow at a given volume are *smaller*, so measurements are less dependent on the subject's effort and plateau conditions for expiratory flow may be achieved throughout the vital capacity. FLS may be less centrally placed than in normal subjects.

Maximal inspiratory flow

In normal subjects, on forceful inspiration via the mouth intrathoracic airways are progressively distended by increases in transairway pressure as alveolar pressure becomes more negative (Figure 1.3c), so no intrapulmonary airflow limitation develops, and flows generated are always dependent on the dynamic intrathoracic pressure achieved (Figure 1.4). This remains the case when there is intrathoracic airways obstruction, but inspiratory dynamic narrowing can occur with disease of the extrathoracic airways or when breathing via the nose, as discussed below.

- Increasing expiratory effort at any lung volume at first increases expiratory flow, but at most lung volumes a plateau of flow is reached.

- The plateau of expiratory flow develops because, above a critical level, the increase in alveolar pressure produced by increasing pleural pressure is exactly counterbalanced by compression of large intrathoracic airways, which act as flow-limiting segments.

- The plateau of expiratory flow makes flow independent of the precise maximum effort applied, except for peak expiratory flow.

- When there is intrathoracic airflow obstruction, maximum expiratory flows are achieved with lower pleural pressures (less expiratory effort) than in healthy subjects.

- Inspiratory efforts dilate intrathoracic airways, so maximum inspiratory flow is effort dependent when breathing via the mouth.

TECHNICAL ASPECTS

Performance of the forced expiratory vital capacity maneuver

Forced expiratory vital capacity maneuvers started from total lung capacity (TLC) are the standard means of assessing the mechanical function of the lungs. Although it is an artificial maneuver, quite unrelated to normal tidal breathing, values are highly repeatable with proper attention to technique. Most of our knowledge of the natural history and prognosis of diseases associated with airway obstruction has been obtained using this simple technique.

The same technical requirements apply for spirometry and for obtaining maximum flow-volume curves. Indeed, visualizing the MEFV curve provides excellent quality control for obtaining reliable measurements of FEV_1 and FVC. Forced expirations should be started immediately after a rapid inspiration to TLC; they should commence rapidly and forcefully and be continued until flow ceases. In young normal subjects, forced expiration is usually complete in three seconds. In older normal subjects a slow expiratory flow may persist for many seconds and termination of the maneuver reflects persistence and breath-holding ability; this is even more the case in subjects with airway disease in whom the maneuver may also provoke coughing towards end expiration. Forced expirations should be continued for a minimum of 6 s and preferably 12 s. In the presence of airway disease, FVC is systematically smaller than the slow vital capacity (VC). In analyzing the MEFV curve and in obtaining maximum mid-expiratory flow or mean transit time from the spirogram, FVC must be used, but FEV_1 may be expressed as a ratio of either FVC or a slow VC obtained in a separate maneuver. Once a complete forced expiration has been performed for initial assessment, follow-up may require only FEV_1. If PEF alone is to be measured, the forced expiration need only be sustained for about 1 s.

The large expiratory airway pressures generated during forced expiration normally result in apposition of the soft palate to the posterior pharyngeal wall, so that a nose clip is usually not necessary. Values are similar in the sitting and standing positions, but prolonged expirations sustaining a high intrathoracic pressure reduce cardiac output and cerebral blood flow so the test is best performed seated, particularly in patients.

Dependence on effort [4]

Although there is usually a plateau of expiratory flow at a given lung volume over a wide range of pressures, sometimes there is a gradual reduction from maximum levels as the expiratory driving pressure is increased ('negative effort dependence') (Figure 1.4) . Furthermore, during a forced expiration lung volume decreases not only because of the volume of gas expired at the mouth, but also from compression of alveolar gas by the positive intrathoracic pressure (which may result in > 10% reduction in lung volume). Alveolar gas compression is not detected by measurements at the mouth using a pneumotachograph (or spirometer) but when the maneuver is performed expiring to atmosphere while seated within a body plethysmograph, the change in thoracic gas volume (TGV) is due to both factors. For precise analysis of lung mechanics in research studies maximum expiratory flow should be measured at a known TGV, particularly when there is airways obstruction which reduces the expiratory flow at the mouth, while allowing the generation of high intrathoracic pressures at large lung volumes.

The practical outcome of 'negative effort dependence' and thoracic gas compression is that the volume expired in 1 s may be greater with a relaxed or submaximal effort than with a maximum effort, particularly when there is severe airways obstruction. This may partly account for exercise performance being better than predicted from the FEV_1. Although a few laboratories have attempted to measure the largest volume expired in 1 s, this measurement requires a large number of efforts and considerable coaching and has not proved repeatable; furthermore the large database available on spirometry has always been obtained with a maximum expiratory effort.

Quality control using MEFV curves[5]

With some untrained or uncooperative subjects, inadequate or erratic expiratory effort can be detected by non-repeatability of the MEFV curve. Real-time visualization of the MEFV curve provides excellent quality control of depth of inflation and effort applied during a forced expiration and may become a routine criterion for accepting spirometric tests.

The most common problems on expiration are a slow start, visualized on the MEFV curve as failure to achieve the highest PEF, and 'dropping off' of the MEFV curve at small volume (Figure 1.5). The details of the MEFV slope should be highly repeatable.

If the preceding inspiration is slow or there is a significant pause at TLC (Figure 1.6), values of expiratory flow are reduced.

Instruments

Flow must be measured with a fast-responding device able to record accurately up to $12 \, L.s^{-1}$. For MEFV and maximum inspiratory flow-volume (MIFV) curves this can be done with a pneumotachograph or other flow measuring device or alternatively by differentiat-

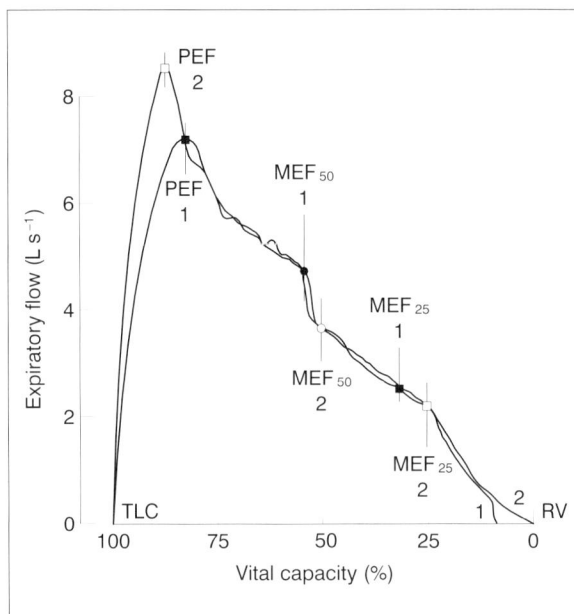

Figure 1.5 Common errors in obtaining MEFV curves

The two most common faults (shown on curve 1) are (a) a slow start to forced expiration resulting in peak expiratory flow (PEF) being achieved later and at a smaller lung volume and so being lower than on repeat curve 2, and (b) failure to complete forced expiration to RV ('dropping off curve' with flow still continuing); this will result in inaccuracies in measuring MEF at 50% and 25% FVC, as shown by the difference in MEF_{50} measured from curve 1 and from the correct curve 2 (which in this normal subject is particularly large because of the large decline in MEF over a small change in volume). The differences in PEF and FVC have no significant effect on FEV_1.

The descending limb of the MEFV curve may show considerable detail which is repeatable in an individual but variable between normal individuals, contributing to the wide range of reference values for MEF_{50} and MEF_{25}.

ing the rate of volume change in a rapid-response flow-volume spirometer. The latter method has the advantage that it does not have to be recalibrated for changes in gas density or viscosity, as may occur with helium-oxygen breathing or even with increased concentrations of inspired O_2. The resistance of the apparatus should be low, particularly for measuring values of peak expiratory flow. Simple devices for measuring PEF may give significantly different values from those obtained with apparatus used for MEFV and MIFV curves.

In contrast, the best instruments for recording the spirogram are still direct volume recording devices; although pneumotachographs and other flow measur-

Figure 1.6 Effect of preceding inspiration and pause at full inflation

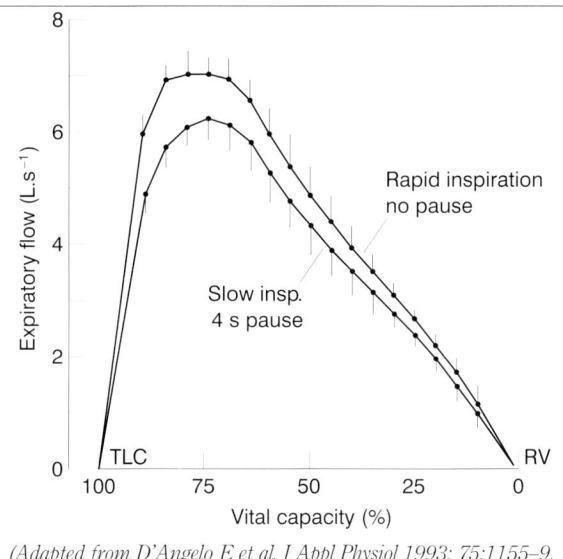

(Adapted from D'Angelo E et al. J Appl Physiol 1993; 75:1155–9, with permission)[6]

ing devices have a rapid response time and are easier to clean, methods integrating flow at the mouth are less robust and are influenced by density of the gas, dirt or water droplets increasing the resistance of the device, and limits to their linearity. The dynamic resistance of spirometers is high during forced expirations but this mainly affects PEF and does not have a significant effect on the FEV_1.

Temperature control is a problem both for spirometers and flow measuring devices – the latter are usually heated. For spirometers it is usually assumed that warm expired gas instantly adopts the ambient temperature although a few spirometers have a rapidly responding internal thermometer. Internal spirometer temperature can rise with frequent expiratory use at short intervals.

Spirometers are subjected to careful checks before being sold commercially, but rigorous tests are not yet consistently applied to other devices, such as PEF monitor gauges. Extensive recommendations on instrumental characteristics are available.[1,7]

Selection of 'best' tests and repeatability

The FEV_1, FVC, and VC all depend on maximum effort, so that variation in obtained values is biased by submaximal efforts (whereas with measurements of many other tests over- and under-estimates are equally likely). As a result most experts suggest that maximum values from three technically satisfactory attempts should be used, provided the second best test is within 100 ml or 5%; others have recommended that the mean of the three best tests should be used. The best FEV_1 and best FVC can be taken from separate maneuvers. In practice, no important discrepancy has been attributed to which of these techniques has been used. For PEF the largest value from three technically satisfactory attempts is also recommended; the second best value should be within 30 L.min^{-1}. Selection of the best MEFV curve is less standardized. The American Thoracic Society recommends the largest sum of FEV_1 and FVC,[1] while the European Respiratory Society suggests that the best three technically satisfactory maneuvers should be superimposed at TLC and the largest values on the composite envelope recorded.[2] Another possibility is the use of a combination of PEF and FVC to select the single best MEFV curve. No recommendations have been developed for MIFV curves.

If tests are poorly repeatable there is no point in repeating them too often: in a few asthmatic subjects, increased airway narrowing may be provoked. Repeatability may be different between normal subjects and those with disease and it is obviously desirable for each laboratory to repeat measurements in their own subjects and so establish their own laboratory standards. Adequate standards have so far only been developed for conventional spirometry, which is more repeatable than PEF, which in turn is more repeatable than other values of maximum expiratory flow taken from the MEFV curve.

Variation in the normal population and reference values[1,2,8]

There is a large between-individual variation in maximum expiratory flow even when the maneuver is performed with good technique and after allowing for height, age, and gender; this probably reflects a true difference in airway geometry for a given size of lungs. While the most common normal shape of the MEFV curve has a well defined peak flow followed by a fairly linear decline in flow to residual volume, there is sometimes a near-plateau of maximum flow over a considerable part of the vital capacity followed by a rapid decline over the remaining vital capacity that is similar to the normal canine MEFV curve and is found particularly in healthy young adults (Figure 1.2). The pattern is believed to indicate the presence of FLS in the trachea over the near-plateau followed by a 'jump' to more peripheral sites of flow limitation at the 'shoulder' of the curve.

In normal subjects, such a high proportion of the FVC is expired in the first second that these large variations in flow-volume contour have little effect on values of FEV_1 which show much less variation in the normal population.

Reference values are available for PEF, maximum expiratory flow at 50% of FVC and when 25% of FVC remains to be expired (MEF_{50} and MEF_{25}), the last showing a particularly wide range. Reference values for spirometry are much more developed and are based on age, sex, height, and ethnic group; recent reference values are derived from non-smokers without particular exposure to environmental pollution. With current predicted values there is still a considerable residual variation between individuals so that 1 SD for FEV_1 and VC is about 10–15% of the mean value. Men have a larger FEV_1 than women even when height is taken into account. At a given height and age Caucasians have larger FEV_1 than Asians (Indians or Chinese) while Africans have intermediate values.

Airway function probably reaches a maximum between 18 and 23 years but decline with age cannot be demonstrated definitely until the late twenties in healthy never-smokers. Thus reference values in adults 18–25 years are assumed to be unchanged. Individuals who start smoking in adolescence before lung growth is complete may show slightly reduced maximum values, and also show decline in FEV_1 in their early twenties. In middle age healthy never-smokers show an average decline of ~30 ml.yr^{-1}, with smokers at this age showing mean declines of 45–60 ml.yr^{-1}.

Performance of the forced inspiratory vital capacity maneuver

Flows generated during forced inspiratory vital capacity maneuvers started from RV are dependent on the dynamic intrathoracic pressure achieved and generally require more training before the best flow-volume curves are obtained.

A common problem in trial efforts is a smooth 'bite' out of the ascending curve as flow increases; this is due to partial collapse of the extrathoracic airway (presumably tongue and pharynx) induced by the accompanying subatmospheric airway pressure (Figure 1.7). With repeated efforts this is lost as the subject learns to activate the upper airway muscles during the forced inspiratory vital capacity maneuver but repeatability is still less than for the MEFV curve. A pattern in which maximum inspiratory flow is rather low in the upper 30% or so of the VC is common. If this pattern is seen efforts should be made to encourage the subject to increase and sustain inspiratory effort.

Measurements from the MIFV curve are not well standardized. Peak inspiratory flow (PIF) occurs at a varying volume in the middle third of the VC. MIF may be compared with MEF at 50% of the expiratory vital capacity. Timed volume measurements from the forced inspiratory spirogram are not very useful because, in normal subjects and those with moderate impairment of MIF, the forced inspiratory volume in one second (FIV_1) is a very high proportion of the inspiratory VC and there are few data on $FIV_{0.5}$. In general, normal values of MIF and PIF are related to the size of the VC but there are no reference values available. This is surprising because tidal inspiratory flow may be a high proportion of MIF during exercise in patients with COPD or respiratory muscle weakness.

Figure 1.7 Effect of pharyngeal collapse on MIFV curve.

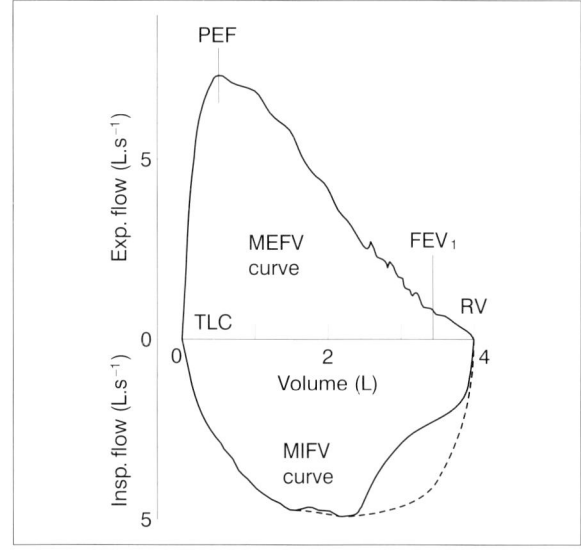

- Standard forced expiratory maneuvers require a full inflation to TLC, a minimum pause at TLC, and a rapid generation of large expiratory pressures; forced expirations should be continued if possible until flow (volume change) ceases.

- In some patients, large expiratory pressures may produce flows (and volume change) which are slightly less than those achieved with smaller pressures (negative effort dependence); however, maximal expiratory efforts should be used to measure FEV_1 and MEFV curves.

- The shape of the descending limb of the MEFV curve varies widely between normal individuals, resulting in a much wider range for reference values than is found for FEV_1.

- Airway function, as measured by FEV_1, begins to decline in young adults at a younger age in smokers than in healthy never-smokers.

MAXIMUM EFFORT FLOW-VOLUME CURVES

Maximum flow-volume curves are commonly used as a supplement or alternative to similar information provided by spirometry (severity of airflow obstruction, etc.), but there are also more specific applications where they provide important information which cannot be obtained from spirometry:

Distinctive patterns
- Intrathoracic obstruction:
  – changes in mild disease
  – two-compartment emptying
- Extrathoracic obstruction:
  – fixed
  – dynamic
- Respiratory muscle weakness

Localization of intrathoracic obstruction
- Helium-oxygen breathing
- Comparison of isovolume flow on maximal and partial expiratory curves

Flow limitation
- Expiratory: in intrathoracic obstruction
- Inspiratory: in nasopharyngeal obstruction

Standard techniques

Although the detailed shape of the maximum effort flow-volume curve is highly reproducible within an individual (Figure 1.5), there are large differences in absolute values of flow between healthy individuals. Hence maximum effort flow-volume curves are often used only for qualitative pattern recognition, unless an intra-subject comparison is available (e.g. before and after bronchodilators, deep inflation, etc.).

Intrathoracic airways obstruction

The characteristic change is the development of curvilinearity, convex to the volume axis, in the maximum expiratory flow-volume (MEFV) curve (Figure 1.8). Obtaining MEFV curves is particularly useful:

1. In mild obstruction when pronounced curvilinearity is present when other values are only slightly abnormal.
2. When there is some doubt about the significance of a low FEV_1 - for instance when the FEV_1/VC ratio is relatively preserved but there is a suspicion that the effort has not been sustained to the true RV.

With intrathoracic airway obstruction, increased tidal expiratory pressure enhances dynamic compression but the more negative tidal inspiratory pressure distends the airways so tidal differences between inspiratory and expiratory airway dimensions are enhanced. This is true also of MEFV and maximum inspiratory flow-volume (MIFV) curves, the MIFV curves being less severely impaired and retaining their smooth shape. There have been suggestions that the contrasts between PEF and flows at small volume on the MEFV curve and between MEFV and MIFV curves are greater in emphysema than in asthma but these group differences are not useful in diagnosis in

Figure 1.8 Intrathoracic airways obstruction

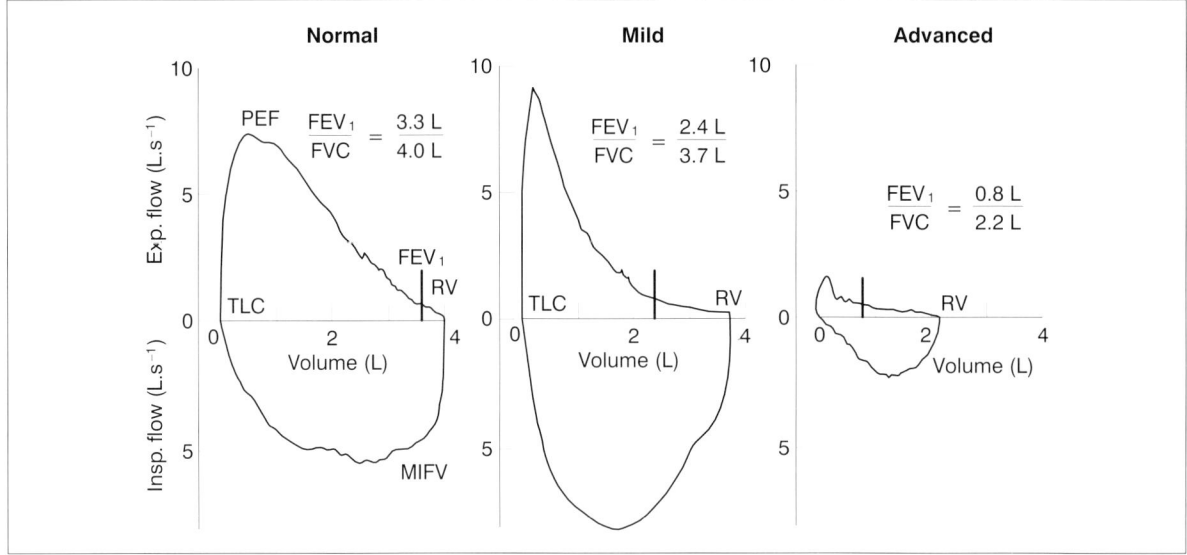

an individual. In normal subjects, PEF reflects the characteristics of the largest intrathoracic airways, while MEF_{50} and especially MEF_{25} are more influenced by the smaller airways. But when airflow resistance is increased by disease – whether it is in large or small airways – PEF, MEF_{50}, and MEF_{25} are all reduced. There is no distinctive pattern of MEFV curve that reflects small airway disease, such as bronchiolitis, but airway closure may be enhanced leading to particularly large increases in RV and decreases in VC and FVC.

A distinctive but rare pattern is 'two compartment' filling and emptying of the lungs, when one lung is normal and the other severely obstructed (Figure 1.9). This occurs after single lung transplantation for emphysema, or when a main bronchus is blocked by tumor.

Extrathoracic airway obstruction

Transairway pressures in the extrathoracic airway show a completely different pattern on forced maneuvers because extra-airway pressure is close to atmospheric pressure and is not influenced by inspiratory or expiratory efforts. On expiration, airway pressures within the extrathoracic airway are above atmospheric pressure and maintain the airway open: on inspiration, the subatmospheric pressure in the extrathoracic airways narrows the airway unless it is supported against collapse by activation of the surrounding muscles. In practice, during forceful inspiratory efforts through the mouth held open by a mouthpiece in normal subjects, there usually is no significant extrathoracic airway narrowing once initial practice maneuvers have ensured adequate co-activation of upper airway muscles of the tongue and pharynx (see Figure 1.7).

Distinctive patterns in flow-volume curves are found which reflect differences in the transmural pressure developed during forceful maneuvers in the extrathoracic and intrathoracic airways. As already

Figure 1.9 Two compartment filling and emptying

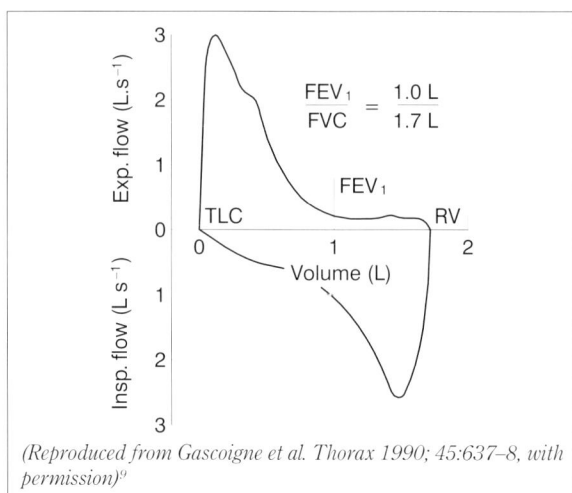

(Reproduced from Gascoigne et al. Thorax 1990; 45:637–8, with permission)[9]

discussed, dimensions of the *intrathoracic* airways at a given lung volume tend to enlarge on forced inspiration, but dynamic compression of central intrathoracic airways develops on forced expiration (Figure 1.3). In contrast, dimensions of the *extrathoracic* airway are maintained on forced expiration but tend to narrow on inspiration.

A distinction may be made between fixed obstruction of the extrathoracic airways which leads to a relatively symmetrical pattern of maximum expiratory and inspiratory flow, and a pattern where there is dynamic narrowing of the extrathoracic airways which reduces maximum inspiratory flow, but in extreme cases may not affect maximum expiratory flow.

Tracheal stenosis and laryngeal paralysis are examples of conditions which give a 'fixed' obstruction pattern; dynamic narrowing may be associated with weakness of the muscles surrounding the supralaryngeal airway such as may occur in some patients with obstructive sleep apnea even when awake, with laryngeal polyps or tumors, and weakening of the tracheal wall, either primary or following surgery or intubation.

FEV_1 may be well preserved with extrathoracic airway obstruction: this is because any reduction in maximum expiratory flow is confined to the upper part of the vital capacity or may even be absent. The pattern shown in Figure 1.10 (left) can be detected by finding a reduction in PEF which is greater than the reduction in FEV_1. The best measurements to make however are complete maximum expiratory and inspiratory flow-volume curves.

Various attempts have been made to diagnose abnormalities predisposing to obstructive sleep apnea (OSA). OSA is caused by repetitive collapse of the pharyngeal airway in response to the subatmospheric pharyngeal pressure during tidal inspiration. Thus factors which increase collapsibility of upper airway muscles (decreased neural activation, increased muscle compliance) or enhance tidal subatmospheric pharyngeal pressure (small dimensions of pharynx, increased nasal resistance) predispose to OSA.

Oral maximum effort flow-volume curves in awake, seated subjects sometimes show a low maximum inspiratory flow/maximum expiratory flow ratio suggesting a small oropharyngeal airway; alternatively sawtooth inspiratory flow oscillations indicating instability of the upper airway have been observed.

Both changes are claimed to be of high specificity but very low sensitivity; this probably reflects that the changes have to be severe before they are detected by tests performed in such different circumstances (oral breathing, maximum effort, sitting and awake) from spontaneous occurrence during sleep. Tests of breathing via the nose when supine and asleep are more promising (see page 22 and Chapter 10).

'Functional' obstruction of the extrathoracic airway when the patient is awake presents a particular problem: it is characteristically episodic and may mimic acute asthma, and airway function tests may be highly variable. Two distinct patterns have been

Figure 1.10 Extrathoracic airway obstruction

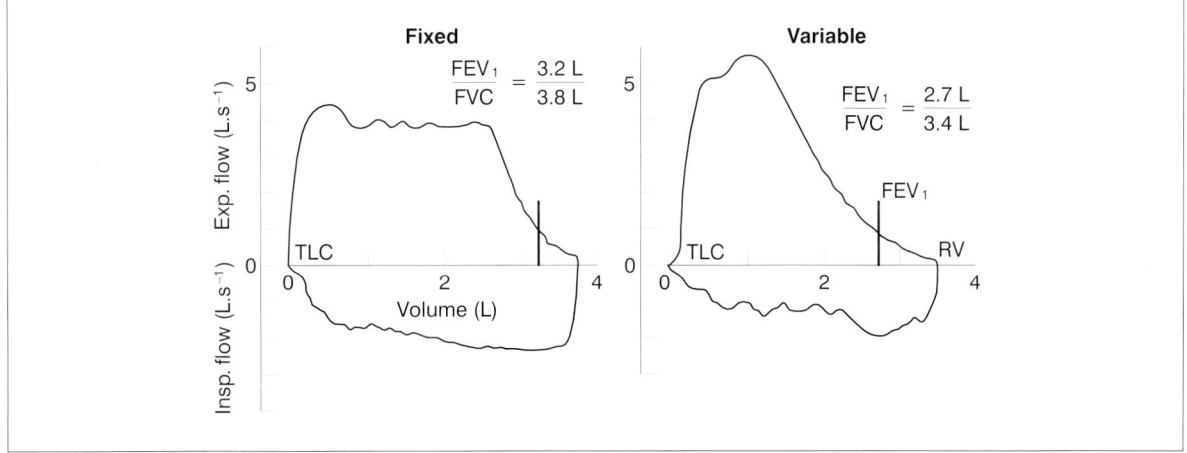

described. Most commonly, inspiratory stridor is associated with reduction in maximum inspiratory flow throughout the vital capacity and normal maximum expiratory flow; sometimes however there is reduction in both maximum inspiratory and expiratory flow. Limited endoscopic examinations suggest that the obstruction is in the larynx. Typically patients are young women with recurrent attacks of noisy acute breathlessness. The second type of functional wheezing is mainly expiratory and is produced by forceful breathing close to residual volume. This is associated with completely normal maximum flow-volume curves; the wheeze probably arises from excessive tidal narrowing of central intrathoracic airways during expiration. Curves are often poorly repeatable. Other aspects of lung function such as blood gases, single-breath N_2 test, and functional residual capacity are usually normal.

Attempts to detect nasal obstruction or abnormalities of the pharyngeal airway in obstructive sleep apnea have included measuring nasal as well as mouth MEFV and MIFV curves; these are discussed in a later section.

Respiratory muscle weakness

Characteristic changes are a reduction in PEF, which is achieved later in expiration at a smaller lung volume, and a reduction in flow throughout the MIFV curve (Figure 1.11). These changes reflect a reduction in the pressures achieved and also a slower rise of pressure at the onset of a forced expiration and a smaller TLC and VC. As with extrathoracic airway obstruction, FEV_1/FVC is often well preserved. In severe expiratory muscle weakness the effectiveness of cough may be impaired. This may be suspected by comparing the standard MEFV curve with curves obtained with successive coughs during expiration; normally cough results in transient spikes of expiratory flow above the standard MEFV curve (see below, Figure 1.17). These spikes are reduced or lost with expiratory muscle weakness.

Restrictive lung disease

Although TLC and VC are reduced, there may be an increase in lung recoil and preserved or even relatively enlarged airway dimensions.

The consequence is that although PEF is reduced, the slope of MEF versus expired volume may be increased and forced expiratory emptying accelerated (Figure 1.12), resulting in an abnormally high FEV_1/VC ratio.

On inspiration the increase in lung recoil might be expected to decrease maximum inspiratory flow but in practice changes in inspiratory curves are not distinctive.

Figure 1.11 Respiratory muscle weakness

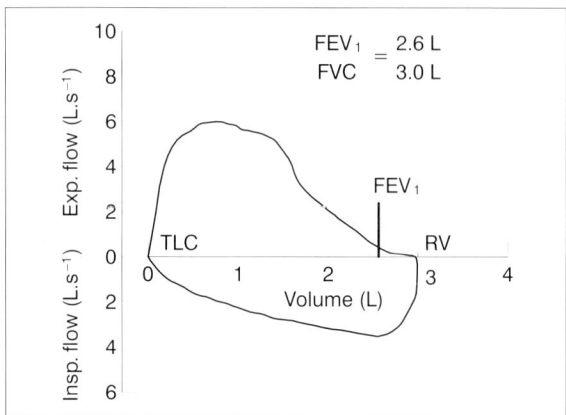

Figure 1.12 Sarcoidosis before and after treatment

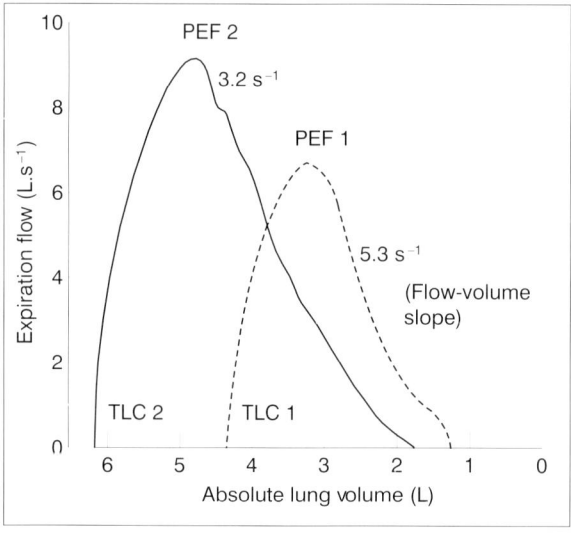

MEFV curves before (-----) and after (——) corticosteroid treatment in a patient with sarcoidosis. Before treatment (1) TLC, PEF, and FVC were reduced but the flow-volume slope was super-normal (5.3 s^{-1}) indicating accelerated emptying of the lungs. After treatment (2) TLC, PEF, and FVC all increased and the flow-volume slope fell.

- Curvilinearity of the MEFV curve is a good indicator of mild *intrathoracic* airflow obstruction.
- *Fixed* and *dynamic* obstruction of the extrathoracic airway can be detected by distinctive patterns of MEFV and MIFV curves.
- Respiratory muscle weakness produces distinctive changes in MEFV and MIFV curves.

Special techniques

Additional techniques have been developed to assess the site and mechanism of intrathoracic airflow obstruction, to assess nasal function and cough, and to detect expiratory and inspiratory flow limitation.

Role of lung recoil pressure in reducing maximum expiratory flow

Lung recoil pressure (P_L) (see Chapter 3) is a major determinant of maximum expiratory flow (MEF), acting as an important component of the total driving pressure for expiratory flow and as an indication of the forces distending the intrathoracic airways via alveolar attachments to their perimeter. In emphysema, but not in asthma, there are large reductions in lung recoil pressure which contribute to the reduction in maximum expiratory flow. This contribution can be examined by plotting maximum expiratory flow versus static lung recoil at different lung volumes (Figure 1.13). The possible abnormalities are shown schematically.

In practice a reduction in maximum expiratory flow caused solely by loss of lung recoil pressure is rarely found except in the mild airway obstruction of early emphysema. The ratio MEF/P_L is sometimes called 'upstream' conductance; this indicates the dynamic conductance of all the parallel airways from the alveoli to the points in the airways where the intra-airway pressure has fallen to a value equal to Ppl ('equal pressure points') (Figure 1.3). This ratio remains normal when reduction in maximum expiratory flow is solely due to loss of P_L. Although 'upstream' conductance for maximum expiratory flow only measures the conductance of part of the total tracheobronchial tree, while plethysmographic and other techniques measure the total conductance of

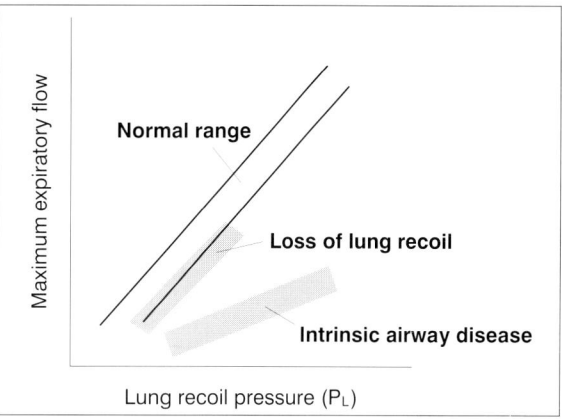

Figure 1.13 Role of loss of lung recoil pressure in reducing maximum expiratory flow (MEF)

In a few patients with emphysema, loss of lung recoil pressure may entirely account for reductions in MEF by truncation of the curve. Intrinsic airway disease leads to reduced $\Delta MEF/\Delta P_L$ slope. Most commonly in COPD there is a combination of loss of lung recoil and intrinsic airway disease, resulting in a reduced $\Delta MEF/\Delta P_L$ slope.

'upstream' and 'downstream' airways, maximal flow 'upstream' conductance may actually be lower than total conductance measured during quiet breathing or panting because of the different measuring conditions which lead to dynamic changes in airway dimensions and large pressure losses within the flowing gas.

Localization of site of airflow obstruction

Comparison of maximum effort curves breathing air and He-O$_2$ Substitution of a low density 80% helium/20% oxygen mixture for air reduces the pressure losses in the large airways where the gas flow velocity is greatest and airflow pattern turbulent. In normal subjects this results in an approximately 60% increase in maximum expiratory flow throughout the VC (Figure 1.14).

In many subjects with intrathoracic airflow obstruction – usually due to asthma or COPD – the increase in maximum expiratory flow when breathing an He-O$_2$ mixture is much reduced or absent; this suggests that the site of flow limitation is no longer in the central intrathoracic airways, as in normal subjects, but has moved to more peripheral airways where flow is presumed to be more laminar and independent of density. This change is usually attributed to increased frictional losses in narrowed peripheral airways, but

Figure 1.14 Density dependence of MEFV curves

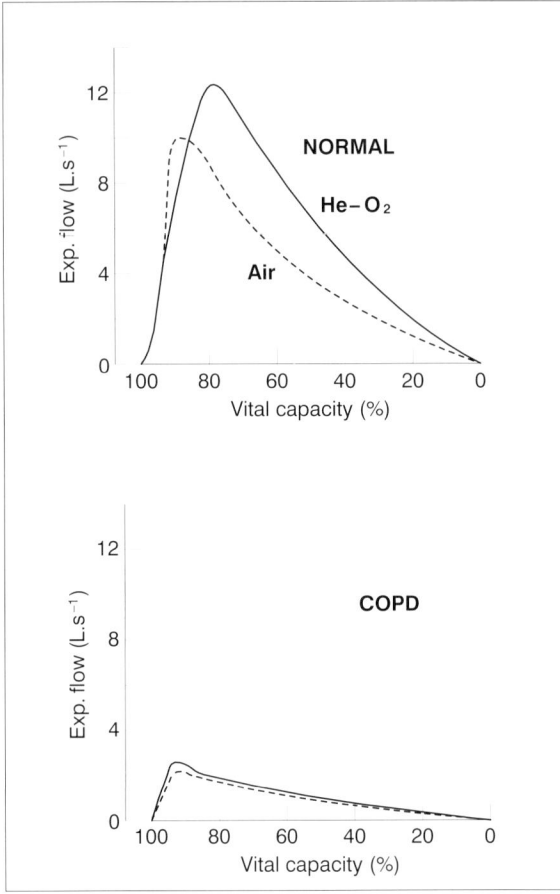

reduced density dependence should not be interpreted as indicating that *only* peripheral airways are narrowed even if they are the site of expiratory flow limitation. The method depends on changes in the airways between the alveoli and the sites of flow limitation (FLS) but animal experiments have shown that relatively small changes in the geometry and location of choke-points could profoundly affect the size of the responses to the He-O_2 so that the technique is now rarely used.

In practice the method is simple; substituting the He-O_2 for air can be achieved sufficiently by taking three VC breaths of the He-O_2 mixture. Care must be taken in measuring flow – the lower density of He-O_2 compared to air means that pneumotachographs have to be recalibrated for He-O_2. It is simpler to use a flow-volume spirometer in which flow is measured by differentiating the rate of volume change.

Alternative related techniques are to *increase* density by substituting a sulfur hexafluoride (SF_6)-oxygen mixture for air, or to measure resistance (usually by the esophageal balloon or forced oscillation technique) when breathing He-O_2. Neither method has been established as useful in pulmonary function laboratories.

Comparison of flow at isovolume on maximum effort partial and complete curves[10] For many years it has been known that a deep inflation (DI) not only immediately distends the airways but may transiently alter airway dimensions subsequently when tidal breathing is resumed. This phenomenon has been used to explain discrepancies between 'large-breath' tests such as the FEV_1 and complete MEFV curve, and 'resting breathing' tests such as airways resistance. To avoid this effect, tests of forced expiration can be commenced from smaller lung volumes at, or a little above, the volume at the end of a tidal inspiration. The effects of a DI can then be studied simply by comparing maximum expiratory flow at 30–40% vital capacity above residual volume from forced expirations begun from the end of a tidal inspiration (partial curve, P) with isovolumic flow during forced expirations started conventionally from total lung capacity (TLC) (maximal curve, M).* From these two forced expirations the results are expressed as M-P ratios. In normal subjects under basal conditions M-P ratios are a little greater than 1.0. In spontaneous episodes of asthma (Figure 1.15a) M-P ratios are < 1.0 (airway function worse after DI) and tend to fall as impairment of FEV_1 progresses. Using a model which examines the response to DI in terms of the relation between parenchymal and airway hysteresis this change has been interpreted as indicating an important obstruction of the most peripheral airways. When acute obstruction is induced by challenge with inhaled drugs, exercise, or hyperventilation M-P ratios rise (Fig. 1.15b), indicating that DI removes the induced obstruction. This has been interpreted as indicating that narrowing has been induced in larger, conducting airways. These interpretations are based on indirect data and the response to DI is complicated by the possibility of inducing changes in airway smooth muscle and/or a change in the compliance of the airway wall.

---

* The terminology is slightly confusing. Both flow-volume curves are maximum effort curves; sometimes they are distinguished as partial and complete (i.e. commenced from total lung capacity).

Figure 1.15 Maximum (M) and partial (P) expiratory flow-volume curves

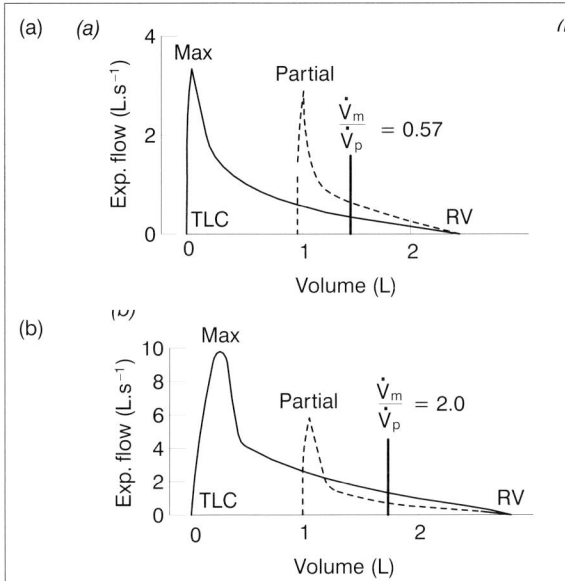

(From Lim TK, Pride NB & Ingram RH. Effects of volume history during spontaneous and acutely induced air-flow obstruction in asthma. American Review of Respiratory Disease 1987; 135:591–6. © American Lung Association)[10]

(a) Effects of spontaneous attack of asthma with flow on MEFV curve less than on PEFV curve, $\dot{V}m/\dot{V}p$ ratio 0.57, and (b) effects of histamine induced obstruction with flow on MEFV curve greater than on PEFV curve ($\dot{V}m/\dot{V}p$ ratio 2.0). The $\dot{V}m/\dot{V}p$ ratio should be measured at a volume level below the transient spike of flow on the PEFV curve.

Maximum effort flow-volume curves via the nose[11]

Oral MEFV and MIFV curves can be used to assess the function of the lower airways, because the mouth (when held open by a large mouthpiece) and the oropharynx (when the surrounding muscles are activated) have a relatively low resistance. When MEFV and MIFV curves are performed through the nose, the usual factors determining oral curves (muscular force applied, pulmonary mechanics) are modified by the additional higher resistance of the nose. Hence comparison of oral and nasal curves can be used to assess nasal patency. Nasal resistance is usually higher than oral resistance, and so nasal maximum flow-volume curves are more dependent on adequate pressure generation than oral curves.

Significant pressures are dissipated across the nose on forced expiration at larger lung volumes, flow limitation becoming intrathoracic at smaller lung volumes when flows via the nose coincide with those expiring via the mouth.

The extent of the difference between nasal and oral maximum expiratory flow-volume curves depends on the nasal airflow resistance. In some normal subjects there are considerable reductions in maximum expiratory flow via the nose, and the curves are similar to oral MEFV curves when there is a fixed laryngeal or tracheal obstruction (Figure 1.10, left), but in others the nasal curve may approach that via the mouth although it never appears to exceed it. On inspiration there is reduction in maximum inspiratory flow on the nasal curve compared with the oral curve at all lung volumes, as would be expected from the additional resistance of the nose. In addition, however, there is flow limitation on forceful inspiration once a driving pressure of about –20 cmH$_2$O is developed in the posterior nasopharynx, so that a pressure-independent plateau of maximum inspiratory flow develops; the level of maximum inspiratory flow is relatively constant throughout the vital capacity. The site of flow limitation appears to be in the anterior nose (nasal 'valve'). Differences between maximum inspiratory flow via the nose and mouth vary greatly between individuals; this may reflect differ-

Figure 1.16 Comparison of nasal and mouth MEFV and MIFV curves in a normal subject

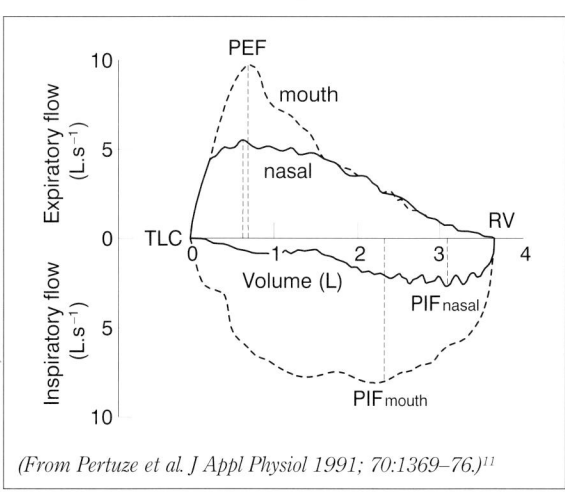

(From Pertuze et al. J Appl Physiol 1991; 70:1369–76.)[11]

The nasal curves resemble oral curves in the presence of fixed tracheal or laryngeal obstruction, indicating that nasal resistance is higher than oral resistance. Instead of measuring complete flow-volume curves, measurements of peak expiratory flow (PEF) and peak inspiratory flow (PIF) can be made with simple peak flow gauges (see page 25–26). Note: nasal and mouth PIF may be at different lung volumes.

ences in the 'valve' but is also influenced by the extent of stabilization of the nasal opening by contraction of the alae nasi muscles.

Both maximum inspiratory and expiratory flow through the nose are increased during exercise (which reduces thickness of the mucosal lining) and by decongestants. Maximum inspiratory flow through the nose can also be increased by activation of the alae nasi muscles which stabilizes the anterior nares. Inspiratory flow limitation facilitates clearance of the nose of foreign particles by permitting these to be moved into the posterior nasopharynx by a sniff which generates a burst of high velocity flow through the nasal valve, in a manner analogous to the expiratory action of cough for the intrathoracic airways. A sniff requires a rapid activation of inspiratory muscles and is used as a 'natural' maneuver to test the pressures generated by these muscles.

Maximum inspiratory flow provides a more specific test of nasal patency than maximum expiratory flow, where reliance is placed on the effects of increased nasal resistance in preventing intrathoracic expiratory flow limitation developing at larger lung volumes. The nose is in series with the lungs and the respiratory muscles, so care has to be taken that reduced flows are not due to inadequate driving pressures (poor cooperation or genuinely weak respiratory muscles) or accompanying lung disease (notably asthma accompanying rhinitis); this can be controlled by comparing nasal and oral curves. Peak expiratory or inspiratory flow via the nose can be measured simply with modified gauges. Proportionate changes in nasal PEF or PIF are smaller than changes in nasal resistance when nasal obstruction is provoked or relieved.

Maximum effort flow-volume curves generated during cough

When a cough is performed below TLC it results in a transient spike of expiratory flow above the flow generated at the same lung volume during a standard MEFV curve started at TLC. This flow is due to the gas expelled from central airways when a large expiratory pressure is generated; after the transient spike of expiratory flow, the remainder of the MEFV curve is superimposed on the standard MEFV curve (Figure 1.17). A similar transient spike of expiratory flow is seen with partial MEFV curves started below TLC (Figure 1.15). Loss of these spikes indicates that there

Figure 1.17 Examples of maximum flow-volume loops with cough efforts superimposed

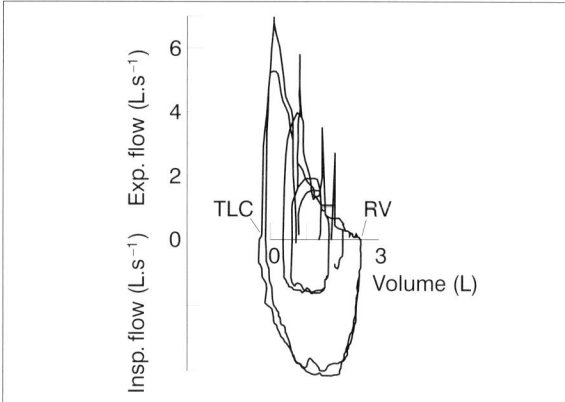

(From Polkey MI, Lyall RA, Green M, Leigh PN, Moxham J. Expiratory muscle function in amyotrophic lateral sclerosis. *American Journal of Respiratory and Critical Care Medicine* 1998; 158:734–41. © American Lung Association)[12]

is poor pressure generation during cough, as occurs with respiratory muscle weakness, but this should be confirmed by direct measurements of maximum expiratory pressures (Chapter 7).

- Low lung recoil pressure (P_L) contributes to reduction in maximum expiratory flow in emphysema.
- Breathing 80% He/20% O_2 instead of air increases maximum expiratory flow in normal subjects. This increase is smaller in most subjects with COPD and asthma.
- A deep inflation to TLC reduces induced airway narrowing in normal subjects but worsens airway narrowing in active asthma.
- Nasal patency can be assessed by comparing nasal and mouth maximum flow-volume curves.

Tidal flow-volume curves

Tidal flow-volume curves have been studied at rest when it is impossible to obtain tests of maximum flow (e.g. infants – see Chapter 11, sleep – Chapter 10). They have also been used to observe how ventilation increases during exercise and to investigate the presence of expiratory flow limitation at rest or during exercise.

Changes in tidal breathing pattern using measurements of tidal volume, breath duration, and mean inspiratory flow are considered in Chapter 7.

Changes between rest and maximum exercise

As intrathoracic obstruction becomes more severe the approximately sinusoidal shape of the resting tidal expiratory flow-volume curve alters, with the highest tidal flow being produced earlier in the breath to be followed by a steep decline in expiratory flow, which may be associated with tidal expiratory flow limitation, and finally interruption of expiratory flow. Changes in tidal flow-volume curves as ventilation is increased during exercise demonstrate the size and position of the tidal volume and the available reserves of inspiratory and expiratory flow when compared with the maximum flow-volume curve (Figure 1.18). In normal subjects, tidal volume is increased both by reducing end-expired lung volume and by increasing end-inspired lung volume. Usually both inspiratory and expiratory flow-volume curves show relatively constant tidal flows on exercise with maximum expiratory flow approached, if at all, only at end expiration. Very fit athletes may approach maximum expiratory and inspiratory flows (using a higher proportion of the available flow capacity) at the end of severe exercise. The exercise pattern in healthy subjects contrasts with that during the 15 s maximum voluntary ventilation test, which is conducted with a small tidal volume closer to TLC and with both inspiratory and expiratory flow reaching the limits of the maximum flow-volume envelope.

In severe airways obstruction, tidal expiratory flow may be maximal at rest; during exercise both end-expiratory and end-inspiratory lung volume increase, allowing an increase in total ventilation. Tidal inspiratory flow also may approach the maximum flow-volume envelope. This dynamic hyperinflation on exercise is an important contributor to the dyspnea of COPD.

Detection of expiratory flow limitation[13]*

In adults during mouth breathing Early studies of expiratory flow limitation during tidal breathing relied on superimposition of tidal and complete expiratory flow-volume curves, the latter usually being performed in the standard way with FVC maneuvers started from TLC. When flow was plotted against

---

* Expiratory flow limitation is used to indicate that maximal expiratory flow is achieved during tidal expiration and is characteristic of intrathoracic airflow obstruction. Some experts use the term chronic airflow limitation as a synonym for COPD to indicate the reduction in maximum expiratory flow that occurs in this disease (and indeed in most other obstructive and restrictive diseases); the latter term does **not** imply that expiratory flow limitation actually occurs during tidal breathing.

Figure 1.18 Schematic tidal flow-volume curves at rest and during maximum exercise, compared to MEFV and MIFV curves in a normal subject and a patient with COPD and moderate airflow obstruction

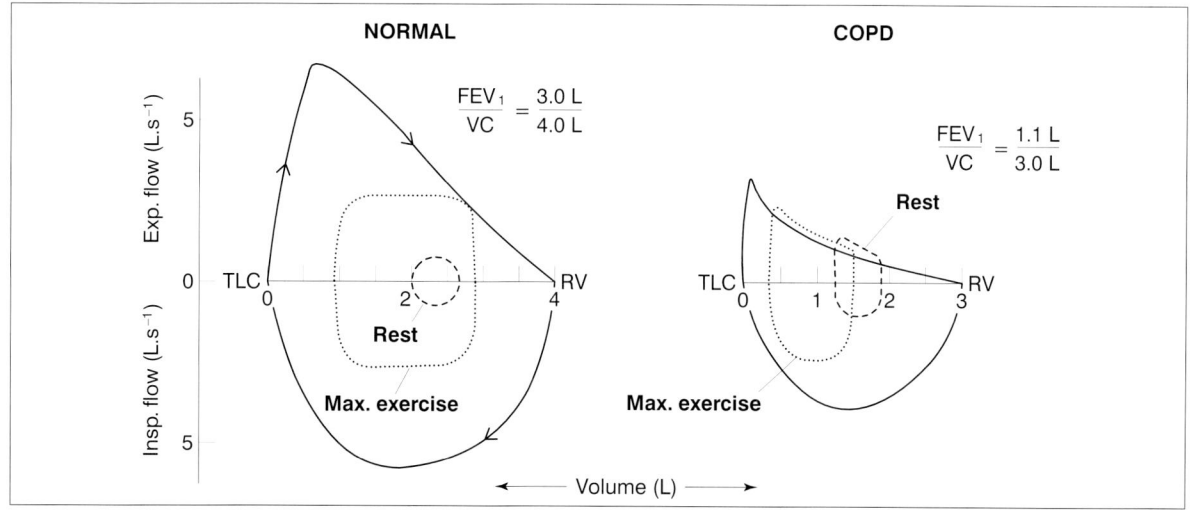

Figure 1.19 Detection of expiratory flow limitation

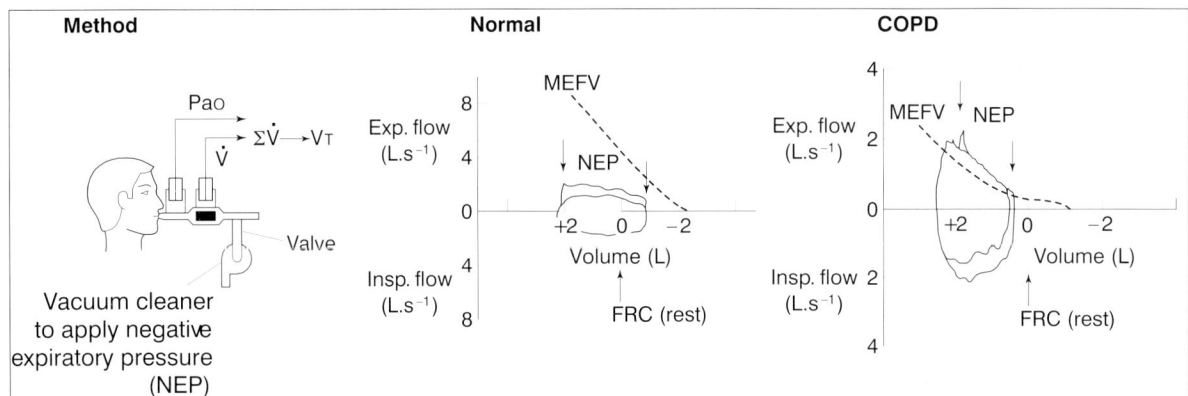

The subject breathes tidally through a pneumotachograph screen which records flow ($\dot{V}$) which is integrated to obtain tidal volume (V_T). After recording baseline V_T, NEP of -5 cmH_2O is applied during the next V_T in which pressure at the airway opening (Pao) is reduced by 5 cmH_2O.

(Adapted from Koulouris NG et al. J Appl Physiol 1997; 82:723–31, with permission)[13]

Both results were obtained during moderate intensity exercise. In the normal subject expiratory flow increases but apart from a transient spike of flow there is no change in a patient with COPD.

The flow and volume scales are different in the two panels. Note the rectangular shape of tidal flow-volume curve in the normal, contrasting with the shape in COPD. Change in volume is referred to end-expired lung volume at rest: note the decrease in normal and increase in COPD during exercise (cf. Figure 1.18). The dashed diagonal lines show the position of the complete MEFV curves. There are considerable reserves of expiratory flow capacity in the normal subject. In the COPD subject at baseline, tidal expiratory flow considerably exceeds that on the MEFV curve at the same volume.

volume expired at the mouth, tidal flow could often exceed that on the concurrent standard MEFV curve in patients with airways obstruction. For research studies tidal expiratory flows were compared with maximum expiratory flows obtained breathing out from a body plethysmograph with varying efforts to achieve true maximum expiratory flows, avoiding the effects of 'negative effort dependence' and thoracic gas compression discussed earlier but still entailing a different volume history.

A much simpler and more accurate method to detect expiratory flow limitation is to apply a small negative expiratory pressure (NEP) (usually -5 cmH_2O) at the mouth during a tidal expiration. This increases the driving pressure for expiratory flow (difference between alveolar pressure and pressure at the airway opening) by 5 cmH_2O and will increase the expiratory flow if this is not maximum (Figure 1.19). This method has the great advantage that it allows for all the effects discussed above, including variations due to the precise volume and time history, and for any change that may occur in airway tone. The negative pressure usually leads to an increase in tone of the muscles surrounding the upper airway, preventing their collapse which could oppose the imposed increase in driving pressure.

In infants during nasal breathing In this technique flow is measured during tidal breathing via a pneumotachograph in a nasal mask and compared with the flow produced at the same volume when intrathoracic pressure is increased by a 'squeeze' around the chest wall within a jacket/body plethysmograph. Maximum flow is measured in the lower part of the VC where the extra resistance provided by the nose is not sufficient to prevent expiratory flow limitation in intrathoracic airways. The supine position and sedation do not appear to cause collapse of the tongue into the pharynx. Further details are discussed in Chapter 11.

Detection of inspiratory flow limitation

In sleeping patients with obstructive sleep apnea, inspiratory flow limitation may develop during nasal tidal breathing before complete obstruction develops. This is recognized by replacement of the normal sinusoidal flow-volume curves by a plateau of inspiratory flow (see Chapter 10) and presumably is caused by pharyngeal narrowing. In contrast to expiratory flow limitation, which is highly dependent on lung volume, inspiratory flow limitation due to upper airway obstruction is similar throughout the VC. Absolute values of maximum inspiratory flow through the nasopharynx are labile because they depend on the activation of tongue and pharyngeal muscles.

- During exercise, normal subjects usually do not reach the limit of the MEFV-MIFV 'envelope', even though the end-expired lung volume decreases.
- When airflow obstruction is severe in COPD, there may be expiratory flow limitation at rest and end-expired lung volume increases during exercise (dynamic hyperinflation).
- Expiratory flow limitation during tidal breathing can be detected by failing to find an increase in expiratory flow when a negative pressure of -5 cmH$_2$O is applied at the mouth.
- Inspiratory flow limitation is indicated by a plateau of inspiratory flow during tidal breathing through the nose.

PEAK EXPIRATORY FLOW

Peak expiratory flow (PEF), like other tests of maximum expiratory flow, was introduced to clinical medicine on an empirical basis. PEF is defined as 'the maximum flow achieved during an expiration delivered with maximal force starting from maximal lung inflation (TLC)'. Its main use is for monitoring airways obstruction in circumstances where spirometry is not available but it has been used also to characterize lung function in epidemiological studies.

Physiological basis[7]

The factors determining PEF are less well understood than for maximum expiratory flow at smaller lung volumes. Conventionally it has been regarded as effort-dependent in healthy subjects, the chief evidence for this being that any added resistance at the mouth reduces the value of PEF. Recent studies have highlighted that values of PEF are more sensitive to the resistance of the measuring instrument and to details of technique than other tests of maximum expiratory flow. To obtain the highest values of PEF, the forced expiration should be started after the shortest possible pause at TLC, and the expiratory pressure increased as rapidly as possible. The PEF achieved will be influenced by the lung volume at which it is achieved; the larger the volume the higher the flow because lung recoil pressure and airway dimensions are larger. In some normal subjects wave speed may be achieved at PEF, but, because PEF is not measured at a fixed lung volume, it remains effort-dependent because with faster rise time of pressure and flow, PEF will be achieved at a larger lung volume. Conversely an added resistance will delay the rise time of pressure and flow and dissipate some of the driving pressure, reducing PEF. An important consequence is that PEF measured with a meter will not be identical with that measured with a pneumotachograph or by differentiating a volume signal.

In normal subjects, PEF is determined by the size of the lungs, lung elasticity, the dimensions and compliance of the central intrathoracic airways, and the strength and speed of contraction of the expiratory (chiefly abdominal) muscles. Frictional resistance of the airways, and particularly of the smaller airways, only makes a small contribution.

Technical aspects

In contrast to other tests of maximum flow, PEF is recorded in L.min^{-1}, following the original instruments. The highest value of three correctly performed blows is recorded at any session; additional blows should be performed if the second best value in a normal subject is > 30 L.min^{-1} lower than the best. A nose clip is not required, but spuriously high values of PEF can be obtained if pressure is built up beneath a closed glottis or behind the tongue pressed into the mouthpiece. Flexion or extension of the neck should be avoided. Forced expiration only has to be sustained for approximately 1 s. Intra-subject variability is greater for PEF than for FEV$_1$. Reference values are less developed, in part because there have been problems with linearity of the scales for mini-meters[14].

Diurnal variation in subjects without respiratory disease has an amplitude of < 10% of the mean value.

Applications

Intrathoracic airways obstruction

PEF is reduced by a variety of respiratory diseases, most commonly obstruction of the intrathoracic airways. In these diseases the increased frictional resistance in smaller airways contributes to the reduced value, allowing PEF to be used to monitor airway function in asthma. The frequent statement that PEF reflects predominantly the caliber of large airways is true only for healthy subjects. In severe airways obstruction a contribution to PEF comes from dynamic narrowing of the central intrathoracic airway at the start of forced expiration, particularly in COPD. In mild airways obstruction the first changes are development of increased curvature of the flow-volume curve with preservation of PEF (Figure 1.8, middle). With more severe airways obstruction in asthma and COPD, PEF is probably less dependent on effort than in normal subjects, with a plateau of maximum flow being achieved even at large lung volumes. PEF will still be larger however when the speed of contraction of the expiratory muscles is increased; characteristically PEF occurs earlier after the start of forced expiration and at a volume closer to TLC in patients with intrathoracic airways obstruction than in healthy subjects.

A reduced PEF does not itself indicate airways obstruction and the diagnosis should always be confirmed by spirometry. Reductions in PEF are relatively less than in FEV_1 as airways obstruction progresses (particularly in COPD) and in general changes with bronchodilator and bronchoconstrictor challenge are proportionately smaller. Despite this lack of sensitivity and the other limitations discussed above, once the initial diagnosis has been made, PEF is of great value for monitoring variation in airway function occurring spontaneously, or with treatment, or occupational and environmental exposure to suspected constrictor agents.

Extrathoracic airways obstruction

PEF is reduced in the fixed type of obstruction (Figure 1.10). A reduced PEF with relatively well preserved FEV_1 is characteristic but complete maximum effort flow-volume curves on expiration and inspiration provide the best diagnostic information.

Restrictive lung disease

PEF is reduced when TLC is reduced (lobectomy, pneumonectomy, pleural effusion, etc.) but the extent of the reduction may be modified by changes in lung elasticity or respiratory muscle strength. In fibrosing alveolitis (idiopathic pulmonary fibrosis) an increased lung recoil pressure at TLC tends to preserve PEF, while in respiratory muscle weakness the slow increase and reduced level of expiratory pressure results in PEF occurring later in expiration and further from TLC than in normal subjects (Figure 1.11), augmenting the reduction in PEF due to a reduced TLC. These factors suggest that PEF is likely to be unreliable in monitoring the acute respiratory muscle weakness that occurs in myasthenia gravis or Guillain-Barré syndrome. In general, PEF is not of value in assessing restrictive lung disease but small lungs should always be considered as an alternative cause of a reduced PEF.

Nasal peak inspiratory and expiratory flow

Maximum flow through the nose can be used to assess nasal obstruction (Figure 1.16). A simple method is to fit an oronasal or nasal face mask to a peak flow meter or mini-gauge and measure nasal peak expiratory flow (nPEF) or, by attaching the mask to the exit of the gauge, nasal peak inspiratory flow (nPIF). Probably nPIF is the more useful of these two measurements. The technique is suitable for home monitoring of nasal obstruction, but little work has been done on this. Changes in nPEF and nPIF are smaller than those in nasal resistance when obstruction is induced or decongestants used. The nose is in series with the lungs, so nPEF and nPIF may be reduced by intrathoracic disease or inadequate effort; nPEF and nPIF should therefore always be compared with values of oral PEF and PIF.

- Peak expiratory flow (PEF) in normal subjects is determined by lung size and elasticity and central airway dimensions.

- In airway disease, PEF is reduced whether obstruction is in large or small airways, so making it suitable to monitor airway function in asthma.

- A reduced PEF by itself does not indicate airflow obstruction as it can be caused by other lung disease: confirmation by spirometry is required.

References

1. American Thoracic Society. Standardization of spirometry. 1994 update. *Am J Respir Crit Care Med* 1995; **152**: 1107–36.
2. European Respiratory Society. Standardized lung function testing. Lung volumes and forced ventilatory flows. 1993 update. *Eur Respir J* 1993; **6**(suppl 16): 5–40
3. Dawson SV & Elliott EA. Wave-speed limitation on expiratory flow – a unifying concept. *J Appl Physiol: Respirat Environ Exercise Physiol* 1977; **43**: 498–515.
4. Krowka MJ, Enright PL, Rodarte JR, Hyatt RE. Effect of effort on measurement of forced expiratory volume in one second. *Am Rev Respir Dis* 1987; **136**: 829–33.
5. Enright PL, Johnson LR, Connett JE, Voelker H, Buist AS. Spirometry in the Lung Health Study. 1. Methods and quality control. *Am Rev Respir Dis* 1991; **143**: 1215–23.
6. D'Angelo E, Prandl E, Milic-Emili J. Dependence of maximal flow-volume curves on time course of preceding inspiration. *J Appl Physiol* 1993; **75**: 1155–9.
7. Lebowitz MD & Quanjer Ph.H (eds). Peak expiratory flow. *Eur Respir J* 1997; **10**(suppl 24): 1–74S.
8. American Thoracic Society. Lung function testing: selection of reference values and interpretative strategies. *Am Rev Respir Dis* 1991; **144**: 1202–18.
9. Gascoigne AD, Corris PA, Dark JH, Gibson GJ. The biphasic spirogram: a clue to unilateral narrowing of a mainstem bronchus. *Thorax* 1990; **45**: 637–8.
10. Lim TK, Pride NB & Ingram RH Jr. Effects of volume history during spontaneous and acutely induced air-flow obstruction in asthma. *Am Rev Respir Dis* 1987; **135**: 591–6.
11. Pertuze V, Watson A & Pride NB. Maximum airflow through the nose in humans. *J Appl Physiol* 1991; **70**: 1369–76.
12. Polkey MI, Lyall RA, Green M, Leigh PN, Moxham J. Expiratory muscle function in amyotrophic lateral sclerosis. *Am J Respir Crit Care Med* 1998; **158**: 734–41.
13. Koulouris NG, Dimopoulou I, Valta P *et al*. Detection of expiratory flow limitation during exercise in COPD patients. *J Appl Physiol* 1997; **82**: 723–31.
14. Pederson DF, Miller MR, van der Mark TW. Performance testing new peakflow meters. *Eur Respir J* 1998; **12**: 261–62.

2 Airflow Resistance
N B Pride

- **PHYSIOLOGY**
  Components of total airflow resistance
  Dependence on phase of breathing, flow and lung volume.
  Variations in airway tone
- **METHODS FOR MEASURING AIRFLOW RESISTANCE**
  Body plethysmography to measure airway resistance (Raw)
  Changes in resistance with changes in lung volume
  Esophageal balloon catheter technique to measure total lung resistance (R$_L$)
  Forced oscillation techniques to measure total respiratory resistance (Rrs)
  Airflow interruption technique (Rint)
- **COMPARISON OF DIFFERENT METHODS FOR ASSESSING AIRFLOW RESISTANCE**
- **REFERENCE VALUES**
- **DISTRIBUTION OF RESISTANCE: SEGMENTAL RESISTANCE**
  Normal subjects
  Chronic obstructive pulmonary disease
  Asthma
  Upper airway resistance
  Nasal resistance
  Oro- or nasopharyngeal resistance
  Resistance of lung tissue and chest wall
- **OTHER TECHNIQUES FOR ASSESSING AIRWAY DIMENSIONS**
- **COMPARISON OF TESTS OF MAXIMUM EXPIRATORY FLOW AND RESISTANCE**

PHYSIOLOGY

Components of total airflow resistance

During tidal breathing the elastic and resistive properties of the total respiratory system determine the pressure required to inflate the lungs. This pressure (ΔP) can be divided into its elastic component (pressure required to change volume, V) and resistive component (Pres, pressure required to generate flow, $\dot{V}$) by the simplified equation of motion of the lungs:

$$\Delta P = E \cdot V + R \cdot \dot{V},$$

where E is elastance (the reciprocal of the more commonly used compliance) and R is resistance. The relevant elastic properties can be divided into two components, those of the lungs and those of the chest wall, which are arranged in series (see Chapter 3). Similarly the resistive pressure can be defined as the total pressure drop in phase with flow through the separate segments of the tracheobronchial tree and across the lung tissue and chest wall, which are arranged in series. While the pressure drop through the airways is a classic ohmic resistance and propor-

Figure 2.1 Serial distribution of total respiratory resistance in a normal young man breathing quietly at rest

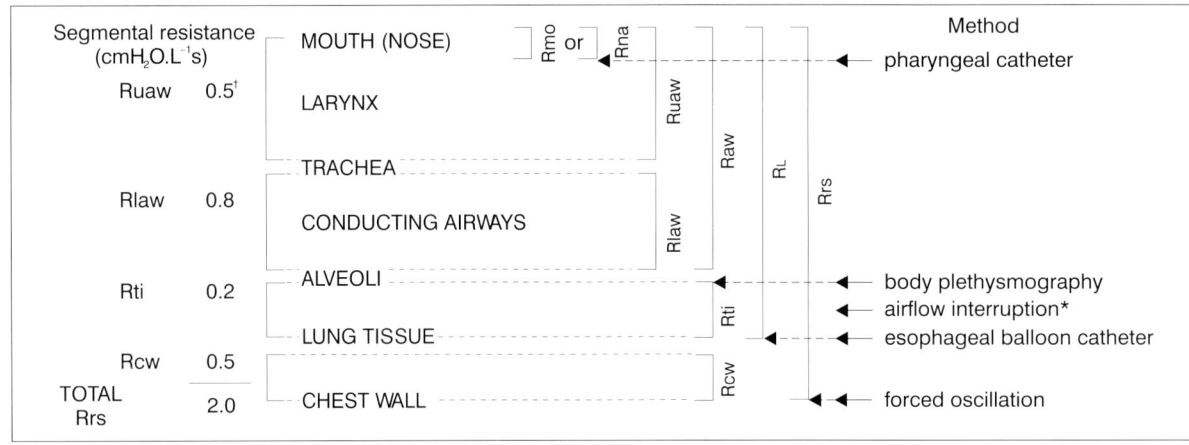

Abbreviations: Rmo – oral airway resistance; Rna – nasal airway resistance; Ruaw – airway resistance above the upper end of the trachea; Rlaw – airway resistance of intrathoracic airways (alveoli to trachea); Raw – total airway resistance; R_L - total pulmonary resistance; Rti – lung tissue resistance; Rcw – flow resistance of chest wall; Rrs – total respiratory resistance.
The total resistance is the sum of all the segments arranged in series.
† *Value when breathing through a large caliber mouthpiece. During nasal breathing Ruaw would be 1–2 $cmH_2O.L^{-1}s$ higher.*
* *Values are usually higher than for Raw but in some circumstances measure Raw accurately.*

tional to flow, pressure drops across the lung tissue and chest wall are not proportional to flow, but rather depend on lung volume, tidal volume, and frequency. Although usually regarded as small in normal subjects, they are included in measurements of total lung resistance (R_L) or total respiratory resistance (Rrs) (Figure 2.1).* Resistance of some of the individual airway segments can be measured by catheters or needles but this is rarely done (except for the nose).

Dependence on phase of breathing, flow and lung volume.

Values of resistance are greatly influenced by the physiological conditions at the time of the measurement, making the technique much less robust than spirometry. These variations are predominantly caused by changes in the airway component. Increases in flow ($\dot{V}$) disproportionately increase Pres due to the development of turbulence and eddies within the flowing gas. The resulting increase in resistance (R, which equals Pres ÷ $\dot{V}$) as flow increases can be expressed by Rohrer's equation:

*In this section, cmH_2O is usually used as the unit of pressure; to convert to kilopascals (kPa) multiply by 0.098 (~0.1).

$$R = k_1 + k_2 \dot{V}$$

where k_1 is a constant indicating a minimum value of R at very low gas flow, which is laminar and orderly, so-called Poiseuille flow, and k_2 expresses the increase in turbulence as $\dot{V}$ increases. The increased driving pressure and changes in transmural pressure of the airways required to increase flow also lead to changes in intrathoracic airway geometry, distending the airways on inspiration and accentuating dynamic airway narrowing on expiration (see Figure 1.3, Chapter 1). Thus expiratory resistance tends to be higher than inspiratory resistance even in normal subjects; this difference is accentuated with intrapulmonary airflow obstruction. If possible, measurements of resistance should be made at low flows, minimizing these effects.

Intrathoracic airway dimensions increase as lung volume increases; patients with severe airflow obstruction utilize this effect by breathing at an increased functional residual capacity (FRC). In the laboratory when bronchodilation is induced, FRC usually falls, whereas FRC rises when significant bronchoconstriction is induced. Other examples where absolute volume change is important are in the assessment of postural changes and in obesity, where FRC is characteristically reduced towards residual volume.

A great advantage of body plethysmography is that lung volume is obtained routinely as part of the measurement. With the other techniques the absolute volume during tidal breathing can be estimated by making a full inflation to total lung capacity after the measurement and measuring absolute volume (close to FRC) by a separate technique (body plethysmography, multibreath helium dilution, or, in the absence of airway obstruction, a single-breath gas dilution technique). Total lung capacity (TLC) does not appear to change with bronchodilation or bronchoconstriction; a small fall – about 100 ml – occurs in the supine position and is similar in normal and diseased lungs.

In measuring airflow resistance the introduction of a large caliber mouthpiece reduces oral resistance; panting, as used in the plethysmographic technique, reduces glottic resistance. These reductions in extrathoracic resistance help to make the measurements sensitive to changes in intrathoracic resistance. With ordinary tidal breathing via the nose, about half the total pressure drop is in the nose; 'natural' oral resistance is also greater than in laboratory conditions. During the high flows of exercise, extrathoracic resistance is minimized by breathing through both the nose and a widely opened mouth. In addition there is an increase in nasal dimensions due to activation of the alae nasi muscles and mucosal vasoconstriction, and dilatation of intrapulmonary airways, mainly because of reduction in vagal tone of airway smooth muscle.

Variations in airway tone

The caliber of the airways is under the control of the autonomic nervous system; most normal subjects have some bronchomotor tone, mediated by vagal efferent nerves, which is reduced during exercise. At rest this tone can be removed by muscarinic antagonists (e.g. atropine or ipratropium) or β_2-adrenoceptor agonists, reducing airflow resistance by about 30%. The tone of the intrathoracic airways shows a circadian rhythm, peaking at about 4.00 hours, when resistance is highest, and being least at about 16.00 hours. Sequential tests of airway pharmacology should therefore have similar starting times on each day of study. Tone can be briefly increased by many inhaled stimuli such as cold air, cigarette smoke, dusts, and air pollutants. In asthma the circadian rhythm has a similar timing, but variation is amplified and may be detected by measuring peak expiratory flow or FEV_1 as well as by changes in resistance.

METHODS FOR MEASURING AIRFLOW RESISTANCE

There are four methods in clinical use which have different strengths and weaknesses and measure slightly different parts of the total resistive pressure drop (Figure 2.1).

Body plethysmography to measure airway resistance (Raw)[1]

The body plethysmograph is the only available method for directly measuring airway resistance in humans and has the added advantage that absolute lung volume can readily be measured, allowing the calculation of a volume corrected (specific) resistance or its reciprocal, conductance. The technique has been particularly valuable for studies of airway pharmacology in normal subjects and subjects with mild asthma, and, suitably modified, in infants (see Chapter 11). Its disadvantages are its bulk and expense and a relative difficulty in using it for different maneuvers or breathing different gas mixtures.

Method and analysis. (See following page)

Technical problems   The assumption that Pmo = Palv during airway occlusion is valid in normal subjects, but Pmo can underestimate Palv (and hence Raw) in the presence of airways obstruction which delays equilibration at the mouth. This problem can be overcome by panting against the closed shutter at 1 Hz or less, or by measuring change in esophageal pressure instead of ΔPmo.[2]

Body plethysmograph measurements of Raw also measure the thoracic gas volume (TGV) because TGV is obtained during the second stage of the procedure, panting against a closed shutter, from the slope ΔPbox/ΔPmo. The results can then be expressed as specific airway resistance (sRaw = Raw × TGV) or, more commonly, its reciprocal specific airway conductance (sGaw = 1/sRaw). Measurements of sRaw or sGaw at FRC are the best method of normalizing for differences in lung size between normal subjects.

If there is poor transmission of Palv to the mouth during panting against the closed shutter, TGV is overestimated. Because poor transmission of Palv to the mouth leads to identical proportionate underestimates of Raw and overestimates of TGV, there is no effect on sRaw or sGaw.

Body plethysmography – method

Principle The subject, seated in a whole-body plethysmograph ('box') breathes through a pneumotachograph back into the box ($\dot{V}$). Mass movement of gas from lungs to box itself results in no change in total volume (provided there are no changes in temperature), and so the change in box pressure (Pbox) during breathing is due to volume change of the lungs caused by compression and rarefaction of alveolar gas; if the volume of alveolar gas is known, the observed change in box pressure can be calibrated in terms of change of alveolar pressure. Dividing change in alveolar pressure by change in flow at the mouth gives airway resistance (Raw).

Method and analysis The body plethysmograph most commonly used has a constant volume, so that any change in thoracic volume which is not simply due to mass transfer from lungs to box results in reciprocal changes in box pressure (i.e. box pressure rises if there is rarefaction of alveolar gas). To calibrate changes in box pressure in terms of change in volume, a pump is used to inject and withdraw repetitively a small volume of gas into the box, while the subject to be studied holds his breath. (A large subject occupies more of the plethysmographic volume, so that a standard pump volume results in a bigger box pressure change than when a small subject is studied.) Alternatively a correction based on subject's body weight can be used and the box calibration performed when empty.

Changes in box pressure on expiration can occur, mainly because of cooling of expired air transferred from lungs to box.* This is minimized *either* by shallow panting through a heated pneumotachograph (this also has the advantage of abducting the cords and minimizing glottal resistance) *or* by rebreathing into a bag heated to 37° (as used in infants, Chapter 11), *or* with computerized simulated correction for the change in temperature and humidity as gas is transferred from lungs to box during tidal breathing.

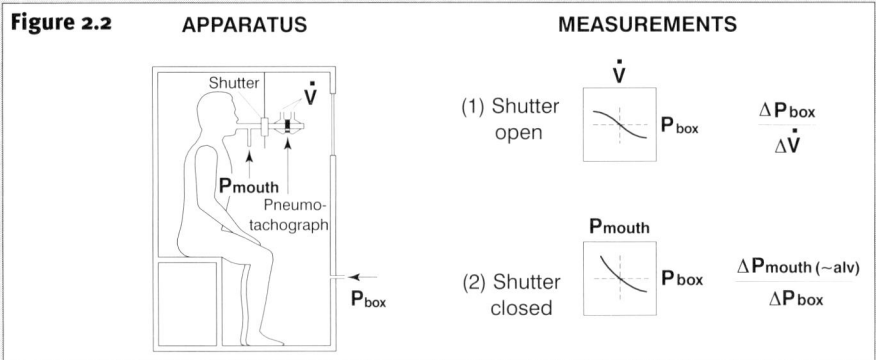

Figure 2.2

The subject is connected by a large caliber mouthpiece to the pneumotachograph shutter assembly (Figure 2.2). In the first part of the procedure changes in box pressure are plotted against flow rate on an oscilloscope, and the angle (ΔPbox/$\Delta\dot{V}$) measured usually around zero flow or from 0 to 0.5 L.s^{-1} inspiratory flow. The shutter is then closed to allow 'calibration' of the Pbox signal in terms of Palv, by measuring Pmo during panting against an occlusion (when it will normally equal Palv) and plotting this against Pbox on an oscilloscope, and measuring the ΔPmo(alv)/ΔPbox slope. Then multiplying the two slopes:

$$\frac{\Delta \text{Pbox}}{\Delta \dot{V}} \times \frac{\Delta \text{Palv}}{\Delta \text{Pbox}} = \frac{\Delta \text{Palv}}{\Delta \dot{V}} = \text{Raw}$$

* Instability of box pressure can be caused by heating of box air after the subject enters. Some plethysmographs are air-conditioned to hold the temperature more stable. there are also small effects from the respiratory exchange ratio being < 1.0.

The relation between resistive pressure and flow is alinear, particularly on expiration, even in normal subjects. Hence, during panting, analyses which are based on defining slopes on oscilloscope traces restrict the flow range to between zero and an inspiratory flow of 0.5 L.s^{-1}. Computerized methods have few samples in early inspiration and tend to be based on the whole panting maneuver so it is important to ensure that peak-to-peak flows are not too large, increasing the value of resistance. Some subjects have difficulty in panting with appropriate flows and a small tidal volume. When there is intrathoracic airway obstruction, expiratory resistance is higher than inspiratory resistance and there is considerable 'looping' of the Pbox vs $\dot{V}$ trace, making it difficult to select an average value with manual methods and affecting the weighting of a value averaged throughout a breath. Unexpectedly (because the laryngeal component should be less), values of resistance during panting are not consistently lower than those obtained during tidal breathing.

Applications The major uses of body plethysmography are in the assessment of airway pharmacology in normal subjects (where there is a much larger signal than with tests of maximum flow started from TLC) and in the assessment of airways obstruction, although, as discussed above, when this is severe it is difficult to define a single value for Raw. A further strength of the method when studying bronchodilator or bronchoconstrictor responses is that it is easy to obtain a concurrent measurement of FRC.

Changes in resistance or conductance with change in lung volume[3,4]

Measurements made by panting at different lung volumes in a body plethysmograph have shown that whereas Raw has a curvilinear relation to lung volume, increasing greatly as residual volume (RV) is approached, its reciprocal conductance (Gaw) decreases linearly with decreases in lung volume with an intercept at RV (Figure 2.3). Hence, for studies in which lung volume (V_L) changes or measurements are made over a range of V_L, it may be more informative to present results as Gaw rather than Raw. However, because of the intercept of the ΔGaw/ΔV_L slope on the volume axis at RV, sGaw in an individual subject falls as V_L is reduced towards RV. In COPD and asthma with airflow obstruction the ΔGaw/ΔV_L slope is reduced and its intercept on the volume axis is increased, corresponding to the increase in RV. The reduced ΔGaw/ΔV_L slope may be caused by reduced expansion of the airways as lung volume is increased. A further analysis can be made by plotting Gaw also against lung recoil pressure (P_L); in some patients with emphysema the ΔGaw/ΔP_L slope may be normal but truncated by loss of P_L, but most patients with COPD (and all with asthma) have both a reduced ΔGaw/ΔP_L slope and a reduced ΔGaw/ΔV_L slope.

When TLC (and FRC) are reduced, as after lung resection, loss of parallel airways leads to a reduction in Gaw but sGaw remains normal; in restrictive lung diseases such as fibrosing alveolitis, if P_L is increased at a reduced FRC, sGaw may be supranormal.

Figure 2.3 Effects of change in lung volume

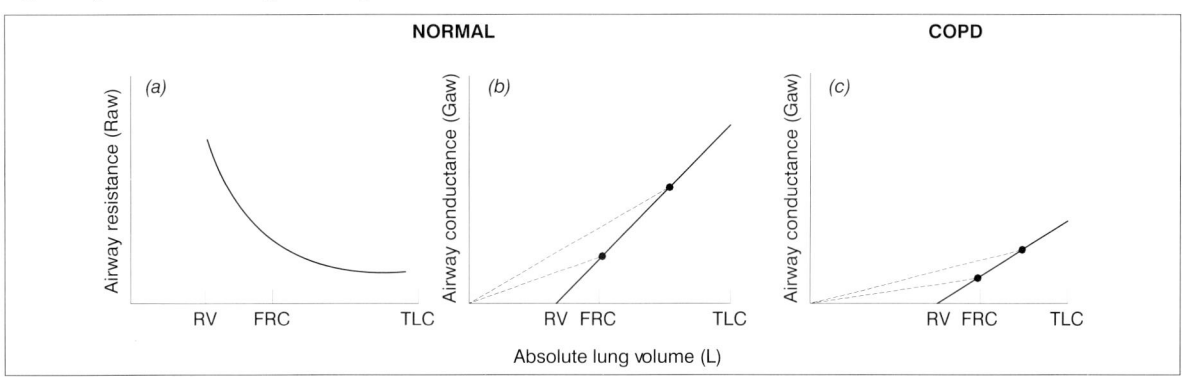

Changes in (a) airways resistance (Raw), and (b) conductance (Gaw) with changes in lung volume in a normal individual. Whereas Raw has a curvilinear relation to lung volume, Gaw shows a linear increase as lung volume is increased from residual volume (RV) to total lung capacity (TLC). Specific airway conductance (sGaw) at any lung volume equals Gaw/V_L, where V_L is the absolute lung volume (L). Because of the intercept of Gaw on the volume axis at RV, sGaw is lower at functional residual capacity (FRC) than at a larger lung volume (as indicated by the dashed lines from the origin). (c) In chronic obstructive pulmonary disease (COPD) Gaw increases less than normal as V_L is increased, and there is a large RV.

Body plethysmography

■ Measures total airway resistance.

■ Strengths:
- most experience is with this technique
- easy to obtain absolute lung volume to measure specific resistance
- possible to measure resistance at different lung volumes.

■ Weaknesses:
- bulky, expensive apparatus
- may require subject cooperation for panting
- in severe airflow obstruction may be slow equilibration of alveolar with mouth pressure
- in severe airflow obstruction resistance varies considerably within a breath.

Esophageal balloon catheter technique to measure total lung resistance (R_L)[5]

Principle Pleural surface pressure can be estimated by placing a small balloon catheter in the lower esophagus. The technical details of obtaining accurate estimates of pleural pressure are described in Chapter 3 in the section on measurement of lung (and chest wall) compliance. During tidal inspiration, changes in pleural (in practice, esophageal) pressure are required to oppose the elastic properties of the lung (measured as dynamic compliance, C_Ldyn) and the resistive properties of the lungs and lung tissue (total lung resistance, R_L). By simultaneous measurement of flow at the mouth ($\dot{V}$) and change in lung volume (ΔV), it is possible to subdivide the change in esophageal pressure into C_Ldyn and R_L.

Method and analysis (see facing page)

Technical problems This is the only method that directly measures intrathoracic pressure, but its invasiveness means that it is not often used solely to measure R_L (and C_Ldyn) in humans, although it is used commonly for this purpose in experimental animals. Once an esophageal balloon catheter has been placed, however, a full analysis of pulmonary mechanics can be made with additional measurements such as the static pressure-volume curve of the lung (Chapter 3) and the mechanical work of breathing on the lungs and chest wall (Chapters 4 and 12).

During quiet breathing in normal subjects, most of the tidal change in pleural (esophageal) pressure is overcoming the elastic properties of the lungs and a much smaller proportion the resistive properties; in addition there is often a notable cardiac artifact on the esophageal pressure trace. As a consequence, measurement of C_Ldyn is more reliable than R_L. One way to improve the signal-noise ratio is to ask the subject to breathe rapidly, with tidal volume similar to that used during quiet breathing; this increase in flow accentuates the resistive component of the total pressure change. The signal-noise ratio for R_L is much better when airways obstruction is present. All calculations of the resistive pressure drop assume dynamic compliance to be constant during the breath and identical on inspiration and expiration. Alinearities in dynamic compliance occur when breathing with large tidal volumes or close to TLC and when dynamic compliance is severely reduced, as in fibrosing alveolitis; these alinearities result in errors in the calculation of R_L.

Measurements of esophageal pressure may be distorted in the supine position because of the effects of gravity on the heart and mediastinal contents and the position of the diaphragm.

Only a few laboratories have sufficient familiarity with the technique to obtain consistent results for R_L. Most laboratories that use the technique frequently find that it is more acceptable to the subjects than

Esophageal balloon catheter – method

An esophageal balloon catheter is positioned in the lower esophagus and connected to a differential pressure transducer which measures the difference between esophageal and mouth pressure (ΔP). The subject, wearing a nose clip, breathes through a pneumotachograph which measures instantaneous flow ($\dot{V}$) which is integrated to give tidal volume (ΔV). Data are collected over at least 10 breaths during quiet breathing (Figure 2.4); in normal subjects it may be useful to breathe also with increased frequency of breathing but with a similar tidal volume because this increases the resistive component of ΔP (Figure 2.5).

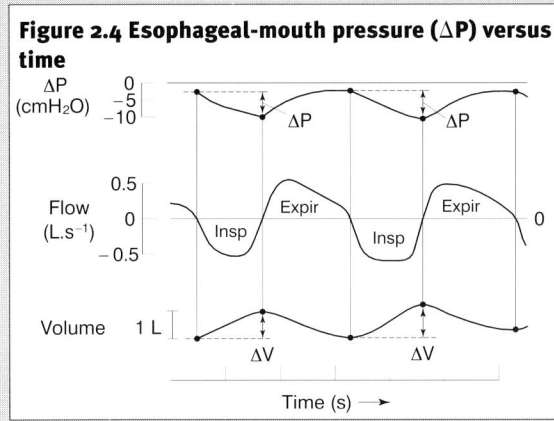

Figure 2.4 Esophageal-mouth pressure (ΔP) versus time

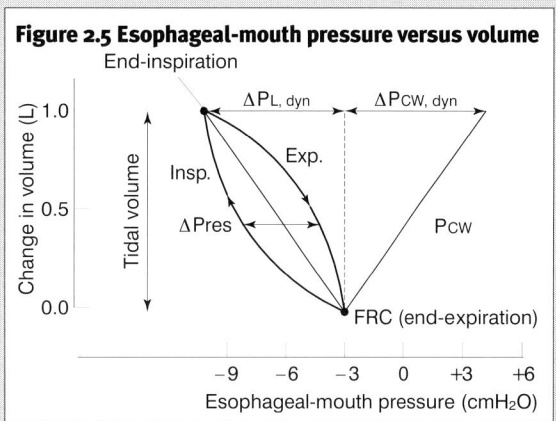

Figure 2.5 Esophageal-mouth pressure versus volume

Analysis of esophageal pressure-volume loop obtained during tidal breathing Although records against time can be used to calculate R_L and $C_L$dyn, the inter-relations between the two measurements and the calculation of work of breathing can be demonstrated better by plotting the relation between pressure and volume during each breath (Figure 2.5). On inspiration pressure becomes more negative until end inspiration. On expiration esophageal pressure rises (becomes less negative).

Dynamic compliance ($C_L$dyn) is obtained by dividing tidal volume (FRC to end inspiration, ΔV) by the difference in esophageal pressure between points of no flow (FRC and end inspiration) (solid circles), distance on pressure axis being equivalent to change in dynamic lung elastic pressure (ΔP_L, dyn).

Total lung resistance (R_L) is obtained by measuring the width of the esophageal pressure-volume loop at iso-volume; this indicates the resistive pressure drop (ΔPres) which can be divided into inspiratory (to left of diagonal line) and expiratory (to right of diagonal line) components and related to the corresponding flow at that volume. Usually however the total ΔPres is used and related to the sum of inspiratory and expiratory flow at this volume, i.e. $R_L = \Delta P\text{res}/(\dot{V}\text{insp} + \dot{V}\text{exp})$. In computerized analysis R_L is calculated from ΔPres at all volumes within the tidal volume and the value for each tidal breath is a time weighted mean, improving the signal-noise ratio. In this example esophageal pressure at the end of a tidal expiration (FRC) is $-3\,cmH_2O$, ΔV is 1.0 L, and ΔP_L, dyn is 7 cmH_2O and $C_L$dyn = 0.143 $L.cmH_2O^{-1}$. At the volume shown ΔPres was 4 cmH_2O and the sum of inspiratory and expiratory flow was 0.8 $L.s^{-1}$ so R_L was 5 $cmH_2O.L^{-1}s$. In normal subjects ΔPres is often 2 cmH_2O or less, resulting in a poor signal-noise ratio.

Work of breathing Inspiratory work is usually measured because expiration is nearly passive, at least at rest. Inspiratory work on the lungs corresponds to the area bounded by the inspiratory esophageal pressure-volume curve, ΔP_L, dyn and the dashed vertical line from FRC. Inspiratory work on both lungs and chest wall is more relevant because it indicates the load on the inspiratory muscles, which corresponds to the whole area bounded by the inspiratory esophageal pressure, ΔP_L, dyn and ΔPcw, dyn and the Pcw versus volume line. The resistive work corresponds to the area to the static left of the diagonal line within the esophageal pressure-volume loop; the largest part of the work is elastic, expanding the lungs and chest wall. The value of Pcw (the recoil pressure of the relaxed chest wall) at different lung volumes is usually assumed for this analysis as it is difficult to measure in most subjects.

anticipated, but the method requires patience and experience to overcome factors distorting esophageal pressure records such as excessive cardiac artifact or esophageal spasm.

Applications and interpretation Values of R_L in normal subjects are usually slightly higher than values of Raw, presumably reflecting tissue resistance of the lungs.[6] When airway narrowing is induced in normal subjects the increment in R_L may be larger than that in Raw; this may be because R_L is measured at a lower breathing frequency than Raw or because R_L also measures an increase in 'tissue resistance' (see later). Few studies have compared values of R_L and Raw in patients with airways obstruction. Although the method is potentially suitable for long-term monitoring of R_L (and $C_L$dyn), in practice this is only used in intensive care units; in the pulmonary function laboratory, forced oscillation is a more acceptable non-invasive technique for monitoring airflow resistance during tidal breathing over long periods. The esophageal balloon – catheter technique is the best method for measuring resistance during the high flows of exercise.

Esophageal balloon catheter technique

- Measures total airway resistance plus lung tissue resistance.

- Strengths:
  - measurements during tidal breathing
  - direct measurement of intrathoracic pressure
  - can be combined with measurement of dynamic and static compliance, work of breathing and respiratory muscle pressures.

- Weaknesses:
  - low signal-noise ratio in normal subjects
  - invasive.

Forced oscillation techniques to measure total respiratory resistance (Rrs)[7,8]

The forced oscillation technique for measuring airflow resistance was introduced in the 1950s at the same time as body plethysmography, but did not become as widely established in clinical physiology because the technical requirements for obtaining accurate pressure and flow signals and the subsequent signal processing were more demanding. Advances in pressure transducer and microcomputer technology have removed earlier problems with signal collection and analysis. Oscillation methods require less cooperation from the subject and less bulky apparatus than body plethysmography, and so the oscillation technique is now becoming more widely used.

Principle Forced oscillation techniques deduce the mechanical properties of the respiratory system from the response to small, externally produced oscillatory forces. From the response – measured as the instantaneous pressure-flow relationship (impedance) – flow resistance and the reactance (the combined effect of elastance and inertance*) of the respiratory system can be computed. These mechanical properties of the lungs are non-linear so it is important that only small external forces (1–2 cmH$_2$O) are applied.

Method and analysis (see facing page)

Applications The main current application in clinical physiology of the forced oscillation technique is as a simple method for obtaining the flow resistive properties of the respiratory system at different frequencies during tidal breathing. Usually results are presented at an oscillation frequency of 4 or 6 Hz and as frequency dependence of Rrs at higher frequencies. There are several modifications of the technique in use in research laboratories which provide a much more elaborate analysis of other mechanical properties or can be used to follow changes in Rrs within a breath.

Airways obstruction In patients with COPD (and asthma) Rrs is increased at the lower applied frequencies but falls with increasing applied frequencies (Figure 2.7: see p. 36). Reactance (Xrs) is lower than in healthy subjects and becomes positive only at higher frequencies, so that resonant frequency is increased. In the presence of inhomogeneity of mechanical properties of the lungs, resistance falls

---

* During quiet breathing the elastic properties (compliance) and resistive properties account for all the pressure required to expand the respiratory system. A third property, inertance, which is related to the pressure required to accelerate flow, is only important in very rapid breaths but becomes significant when oscillation is applied at high frequencies.

Forced oscillation method for measuring input impedance during tidal breathing

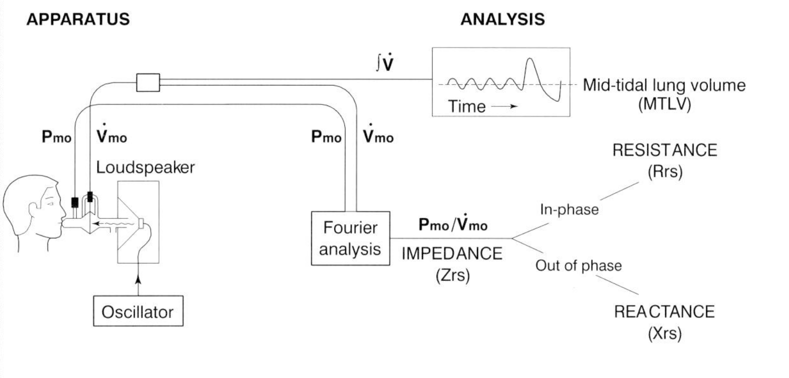

Figure 2.6

Apparatus The loudspeaker may be driven to generate a sinusoidal oscillation at one frequency, a sequential series of sinusoidal oscillations at different single frequencies, or, as in most modern applications, a random noise signal. The flow signal can be integrated to give tidal volume and, at the end of the measurement period, inspiratory capacity.

Analysis Mouth pressure (Pmo) and flow ($\dot{V}$mo) signals are fed into a Fourier analyzer, ensemble averaged over the measurement period (usually 8–16 s), and the component of the Pmo and $\dot{V}$mo signals caused by the applied oscillation distinguished from changes due to tidal breathing. Impedance (Zrs), the instantaneous ΔPmo/$\Delta\dot{V}$mo relationship, is then calculated over a wide range of frequencies. These values are the mean values of inspiratory and expiratory impedance over the several breaths of the measurement period. Impedance is further subdivided into the components of the Pmo signal in phase with $\dot{V}$mo and the out-of-phase signal. The in-phase signal is the resistance (Rrs) of the total respiratory system; it is also known as the *real* part. The out-of-phase signal is called reactance (Xrs) and sometimes the *imaginary* part. Various models can be used for further subdividing reactance in research analyses.

with increasing frequency, but this fall is exaggerated by increased dissipation of the applied oscillatory signal in the upper airway (chiefly the cheeks and floor of mouth). The contribution of the cheeks and mouth (sometimes called upper airway shunt) to total impedance can be reduced, but not eliminated, by firm support of the cheeks and floor of the mouth with the palms and fingers.

Other applications The apparatus can be adapted to make measurements in different postures and with different gas mixtures and can be applied to various airway openings (mouth, nose, tracheostomy, endotracheal tube). Obvious future areas of application include acute respiratory illness, respiratory disease in children, anesthesia, sleep, and intensive care. The method can also be applied to epidemiological surveys because little training of subjects is required. Measurement of the total resistance to breathing is probably the correct measurement to use in external loading studies. The technique has been relatively disappointing in evaluating restrictive disease of the lungs and chest wall.

Figure 2.7 Typical changes in total respiratory resistance and reactance at different applied oscillation frequencies

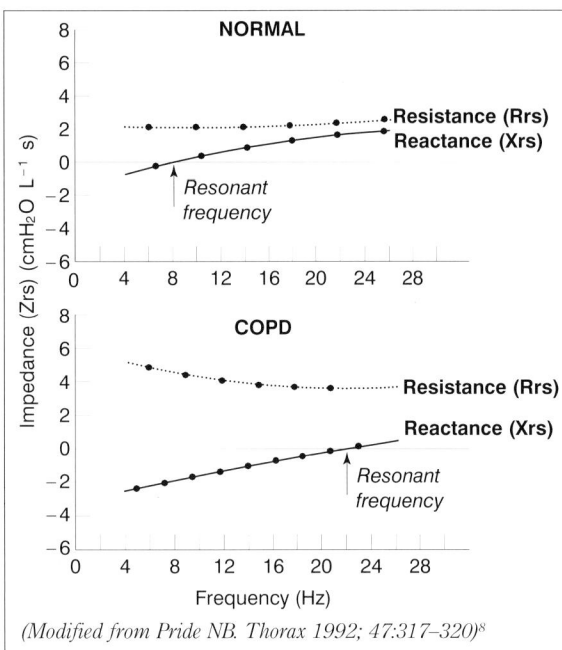

(Modified from Pride NB. Thorax 1992; 47:317–320)[8]

In a patient with airways obstruction resistance is higher at all frequencies than in a normal subject and decreases with increasing frequency; reactance is lower at all frequencies and resonant frequency (frequency at which reactance = 0) is increased. The tidal breathing pattern can be monitored during measurement by integrating V̇mo and absolute volume determined by measuring inspiratory capacity at the end of the measurement period to calculate specific Rrs (Rrs × MTLV).

Forced oscillation

- Measures total airway resistance plus lung and chest wall tissue resistance at different frequencies.
- Strengths:
  - measurement during tidal breathing
  - little demand for subject cooperation
  - easy to measure in different postures, with different gas mixtures
  - potential for use during sleep, anesthesia, intensive care.
- Weakness:
  - underestimates high values of resistance.

Airflow interruption technique to measure resistance (Rint)[6]

Principle The interruption technique is the simplest technique for measuring airflow resistance. Spontaneous breathing is interrupted by occluding the mouthpiece, and the flow immediately before occlusion is related to an estimate of alveolar pressure (Palv) shortly after occlusion which is derived from the trace of mouth pressure (Pmo) (measured on the alveolar side of the closed mouthpiece) versus time. The method requires minimal subject cooperation (the ability to use a flanged mouthpiece), can now be measured by simple portable devices, and does not require full inflation or unusual breathing maneuvers.

Method and analysis (see facing page)

Physiological significance In most comparisons, values of Rint have been higher than those of Raw and of R_L in normal subjects but the precise reasons for this difference were undetermined. More recently it appears that, if Pmo is back-extrapolated to time of half-closure of the valve, then Rint is similar to Raw in normal subjects but is lower than Raw when there is airway obstruction. This underestimate is probably caused by slow equilibration of Palv with Pmo. Interpretation of the later increase in Pmo on the Pmo versus time curve is less clear because it is not possible to distinguish the roles of continuing respiratory muscle activity, stress recovery of lung and chest wall tissues, and redistribution of gas – either between intra-and extrathoracic airways or between parallel intrathoracic airways. Despite these limitations in physiological interpretation, measurement of Rint has proved useful for the empirical detection of airway narrowing.

Applications: *Spontaneously breathing subjects* In comparison with the three other methods of measuring airflow resistance discussed above, the interrupter method is less sensitive in detecting induced airway narrowing. However its simplicity means that it can be applied in situations (e.g. bedside measurements in asthma) and in subjects where it is impossible to apply other methods. The interruption is usually for 100 ms, does not cause subject discomfort, and can be repeated over a number of breaths, either in inspiration or expiration; the disadvantages are that lung volume is not measured and resistance is only

Airflow interruption – method

The subject, with nose clipped, breathes tidally through the interrupter device which comprises a tube with a fast-closing valve and a flow-measuring device, usually a pneumotachograph screen. Valve closure may be triggered at a given flow or randomly and typically lasts 100 ms. Pmo before occlusion (Ppre) is proportional to screen resistance and is used to measure flow.

Apparatus

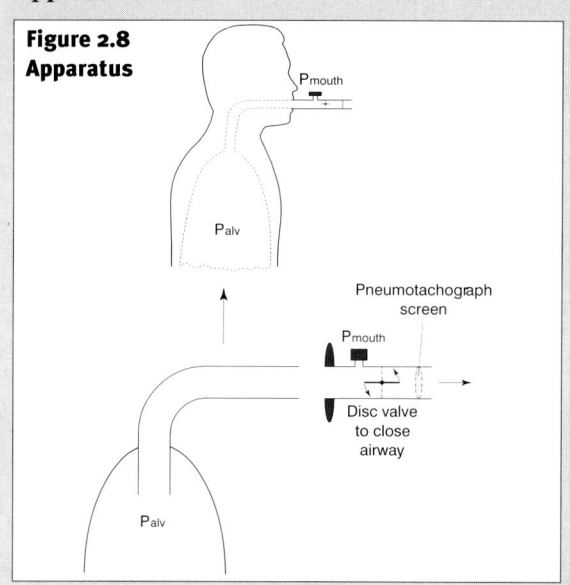

Figure 2.8 Apparatus

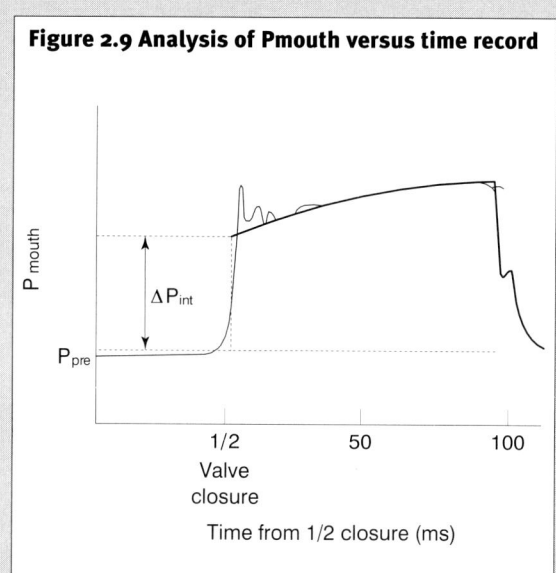

Figure 2.9 Analysis of Pmouth versus time record

Records and analysis   During expiratory flow, mouth pressure (Pmo) is lower than alveolar pressure (Palv) because of the resistance of the airways. Pmo indicates the pressure drop across the pneumotachograph screen (Ppre) and measures flow ($\dot{V}$). When the disk valve closes, flow ceases and Pmo rises rapidly to equilibrate with Palv. Following flow interruption, three distinct phases in the Pmo versus time curve occur: (1) a rapid initial rise in Pmo, (2) pressure oscillations, (3) a secondary slower rise in Pmo. Interruption resistance (Rint) is calculated as the ratio of Palv at interruption (time of half-closure of valve) and the flow measured just before valve closure. The problem is to estimate Palv at interruption; the rapid initial rise in Pmo is amplified by a mechanical overshoot and subsequent oscillations, making it impossible to measure Pmo at the precise moment of closure. After valve closure Palv may change because of continuing respiratory muscle activity, by stress recovery of lung and chest wall tissues, and, in abnormal lungs, by gas redistribution between parallel airways (pendelluft). The most accurate method is to fit a curve extrapolating the Pmo versus time trace back to the time of half-closure of the valve and taking Palv as the difference between this extrapolated Pmo and Ppre just before valve movement (ΔPint) (Figure 2.9). A commercial apparatus[9] back-extrapolates Pmo to 15 ms after valve closure, accepting a small overestimate of Palv.

measured at one point in a tidal breath although, in the past, methods of repetitive interruption have been used. The place of this technique should become clearer with the recent availability of portable equipment to measure interruption resistance.

Intensive care unit, during anesthesia[10]   Many of the problems encountered in analyzing mouth pressure after interruption in spontaneously breathing subjects are absent during positive pressure ventilation with constant flow inflation via an endotracheal tube.

In the absence of respiratory muscle activity and changes caused by compliance of the extrathoracic airway, the immediate change in pressure at the airway opening reflects the airway resistance (Raw) and the subsequent secondary change from stress recovery and pendelluft. Pressure at the airway opening can also be used to assess total respiratory compliance (see Chapter 12).

> **Airflow interruption**
>
> ■ Measures total airway resistance in carefully controlled circumstances.
>
> ■ Strengths:
> - simple apparatus and analysis
> - little demand for subject cooperation
> - full analysis of respiratory mechanics in intubated, ventilated subjects.
>
> ■ Weaknesses:
> - underestimates increases in resistance in spontaneously breathing patients
> - affected by slow equilibration of alveolar with mouth pressure and compliance of upper airway
> - no measurement of absolute lung volume.

COMPARISON OF DIFFERENT METHODS FOR ASSESSING AIRFLOW RESISTANCE

Forced oscillation and airflow interruption are more convenient and require less subject cooperation than esophageal balloon and body plethysmography methods, but unfortunately they are less sensitive than the last two methods and tend to underestimate resistance, at least in the simpler methods used in the clinical laboratory. Only the esophageal balloon catheter directly measures intrathoracic pressure, and the measurement is subject to noise. The other three methods rely on the measurement of Pmo, changes in which tend to be increasingly underestimated as airway obstruction becomes more severe. This is because pressure is dissipated in the compliant extrathoracic airway, which is important in the forced oscillation technique; in addition there is slow equilibration of alveolar and mouth pressure which leads to underestimates of resistance with the airflow interruption technique and, in the plethysmographic method, overestimates of lung volume and consequent underestimates of Raw (measurements of sRaw or sGaw are not affected). Standard techniques for measuring R_L, Raw, and Rrs all average resistance over a whole breath, but Rint is usually derived from a single inspiratory or expiratory measurement.

In normal subjects resistance values are relatively similar with all four methods, although forced oscillation usually gives slightly higher values.

REFERENCE VALUES

A major factor restricting the use of measurements of resistance is that reference values are so undeveloped. From what is known about the growth of the airways and gender differences, resistance would be expected to be related to the size of the lungs, with lower values in tall than in short individuals and, at a given height, lower values in men than in women. However there is remarkably little evidence on these points. Values of Raw in normal adults are in the range 1.5–2.0 $cmH_2O.L^{-1}$ s. Some laboratories merely report a value above which they consider resistance to be abnormal in any adult. Most of the available information has been obtained using body plethysmography, so that results for sGaw and sRaw have been available, which allows for differences in FRC between subjects. Values of sGaw between 0.13 and 0.35 cmH_2O^{-1} s^{-1} are regarded as normal from adolescence to old age in men and women; in contrast to the age-related decline in FEV_1 and maximum expiratory flows, there is no evidence that sGaw falls with increasing age.

DISTRIBUTION OF RESISTANCE: SEGMENTAL RESISTANCE

All these methods measure total airways resistance with variable additional components of lung and chest wall tissue resistance. Limited studies of the serial distribution of serial resistance have been made using intrabronchial catheters[11] and tracheal needles, by comparing values of R_L or Rrs during air and helium-oxygen breathing, and by using an esophageal balloon to subdivide Rrs into lung and chest wall components.

Normal subjects

Total pulmonary resistance (RL) during quiet breathing via a large caliber mouthpiece is approximately equally divided between the extrathoracic airway, major conducting airways, and peripheral airways (less than 3 mm internal diameter) and lung tissue (Table 2.1). The contribution of the small, peripheral airways is low because the reduction in cross-sectional area of the lumen in each individual airway is far outweighed by the large numbers of these airways. The total cross-sectional area available for gas flow is much greater in the small airways than in the trachea, and the progressive increase in total airway cross-section per generation has been likened to the opening out of a trumpet. The tissue resistance of the chest wall probably contributes a further 0.5 $cmH_2O.L^{-1}$ s. Nasal resistance is much higher than oral resistance so that typically extrathoracic resistance would be at least 1 $cmH_2O.L^{-1}$ s higher during nasal breathing.

Chronic obstructive pulmonary disease

Most of the increased total resistance is caused by narrowing of the peripheral airways, with only small increases in resistance of the larger conducting airways. In addition there is much less reduction in resistance and increase in conductance (Figure 2.3) as lung volume is increased, compared to the large changes found in normal subjects. The tissue resistance of the chest wall remains normal and so only makes a small contribution to total Rrs.

Asthma

The distribution of resistance in episodic asthma is uncertain and probably is variable between subjects and at different times in an individual subject. In middle-aged asthmatic subjects with chronic airflow obstruction, the increase in resistance is approximately equally distributed between the major conducting airways and the peripheral airways.[11]

Upper airway resistance

A few measurements have been made of upper airway resistance during tidal breathing using a needle in the trachea (these estimates have been used in Table 2.1). Measurements of nasal and pharyngeal resistance are more commonly measured.

Nasal resistance[12]

It is easy to measure transnasal pressure, and so measuring nasal resistance is the method of choice to assess nasal patency. Changes in resistance are much larger than changes in maximum flow through the nose, as discussed in Chapter 1.

There are three established methods for measuring nasal resistance (Rna).

Active anterior rhinomanometry The subject breathes through one nostril, while the contralateral nasal opening is occluded by tape, through which a small tube is passed to measure pressure in the anterior nose. There is no flow through the occluded nostril, so the pressure measured is the same as that in the postnasal space. Flow through the patent nostril during tidal breathing is measured by a pneumotachograph attached to a tightly fitting nasal or oronasal mask, and is plotted against transnasal pressure (mask pressure – pressure in occluded nostril) (Ptn). Resistance of the patent nostril ($\Delta Ptn/\Delta \dot{V}$) is calculated at a Ptn of 0.15 kPa (1.5 cmH_2O). The nostril that was initially patent is then occluded and used to measure postnasal pressure, and the resistance of the other nostril is measured at the same Ptn of 0.15 kPa. Total Rna is then calculated from the right and nostril values (Rna,r and Rna,l) as:

$$1/Rna = 1/Rna,r + 1/Rna,l$$

Table 2.1 Distribution of total lung resistance (RL)

	Normal ($cmH_2O.L^{-1}$ s) (% of total)	Severe COPD ($cmH_2O.L^{-1}$ s) (% of total)
Extrathoracic airway	0.5 (33)	0.5 (8)
Major intrathoracic conducting airways	0.5 (33)	1.0 (17)
Peripheral airways (< 3 mm diameter) and lung tissue	0.5 (33)	4.5 (75)
Total	1.5 (100)	6.0 (100)

The values are for a typical patient with severe COPD during tidal breathing via the mouth. Extrathoracic resistance would be at least 1.0 $cmH_2O.L^{-1}$ s greater when breathing through the nose.

It is important that Rna,r and Rna,l are measured at a common postnasal pressure; this will be associated with different flow through the two nostrils if there are differences in resistance between the two sides.

Passive anterior rhinomanometry This method also measures unilateral nasal resistance, but during breath-holding with the mouth open and the contralateral nostril patent. A flow controller is attached to an adapter, which also has a lateral port to measure pressure; the adapter is placed in the external nares and sealed to avoid leaks. Flow is then gradually increased up to 0.08 $L.s^{-1}$ through the chosen nostril and resistance calculated as transnasal pressure, which in this method is simply the lateral pressure at the adapter (postnasal pressure is expected to be atmospheric with an open mouth) at an 'inspiratory' flow of 0.05 $L.s^{-1}$. The procedure is then repeated for the second nostril and total Rna calculated as for active anterior rhinomanometry.

Active posterior rhinomanometry This method measures the resistance of both nostrils simultaneously, while the subject breathes normally through the nose with the lips firmly closed around an occluded mouthpiece containing a tube to measure pressure. Flow is measured by a pneumotachograph attached to a tightly-fitted nasal or oronasal face mask. Postnasal pressure is indicated by the tube passed through the mouthpiece, over the top of the tongue, towards the post-pharyngeal wall.

Transnasal pressure is recorded as the difference between pressure in the mask and pressure in the tube passed through the mouthpiece. In this method complete inspiratory and expiratory plots of Ptn versus $\dot{V}$ are obtained, but a common convention is to measure Rna at a Ptn of 0.075 kPa (0.75 cmH_2O).

The major problem with this method is in measuring postnasal pressure accurately. During nasal breathing, the soft palate may be apposed to the posterior of the tongue, so that oral pressure does not reflect pressure in the postnasal space. Alternatively, if the pressure tube extends too far posteriorly, gagging and contraction of pharyngeal constrictor muscles may take place.

Other methods Alternative methods are to measure total resistance sequentially during periods of nasal and oral breathing and to estimate Rna by the difference between the two measurements. This has been done for body plethysmography and for forced oscillation and could be applied also to esophageal balloon catheter and airway interruption methods. In these methods oral resistance is assumed to be negligible and the breathing pattern should be similar during the two measurement periods.

Resistance is often used as a surrogate for dimensions of the nasal cavity; a cross-sectional area-distance function, and hence derived volume, can be obtained simply and quickly by acoustic reflection in which an acoustic pulse is generated at the airway opening. Alternatively nasal volume can be measured directly by instilling warm saline into one nostril with the head flexed, until it enters the nasopharynx and then measuring the volume returned.

Interpretation/applications During quiet breathing via the nose, Rna is in the range 1–2 $cmH_2O.L^{-1}$ s in subjects without nasal disease and so accounts for about half the total airflow resistance. Repeatability of values of Rna is less good than might be expected from the simplicity of the methods. In part this is because of the alinearity of Rna which increases markedly as flow increases, even in normal subjects. The other major factor is that Rna is very sensitive to the extent of vascular congestion of the mucosa, which is affected by temperature, flow, irritants, and many other factors. Much of the pressure dissipation during breathing is in the anterior part of the nose – the so-called 'nasal valve'. Small changes in this region can greatly alter Rna, even when there is little total change in other dimensions of the nasal cavity. Rna drops considerably on exercise, allowing greater nasal flow. Some subjects appear to show spontaneous 'cycling' of nasal resistance, with reciprocal changes in vascular congestion in the two nostrils. Rna is higher in the supine than in the sitting position, probably from vascular congestion when supine. There may also be reflex interactions between the lungs and the nose. All these changes make Rna more labile than airway resistance in normal subjects. Subjects should rest quietly in the laboratory for 15 minutes before measurements are commenced.

Despite these limitations, measurement of Rna is useful in the assessment of many types of nasal disease such as rhinitis, septal deviation, and turbinate hypertrophy, and can be used to assess the results of both medical and surgical treatment. It may be useful in the assessment of obstructive sleep apnea. In the future it will probably be useful to combine the measurement of Rna with the information on nasal cavity geometry obtained with acoustic reflection.

> - Nasal resistance is the best method for assessing nasal patency; several methods are available.
> - Of the established methods only active posterior rhinomanometry assesses resistance during normal tidal breathing.
> - Nasal resistance is highly labile because of variation in vascular congestion of the mucosa.
> - Most of the resistance is in the anterior nose – the nasal 'valve'.

Oro- or nasopharyngeal resistance

Changes in airflow resistance (and compliance) of the pharynx, particularly when asleep, may be important in the genesis of obstructive sleep apnea. Catheters have been placed at various levels in the pharynx to measure resistance during oral or nasal breathing, but care has to be taken to prevent these inducing abnormal contraction of the pharyngeal muscles.

During sleep there is an increase in total R_L measured by an esophageal balloon catheter during nose breathing in normal subjects. When esophageal pressure measurements are combined with measurements from a catheter in the posterior pharynx, the larger part of the rise in R_L has been in the nasopharyngeal segment but there are also increases in resistance of the lower tracheobronchial airways.

Resistance of lung tissue and chest wall

The most familiar part of airflow resistance is the resistive pressure drop between the airway opening (mouth or nose) and the alveoli, which is related to airflow through the airways (Raw). But there are also pressure losses across the lung tissue (the difference between alveolar and pleural pressure) and chest wall (difference between pleural and atmospheric pressure) which are in phase with flow; the pressure drop across lung tissue is included in R_L, and that across lung tissue and chest wall in Rrs measured by forced oscillation.

Chest wall resistance accounts for about 0.5 $cmH_2O.L^{-1}$ s of the total values of Rrs and hardly varies over a wide range of lung volumes in normal subjects. Similar values have been found in COPD, but few studies have been made in other diseases. It is therefore reasonable to assume that changes in Rrs found with change in lung volume or after bronchoconstrictor or bronchodilator drugs reflect changes in properties of the airways or lung tissue.

Lung tissue resistance is greatest when breathing with a large tidal volume and slow breathing frequency, so it makes a bigger contribution to R_L than Rrs. Nevertheless, R_L is only slightly greater than Raw in normal subjects. The importance of lung tissue resistance in disease is less clear. Lung tissue resistance can be measured directly in animals and increases in this component have accounted for a large proportion of the total rise in R_L after inhalation of bronchoconstrictor aerosols. In living humans lung tissue resistance cannot be measured directly, but after inhalation of methacholine the rise in R_L is greater than in Raw at normal breathing frequencies, although the difference is less dramatic than in animals. Excised emphysematous lungs also have increased lung tissue resistance.

OTHER TECHNIQUES FOR ASSESSING AIRWAY DIMENSIONS

Airflow resistance provides an indirect estimate of lumped airway dimensions, used for instance to detect bronchodilator or bronchoconstrictor responses. Imaging by bronchography or computed tomography can be used to obtain more direct information on the dimensions of some of the airways. A promising technique to obtain the dimensions of extrathoracic airways is acoustic reflection, from which an area-distance function can be obtained. At present this technique is most easily applied to the nose; reliable measurements when applied at the mouth require the subject to breathe a helium-oxygen mixture. Total cross-sectional area can be obtained to the carina and the technique has been useful for investigating subjects with obstructive sleep apnea. There are hopes that the technique can be simplified to avoid the need for the subject to breathe a helium-oxygen mixture and to obtain cross-sectional area of the larger intrapulmonary airways.

COMPARISON OF TESTS OF MAXIMUM EXPIRATORY FLOW AND RESISTANCE

Airway caliber is commonly assessed either by tests of maximum flow, particularly FEV_1, or by resistance – most commonly measured in a body plethysmograph. Both types of tests depend on the mechanical properties of the lungs but, because of the different circumstances of measurement, perfect correspondence cannot be expected when assessing airway disease.

The relation between the two types of test can be visualized on an iso-volume pressure-flow curve constructed from a whole series of inspirations and expiration conducted with varying effort (Figure 2.10).

Figure 2.10 Iso-volume pressure-flow curve

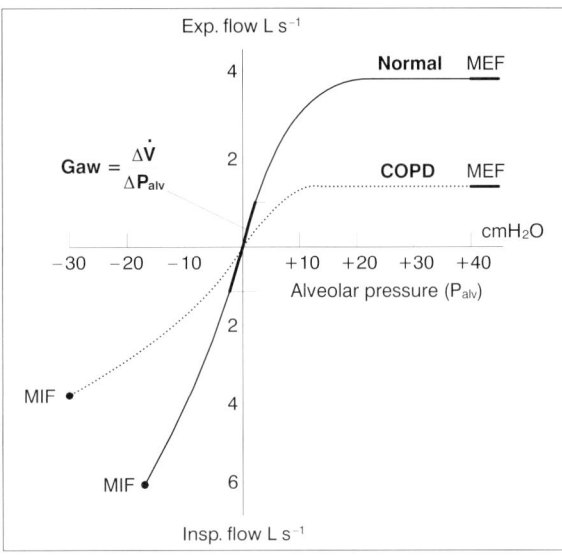

This pressure-flow curve is similar to Figure 1.4 but flow is plotted against alveolar pressure not pleural pressure. The slope around zero flow ($\Delta \dot{V}/\Delta Palv$) is airways conductance, as measured at low flow in the body plethysmograph. The relation between flow and Palv is curvilinear, especially on expiration, so that if panting is conducted with high flows Gaw will be lower (and Raw higher) than with low flow panting. On expiration, flow at first increases as Palv is increased, but reaches a maximum level (MEF) which is not increased by further increases in Palv. On inspiration there is some curvilinearity of the pressure-flow curve but no plateau of flow develops and MIF is determined by the lowest (most negative) Palv. When there is intrapulmonary airflow obstruction (asthma, COPD, etc.) both the initial $\Delta \dot{V}/\Delta Palv$ slope (Gaw) and MEF are reduced, and MEF develops at a lower Palv.

In practice, FEV_1, which is determined by MEF over a wide range of lung volumes, is usually compared to Gaw or Raw. In general, Gaw and FEV_1 are both reduced by airway disease, but proportionate changes may differ. For instance, it has been suggested that at a given reduction in FEV_1, the decrease in Gaw is less in emphysema than in asthma or in upper airway obstruction.

Nasal patency is usually assessed by resistance measurements because of the ease with which posterior nasal or pharyngeal pressure can be measured. For assessing intrathoracic airways however spirometry, peak expiratory flow, and maximum expiratory flow-volume curves are more widely used than resistance in most countries. In some specialized laboratories most emphasis is placed on body plethysmograph measurements. In severe intrathoracic airflow obstruction, however, resistance varies considerably within a breath and there is considerable looping of the trace during panting, so it is difficult to define a representative value of resistance; spirometry is a more robust measurement in these circumstances.

For assessing airway responses (bronchodilatation and bronchoconstriction) a further factor determining the choice of test is that FEV_1 requires an inflation to TLC whereas resistance is usually measured in the tidal breathing range. However, tests of forced expiration can be commenced from smaller lung volumes as discussed in Chapters 1 and 14.

Resistance measurements

■ Advantages:
- well-defined physiological basis
- measured in tidal breathing range
- sensitive to small changes in airway caliber.

■ Disadvantages:
- apparatus usually expensive and bulky
- depends on flow, phase of breathing, and volume
- influenced by normal upper airway.

■ Particular indications:
- airway pharmacology in normal subjects and mild asthma.

Tests of maximum expiratory flow

■ Advantages:
- robust and repeatable
- apparatus widely available
- less influenced by normal upper airways.

■ Disadvantages:
- usually require a full inflation
- less defined physiological basis.

■ Particular indications:
- established intra- or extrathoracic airway disease
- epidemiological studies.

References

1. DuBois AB, Botelho SY & Comroe JH Jr. A new method for measuring airway resistance in man using a body plethysmograph: values in normal subjects and in patients with respiratory disease. *J Clin Invest* 1956; **35**: 327–34.
2. Stanescu DC, Rodenstein D, Cauberghs M, Van de Woestijne KP. Failure of body plethysmography in bronchial asthma. *J Appl Physiol: Respirat Environ Exercise Physiol* 1982; **52**: 939–48.
3. Butler J, Caro CG, Alcala R, DuBois AB. Physiological factors affecting airway resistance in normal subjects and in patients with obstructive respiratory disease. *J Clin Invest* 1960; **39**: 584–91.
4. Briscoe WA & DuBois AB. The relationship between airway resistance, airway conductance, and lung volume in subjects of different age and body size. *J Clin Invest* 1958; **37**: 1279–85.
5. Mead J & Whittenberger JL. Physical properties of human lungs measured during spontaneous respiration. *J Appl Physiol* 1953; **5**: 779–96.
6. Phagoo SB, Watson RA, Silverman M, Pride NB. Comparison of four methods of assessing airflow resistance before and after induced airway narrowing in normal subjects. *J Appl Physiol* 1995; **79**: 518–25.
7. Peslin R. Methods for measuring total respiratory impedance by forced oscillations. *Bull Eur Physiopathol Respir* 1986; **22**: 621–31.
8. Pride NB. Forced oscillation techniques for measuring mechanical properties of the respiratory system. *Thorax* 1992; **47**: 317–20.
9. Chowienczyk PJ, Lawson CP, Lane S, Johnson R, Wilson N, Silverman M, Cochrane GM. A flow interruption device for the measurement of airway resistance. *Eur Respir J* 1991; **4**: 623–8.
10. D'Angelo E, Robatto FM, Calderini E, Tavola M, Bono D, Torri G, Milic-Emili J. Pulmonary and chest wall mechanics in anesthetized paralyzed humans. *J Appl Physiol* 1991; **70**: 2602–10.
11. Yanai M, Sekizawa K, Ohrui T, Sasaki H, Takishima T. Site of airway obstruction in pulmonary disease: direct measurement of intrabronchial pressure. *J Appl Physiol* 1992; **72**: 1016–23.
12. Eiser NM. The hitch-hiker's guide to nasal airway patency. *Respir Med* 1990; **84**: 179–83.

3 Lung Volumes and Elasticity
G J Gibson

- **ELASTIC PROPERTIES OF THE RESPIRATORY SYSTEM, LUNGS, AND CHEST WALL**
  Theory
  Compliance
  Static pressure-volume (PV) curve of the lungs
  Dynamic compliance of the lungs
  Total respiratory (and chest wall) compliance

- **LUNG VOLUMES**
  Measurement of lung volumes
  Inert gas dilution
  Body plethysmography
  Radiographic techniques
  Interpretation and reliability (all methods)

  Determinants of lung volumes
  Functional residual capacity (FRC)
  Total lung capacity (TLC)
  Residual volume (RV)
  Postural effects

  Patterns of abnormality in disease

ELASTIC PROPERTIES OF THE RESPIRATORY SYSTEM, LUNGS, AND CHEST WALL

Theory

The respiratory system is an elastic structure changing volume when pressures are generated by inspiratory or expiratory muscles. If the muscles are relaxed the respiratory system returns to its relaxation volume (Vr) (referred to in the pediatric literature as the elastic equilibrium volume [EEV]), which in normal subjects is the end-expired volume or functional residual capacity, FRC, where alveolar pressure is equal to atmospheric pressure.

When an anesthetist hand-ventilates a paralyzed patient at this volume by applying a positive pressure at the proximal end of the airway and measures the change in volume per unit change in applied pressure ($\Delta V/\Delta P$) the 'stiffness' or compliance of the *total* respiratory system (Crs) is measured (Figures 3.1 and 3.2). Some of the applied pressure inflates the lungs and some the chest wall. Thus, the total respiratory compliance is less than the compliance of either structure individually. For example, if the compliance of the lungs (C_L) is 0.2 $L.cmH_2O^{-1}$ and that of the chest wall (Ccw) is similarly 0.2 $L.cmH_2O^{-1}$, then to increase the volume of both together by 0.2 L requires a total applied pressure of 2 cmH_2O (Figure 3.2). Hence, in this situation the total respiratory compliance (Crs) is 0.1 $L.cmH_2O^{-1}$ or, more generally,

$$\frac{1}{Crs} = \frac{1}{C_L} + \frac{1}{Ccw}$$

Figure 3.1 Static PV curve of respiratory system with maximal pressures generated by respiratory muscles

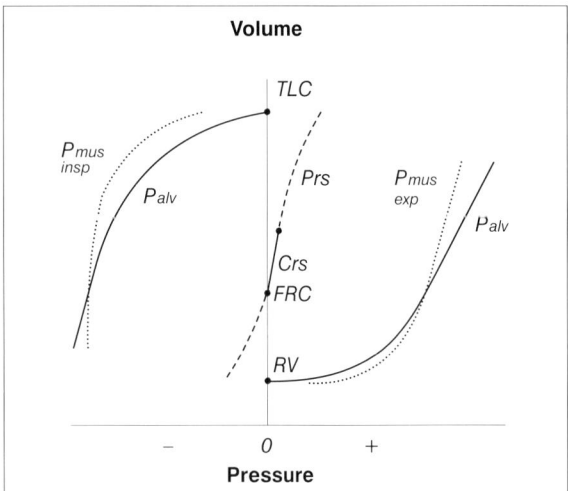

Static PV curve of the total respiratory system (Prs – broken line) compliance in the tidal range (Crs) and functional residual capacity (FRC), and the pressures recorded during maximal inspiratory Pmus insp (left side) and expiratory efforts Pmus exp (right side) at various lung volumes in a healthy young adult (dotted line). Solid lines show alveolar pressure (Palv, i.e. mouth pressure when efforts are made against a closed airway). Palv represents the sum of Prs and Pmus. Total lung capacity (TLC) is set by the balance between Prs and inspiratory muscle effort, i.e. at TLC, Prs is equal and opposite to inspiratory Pmus. Residual volume (RV) is set by the balance between Prs (negative because at low volumes net recoil of the respiratory system is outward) and expiratory Pmus.

Figure 3.2 Static PV curves of respiratory system, lungs, and chest wall

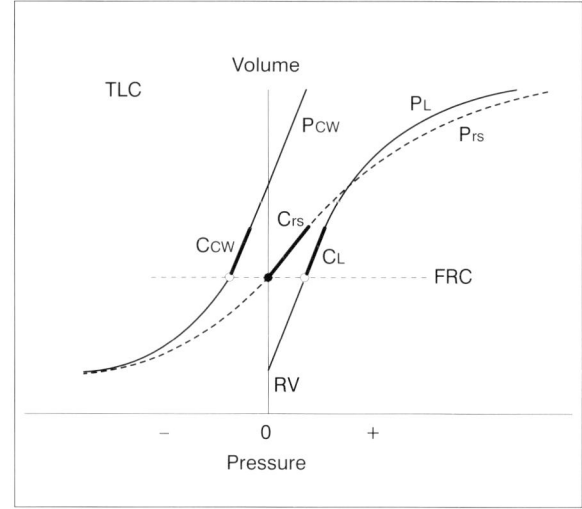

'Rahn diagram'[1] showing how static PV curve of respiratory system (Prs-broken line) shown in Figure 3.1 relates to PV curves of its two components, the lungs and chest wall. Scale on pressure axis is expanded. P_L, Pcw, Prs represent recoil pressures and C_L, Ccw, Crs static compliance of lungs, chest wall, and respiratory system respectively. Compliance is represented by the slope of the respective PV curve over the approximate tidal range (heavy lines). Note: (1) at FRC P_L = –Pcw; (2) Crs is less than either C_L or Ccw alone; (3) P_L increases disproportionately towards TLC; (4) Pcw becomes increasingly negative towards RV; (5) resting volume (Pcw = 0) of chest wall greatly exceeds that of lungs (RV).

Although in health C_L and Ccw are similar in the tidal range, the resting volume (volume when any distending or collapsing force is removed) of the chest wall is much larger than that of the lungs which collapse down to a small volume in the absence of distending forces.

Note that the analysis in Figures 3.1 and 3.2 relates only to gas volume of the lungs and that tissue and fluid volumes are ignored. In some diseases (cardiac failure, adult respiratory distress syndrome) the fluid volume in the lungs increases markedly and may complicate analysis of the balance of pressures across the respiratory system. Similarly the volume of a pleural effusion or a pneumothorax is ignored if only pulmonary gas volume is considered.

- Compliance of the total respiratory system (Crs) has two components – lung compliance (C_L) and chest wall compliance (Ccw).

- Crs is the relationship between volume change (ΔV) and the recoil pressure of the respiratory system (Prs).

- Total lung capacity (TLC) is set by the balance between Prs and inspiratory muscle effort (inspiratory Pmus).

- Residual volume (RV) is set by the balance between Prs and expiratory muscle effort (expiratory Pmus).

- At relaxation volume (Vr) (in healthy subject synonymous with functional residual capacity [FRC]), the elastic recoil of the lung (P_L) is balanced by the outward recoil of the chest wall (Pcw).

Compliance

In most clinical circumstances the compliance of the chest wall is of little importance. Measurement of total respiratory compliance is difficult in the adult conscious subject, and so it is rarely measured in the pulmonary function laboratory.

On the other hand, the static compliance of the lungs is of considerable interest and is frequently abnormal in disease.[2,3] In practice, however, it is measured infrequently because it involves the subject swallowing a tube into the esophagus and lengthy breathing maneuvers and analysis.

Static pressure-volume (PV) curve of the lungs

Method

To construct the static PV relationship of the lungs requires measurement of the difference between alveolar and pleural pressures (transpulmonary pressure) at several lung volumes. This is obtained during breath-holding with a balloon-catheter system or a small pressure transducer in the lower esophagus to approximate pleural pressure. This pressure is compared to the pressure at the airway opening which during breath-holding reflects alveolar pressure. Occasionally, the quasi-static PV curve is measured during a very slow expiration.

Volume change is measured either with a spirometer or with the subject seated in a variable volume body plethysmograph,[8] which allows direct measurement of changing thoracic gas volume. An esophageal balloon or appropriate miniature pressure transducer is swallowed, usually via the nose, into the lower third of the esophagus. When using a balloon-catheter system a small volume of air is introduced with the aim of producing a bubble at the upper end of the balloon. The volume of air used needs to be neither too large to distend the esophagus, nor too small to cause the balloon itself to develop a negative recoil. In practice this is usually between 0.2 and 0.5 ml. The position of the balloon or transducer is adjusted up and down to give the most negative values of pressure at FRC, usually by trial and error. Alternatively the depth of the balloon may be standardized in relation to the height of the subject by using the formula of Zapletal et al,[4] based on which the tip of a 10 cm balloon should be positioned at a depth of (height [cm]/5 + 9) cm from the nostril.

Measurements of transpulmonary pressure (mouth minus esophageal pressure, P_L) at various volumes are usually made during deflation after a standard sequence (volume history) of three full inflations. If expired volume is used, either the subject needs to maintain an inspiratory effort and open airway during breath-holding at each volume or, if allowed to relax against a shutter, a correction to the volume is necessary due to the resulting small changes in thoracic volume associated with the positive pressure which accompanies relaxation (Boyle's law). With a variable volume plethysmograph (with the door closed) no correction is needed as the effects of gas compression are measured directly.

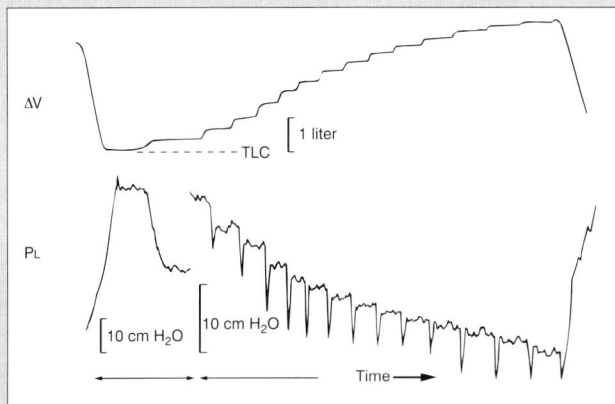

Figure 3.3 Measurement of lung PV curve and compliance

Record against time of volume (ΔV) expired during interrupted expiration from total lung capacity (TLC), and transpulmonary pressure (mouth − esophageal pressure). During breath-holding (plateaux of volume and pressure) mouth = alveolar pressure and thus transpulmonary pressure = lung recoil pressure (P_L). Irregularities on pressure record are due to cardiac pulsation. Gain on pressure amplifier doubled at point indicated by converging arrows.

Figure 3.4a Static lung PV curve

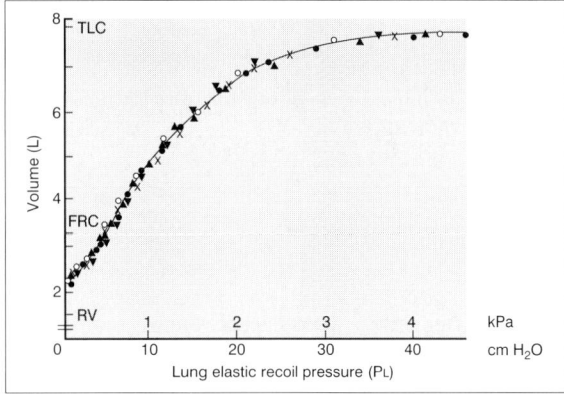

P_L *plotted against absolute lung volume. TLC, measured separately. Different symbols indicate measurements made during five separate interrupted expirations from TLC. At volumes below FRC, the slope of the PV curve becomes shallower. Maximum P_L in this healthy young individual is unusually high at approximately 50 cmH$_2$O.*

Analysis of the PV curve (Figure 3.4b)

Measurements of volume and transpulmonary pressure are plotted and a curve may be drawn by hand.

Figure 3.4b Measurements from static lung PV curve and dynamic lung compliance

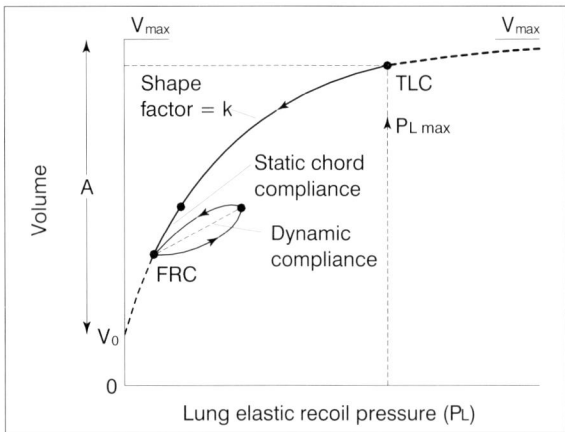

Thick line is a diagrammatic static PV curve of lungs from TLC to FRC with extrapolation to Vmax and Vo (difference = A) to allow calculation of shape factor 'k'.

Also shown is 'chord' compliance measured over tidal breathing range and transpulmonary (mouth-esophageal) pressure recorded continuously during a tidal breath. The slope of the broken line joining points of zero airflow at end expiration and end inspiration represents dynamic compliance. In normal subjects, dynamic compliance is only slightly less than static compliance.

The usual method of expressing static pulmonary compliance is to measure the average slope ('chord' compliance) over the approximate range of tidal breathing (usually between FRC and FRC + 0.5 L.). Another useful index is the maximum lung recoil pressure ($P_L$max), i.e. the value of P_L at TLC. The compliance of lungs becomes progressively less as they are inflated. To allow for this, a monoexponential function can be fitted to the volume (V) and pressure (P) data points to give a curve described by the equation[5]

$$V = Vmax - Ae^{-kP}$$

where Vmax represents the volume asymptote to the curve, A is a constant related to the intercept of the curve on the volume axis, and k is a shape factor which gives a volume-independent index of pulmonary compliance (Figure 3.4b). In general, the greater the value of k, the more distensible the lungs.

Changes in PV curve with disease (Figure 3.5)

With aging in normal subjects both static compliance and k increase while P_L and $P_L$max decline. In general, in patients with emphysema and an increased TLC, static compliance (L.cmH$_2$O^{-1}) and k are both increased and recoil pressures including $P_L$max are reduced. In diffuse pulmonary fibrosis and restricted lung volumes the converse findings are typical, i.e. decreased compliance and k and increased lung recoil pressures.

In some conditions lung expansion is limited by inability to apply a normal distending pressure to the lungs; this occurs, for example, with respiratory muscle weakness or severe scoliosis. As a result, the $P_L$max is less than normal. While a normal static lung compliance over the tidal breathing range might be anticipated, in practice a reduction occurs because of secondary changes in the elastic behavior of the lungs. For this reason a single measurement of chord compliance in the tidal range (Figure 3.4b) alone in a patient with a restrictive ventilatory defect will not distinguish intrapulmonary and extrapulmonary causes of volume reduction. In extrapulmonary volume reduction, the D_{LCO} (T_{LCO}) and especially the D_L/V_A (K_{CO}) are raised and may be helpful (see Chapters 6 and 17).

Figure 3.5 Typical static expiratory PV curves of the lung in various conditions

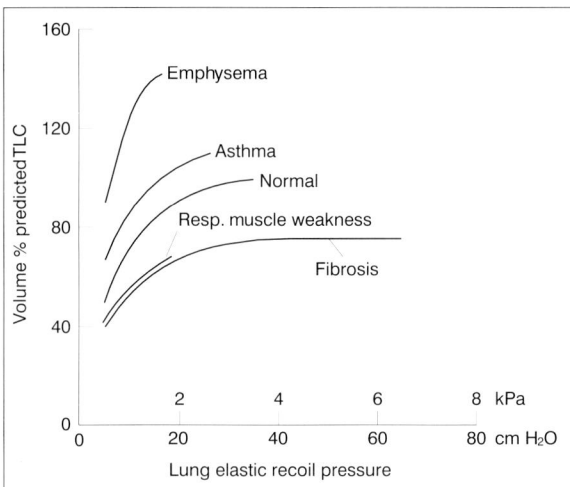

Dynamic compliance

Measurements of transpulmonary pressure and volume can also be recorded continuously during tidal breathing; the so-called 'dynamic compliance' can then be obtained – usually on a plot of pressure versus volume – by measuring the slope of a line joining values of pressure and volume at end expiration and end inspiration as determined by zero airflow at the mouth (Figure 3.4b). In normal subjects, dynamic compliance is only slightly less than static compliance. In patients with airway disease, redistribution of air continues through narrowed intrapulmonary airways even when flow at the mouth ceases. Consequently some of the transpulmonary pressure apparently overcoming elastic forces is being dissipated against resistive forces and the apparent compliance is less than that measured statically. This effect increases as breathing frequency increases so that dynamic compliance falls as frequency increases in patients with diffuse airway disease, even when this is mild.

Total respiratory (and chest wall) compliance

Measuring total respiratory compliance (Crs) requires muscular relaxation and is chiefly done in intensive care units or during anesthesia in adults (see Chapter 12). In infants, muscular relaxation can be more easily achieved and more use is made of the measurement. In conscious adults, it is difficult to relax the muscles; the weighted spirometer technique during tidal breathing has been used on the assumption that relaxation is present at the end of each tidal expiration. In circumstances where muscular relaxation is achieved, use of an esophageal balloon and measurement of both mouth and esophageal pressures allow Crs to be subdivided into C_L and Ccw.

- The pressure-volume curve of the lung is measured with an esophageal balloon (to approximate pleural pressure).

- The static PV curve of the lung has an exponential shape and can be represented mathematically by the shape factor 'k'.

- With aging and in emphysema, static lung compliance and k increase. In lung fibrosis lung compliance and k decrease.

- Dynamic compliance of the lung, recorded during tidal breathing falls as breathing frequency increases in patients with mild airflow obstruction.

- Total respiratory compliance requires complete muscular relaxation and can be measured in the ICU.

LUNG VOLUMES

In contrast to lung compliance, measurements of total lung capacity (TLC) and functional residual capacity (FRC) are an important part of the routine pulmonary function assessment. The role of elastic properties in determining the various subdivisions of lung volume is discussed below. In general, TLC is usually reduced when lungs are 'stiff', while for 'floppy' lungs with increased compliance TLC is usually large.

Measurement of lung volumes

METHODS

a. Inert gas dilution[6]

The subject breathes from a closed circuit a gas mixture containing a measured concentration of an inert gas, usually helium, which equilibrates gradually with the resident gas in the lungs. The helium concentration falls progressively, stabilizing once mixing is complete. During rebreathing, CO_2 is absorbed and oxygen is added continuously to maintain a constant overall volume of the system (equipment + lungs). The normal recommendation is for the subject to continue until the helium concentration falls by < 0.02% over a 30 second period. In a healthy individual this is achieved in 5–10 minutes, but in patients with airway disease mixing is much slower and the end point much less definite. The volume measured is that at which the subject is switched into the circuit; usually [FRC + V_D], where V_D is the sum of the apparatus and anatomic dead spaces. The total amount of helium (He) equals the product of its concentration and the volume (V) in which it is distributed. The initial fractional concentration of He (F_1He) in the circuit (V1) falls after switching, reaching an equilibrium concentration F_2He. The total *amount* of helium is unchanged (an insignificant proportion enters solution in the lung tissues and circulating blood):

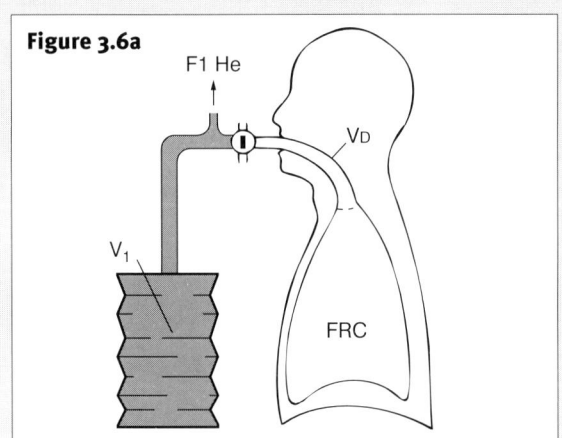
Figure 3.6a

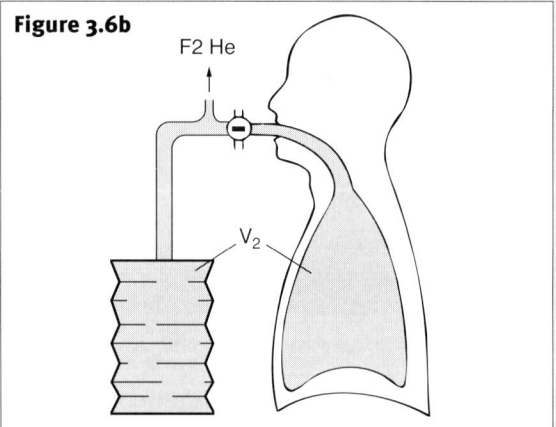
Figure 3.6b

Calculation

Therefore
$$V_1 \cdot F_1He \; (amount\ of\ He) = V_2 \cdot F_2He \; (amount\ of\ He)$$
$$= (V_1 + FRC + V_D) \cdot F_2He$$

whence
$$FRC + V_D = V_1 \left(\frac{F_1He - F_2He}{F_2He} \right) L._{ATPS}$$

Conventionally lung volumes are expressed as L.BTPS (which adds about 10% to the ATPS value).*

At the end of the procedure the subject takes a full inspiration from a spirometer and the inspiratory capacity recorded is added to FRC to give TLC. V_D of the apparatus, but not that of the anatomic dead space should be subtracted.

* For ATPS to BTPS conversion multiply by $(310/273 + t°) \cdot (Pb - P_{H_2O}(t°)/Pb - P_{H_2O}[37°C])$ where t° and 37° are ambient and body temperatures (°C), Pb is barometric pressure, P_{H_2O} is water vapour pressure.

b. Body plethysmography

In Panel I (Figure 3.7) the subject seated within the box is relaxed at FRC with open airway; box, mouth, and alveolar pressure are all atmospheric. A shutter (S) at the mouthpiece is closed transiently (Panel II) and the subject makes gentle inspiratory and expiratory efforts. Since the airway is closed there is no movement of gas in and out of the lungs, but during inspiratory efforts the alveolar pressure still becomes negative (subatmospheric) (see [a], Panel II). According to Boyle's law a reduction of pressure of the gas within the lungs is inevitably accompanied by a small increase in their volume (since P.V product remains constant). Within a rigid plethysmograph the rarefaction of alveolar gas and concomitant increase in thoracic gas volume (TGV) (see [b], Panel II) results in an increase in *box* pressure (see [c], Panel II). (During expiratory efforts against a closed airway – not shown – reciprocal changes occur, i.e. the small increase in alveolar pressure above atmospheric is accompanied by a reduction in TGV and a consequent reduction in pressure within the box.)*

*In the alternative variable volume plethysmograph,[8] increases and decreases in thoracic volume are accommodated by displacement of measured volumes of air out of and into the plethysmograph.

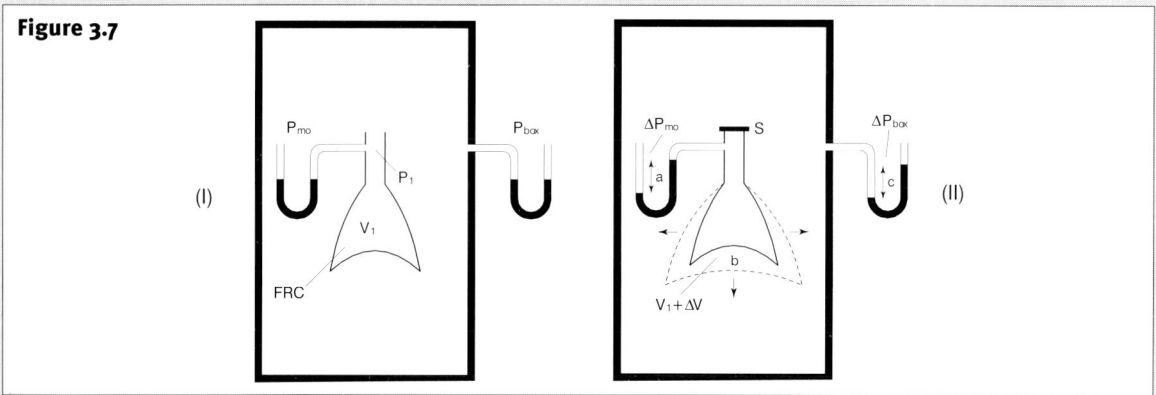

Figure 3.7

Calculation

Panel I – At relaxed end-expiration, mouth and alveolar pressure P_1 equals atmospheric pressure, while $V_1 = FRC$ (the 'unknown')

Panel II – At any instant during an inspiratory effort against the shutter, the new alveolar pressure, P_2, is slightly *less* than P_1 i.e. $(P_1 - \Delta P_{mo})$ *([a])*.

Similarly, the new thoracic gas volume (TGV) is slightly *greater* than V_1 i.e. $(V_1 + \Delta V)$ *([b] in Panel II)*.

Hence: applying Boyle's Law
$$P_1 V_1 = (P_1 - \Delta P)(V_1 + \Delta V)$$
$$= P_1 V_1 - V_1 \Delta P + P_1 \Delta V - \Delta P \Delta V$$

The product $\Delta P \Delta V$ is extremely small and is ignored.

Whence: $V_1 \Delta P = P_1 \Delta V$ So: $V_1 = P_1 . \dfrac{\Delta V}{\Delta P}$

It is assumed that, with a closed external airway, changes in alveolar pressure (ΔP) equal changes in mouth pressure (ΔP_{mo}) and therefore can be measured easily by a transducer connected to the mouthpiece on the subject side of the shutter. Since, in a constant volume plethysmograph, changes in alveolar volume (ΔV) *[b] in Panel II)* are proportional to the change in box pressure (Pbox) *([c] in Panel II)*, the last equation can be written:

$$V_1 \propto P_1 . \frac{\Delta Pbox}{\Delta Pmo}$$

The relationship of $\Delta Pbox$ to ΔV is obtained by introducing a calibrating volume signal from a syringe or sine wave pump. V_1 is then obtained simply from this calibration factor, barometric pressure (P_1) and the slope of the relation between Pbox and Pmo during gentle panting.

If desired, the subject can be asked to inspire fully to total lung capacity (TLC) as soon as the shutter opens, the volume inspired is added to the measured V_1 to give TLC.

c. Radiographic techniques

An alternative approach to measurement of lung volumes is by reconstruction from plain posteroanterior and lateral radiographs. As originally described[9] the method involves dividing the lung fields into a series of elliptical 'slices', the volumes of which are calculated from measurements in two planes. The volume of the heart is subtracted and assumptions are made about the volumes of tissue and blood. While good concordance with physiological measurements is obtainable in healthy subjects, the methods have not been widely applied in disease. X-ray computed tomography can be used in a similar way.

Interpretation and reliability (all methods)

Inert gas dilution.

This technique underestimates absolute lung volumes in patients with airflow obstruction because some areas of lung are insufficiently ventilated to be exposed to the helium. In general, the more severe the airway narrowing the greater this underestimation. An extreme example occurs in the presence of an emphysematous cyst or bulla; this is likely to be virtually unventilated and consequently unreachable by the helium.

An even simpler estimate of absolute lung volume is given by dilution of inert gas during a single breath-hold, as is used during the standard measurement of T_{LCO}. This 'alveolar volume' (V_A) is close to TLC in healthy lungs but in airway disease V_A underestimates TLC to an even greater extent than does the multibreath dilution method.

Body plethysmography

In theory the whole body plethysmograph measures all thoracic gas plus any gas within the body which shares the pressure changes which accompany breathing efforts, e.g. emphysematous bullae, pneumothorax, abdominal gas, etc. However, the important assumption that changes in mouth pressure and alveolar pressure are identical does not apply in all circumstances. This is particularly relevant to patients with airway obstruction. In this situation thoracic gas volume may be overestimated due to dynamic changes in the upper airway during panting in the presence of an increased airway resistance.[10] The error is greater the more severe the airway obstruction. It can be minimized by encouraging gentle panting at a low frequency (< 1 Hz) and by the subject supporting the cheeks and floor of the mouth with the hands in order to reduce the compliance and minimize volume changes of the mouth and pharynx.

Radiographic Technique

The radiographic method, like body plethysmography, will measure all the lung gas volume including that in slowly ventilated spaces such as cysts and bullae. On the other hand, because a subtraction is made for lung tissue and blood volume (a nomogram is used) gas volumes will be overestimated in cardiac and interstitial lung disease when these volumes are increased. Distortion of thoracic shape, as in kyphoscoliosis, may also lead to errors because of the geometric assumptions.

Determinants of lung volumes

Functional residual capacity (FRC)

FRC equals the volume of the lungs at the end of a quiet tidal expiration, often termed the end-expiratory lung volume (EELV). In healthy subjects, who are relaxed and at rest, FRC represents the mechanically neutral position of the respiratory system as a whole (Figure 3.2) and corresponds to the position of the chest during complete relaxation (relaxation volume, Vr, or in the pediatric literature, the elastic equilibrium volume, EEV). Note, however, that at FRC the lungs have a positive (inward) recoil and the chest wall a negative (outward) recoil, i.e. if the chest is opened the lungs deflate while the rib cage springs out. In healthy young adults, FRC is about 50% of total lung capacity. FRC is not always synonymous with the relaxation or mechanically neutral volume of the thorax. For example, in healthy subjects on exercise the end-expiratory level is *lower* than Vr or EEV but it is still referred to as FRC.

In patients with *generalized airway disease* (asthma, emphysema, etc.) the FRC is often markedly increased. In part this results from an alteration in the position of the PV curves of the lungs and chest wall such that the balance of passive forces occurs at a larger volume (static hyperinflation). In addition there may be a variable degree of dynamic hyperinflation, which occurs as an adaptation to the airway narrowing and the consequently severely limited expiratory flow. Greater expiratory flow can be achieved by breathing at higher volumes (see Chapter 1). As a result of the limited flow at lower volumes, tidal expiration is terminated and the next inspiration initiated before the system can deflate to the relaxation volume.[10]

During tidal breathing in normal subjects end-expiration (FRC) occurs with an alveolar pressure of zero, during a gradual transition from positive (expiration) to negative (inspiration). If, however, the airway is occluded immediately prior to inspiration in a patient with dynamic hyperinflation, a positive pressure is recorded as inspiration commences before the lungs and chest wall are allowed to deflate to the relaxation volume of the respiratory system. This positive airway (and alveolar) pressure is known as intrinsic positive end-expiratory pressure (PEEPi).

Total lung capacity (TLC)

A balance of opposing forces also determines lung volume at full inflation. In this case the recoil inwards of the respiratory system is balanced by the outward pull of the inspiratory muscles (Figure 3.1). The effectiveness of inspiratory muscle contraction ('mechanical advantage') diminishes as the length of the muscle fibers shortens. In general the larger the lung volume, the shorter the muscle fibers. Consequently the pressure resulting from inspiratory muscle contraction declines as lung volume increases, until a point (TLC) is reached where it balances respiratory system recoil and further inspiration is impossible.

In conditions such as *pulmonary fibrosis*, where the shrunken lungs have a reduced compliance, this balance is reached at a lower than normal volume and consequently TLC is reduced. At this restricted TLC the mechanical advantage of the inspiratory muscles is greater than at the normal TLC, and so the pressure distending the lungs and consequently the (equal and opposite) lung recoil pressure are greater than normal (Figure 3.5). The converse situation is seen in *emphysema* where lung compliance is greater than normal and the lungs can be inflated to an abnormally large TLC at which the maximum lung recoil pressure is less than normal (Figure 3.5).

Residual volume (RV)

In healthy *young* subjects the position of RV is again dependent on a balance, this time between *outward* recoil of the respiratory system and the force generated by the expiratory (i.e. mainly abdominal) muscles (Figure 3.1). In *older* normal subjects dynamic airway narrowing and closure become important during expiration below FRC. This limits deflation of the lungs and accounts for the progressively rising RV seen with age.[11] This aging effect is exaggerated in patients with diffuse airway narrowing (asthma, COPD), in whom an abnormally large RV (and RV/TLC ratio) is characteristic. For a discussion of Closing Volume, see Chapter 5.

Postural effects

Lung volumes are affected by posture, although in healthy subjects reductions in TLC and VC in the supine posture are small; the largest change is a fall in FRC, mainly due to the gravitational effect of the abdominal contents reducing the relaxation volume (Vr). The most frequently measured postural effect is the fall in VC between upright and supine, which occurs mainly because of the displacement of air by blood pooling in the chest as a result of gravity. The magnitude of this postural change in VC (usually about 200 ml) decreases with age.[12] In disease the effect of posture is of most importance in evaluating diaphragmatic function: diaphragmatic paralysis, especially if bilateral, results in a dramatic fall in VC (> 25% VC, see Chapters 4 and 18) when supine, as the paralyzed diaphragm is unable to resist the effect of gravity on the abdominal contents.

In obese individuals FRC and expiratory reserve volume (ERV = difference between FRC and RV), which are already reduced in the sitting position (see Figure 3.8) may reduce further in the supine posture due to the increased gravitational effects of the large abdomen.

- Inert gas dilution (e.g. helium) techniques may underestimate lung volumes in patients with moderate or severe airflow obstruction.

- Body plethysmographic measurements may overestimate lung volumes in airflow obstruction, but slow and gentle panting with the cheeks supported will minimize the error.

- FRC is increased in patients with airflow obstruction, partly due to changes in elastic properties of the lungs and chest wall, and partly due to intrinsic PEEP.

- RV in normal older subjects rises because narrowing and closure of peripheral airways in dependent zones prevent complete emptying.

- FRC falls when measured in the supine posture; this effect is exaggerated in bilateral diaphragm paralysis.

Causes of reduced total lung capacity

Intrapulmonary: Pneumonectomy
Collapsed lung
Consolidation
Edema
Fibrosis, etc.

Extrapulmonary: Pleural disease:
1. Effusion
2. Thickening
3. Pneumothorax

Rib cage deformity:
1. Scoliosis
2. Thoracoplasty

Respiratory muscle weakness
Gross abdominal enlargement
Severe obesity

Patterns of abnormality in disease

An increase in total lung capacity is seen in emphysema (best measured by body plethysmography) the largest increases occurring when emphysema is associated with large 'giant bullae. Less dramatic increases in TLC may occur with any cause of generalized and severe airflow obstruction, e.g. asthma[13] and COPD. Increases in TLC may go unrecognized in the face of severe airway narrowing if TLC is measured by helium dilution. In occasional patients with *mild* emphysema an increase in TLC is accompanied also by an increase in VC (as might be expected with greater distensibility of the lungs). However, in the vast majority of patients with airway obstruction any tendency for VC to increase by this mechanism is outweighed by the effects of airway narrowing which causes an increase in RV at the expense of VC. Consequently the common pattern of lung volumes in patients with symptomatic airway obstruction is an increase in TLC with a reduction in VC and marked increases in RV and FRC (Figure 3.8). Some cases of acromegaly may have an increased TLC.

Reductions in TLC are usually associated with a reduced VC. With intrapulmonary restriction RV is usually normal so that the RV/TLC ratio is high (and in this context does not necessarily imply airway obstruction) (Figure 3.8).

A mixed obstructive and restrictive ventilatory defect is not uncommon. A mixed pattern is often associated with two different pathologies, such as COPD coincident with fibrosing alveolitis (CFA/IPF). Alternatively, the combination of emphysema and CFA/IPF may result in preservation of TLC in spite of extensive fibrosis.

In the situation of an otherwise typical restrictive defect, a reduced FEV_1/VC confirms coexisting airway narrowing (especially since patients with pure fibrosis often have an FEV_1/VC which is greater than normal). An increase in RV, however, is less specific for airway disease.

In some patients TLC may be within the normal range in the presence of a reduced VC and raised RV

Causes of raised residual volume

Intrapulmonary: Generalized airway obstruction (All causes)
Pulmonary vascular congestion
Mitral stenosis

Extrapulmonary: Expiratory muscle weakness:
1. Spinal injury (disease)
2. Myopathies, etc.

Figure 3.8 Typical changes in lung volume subdivisions in disease

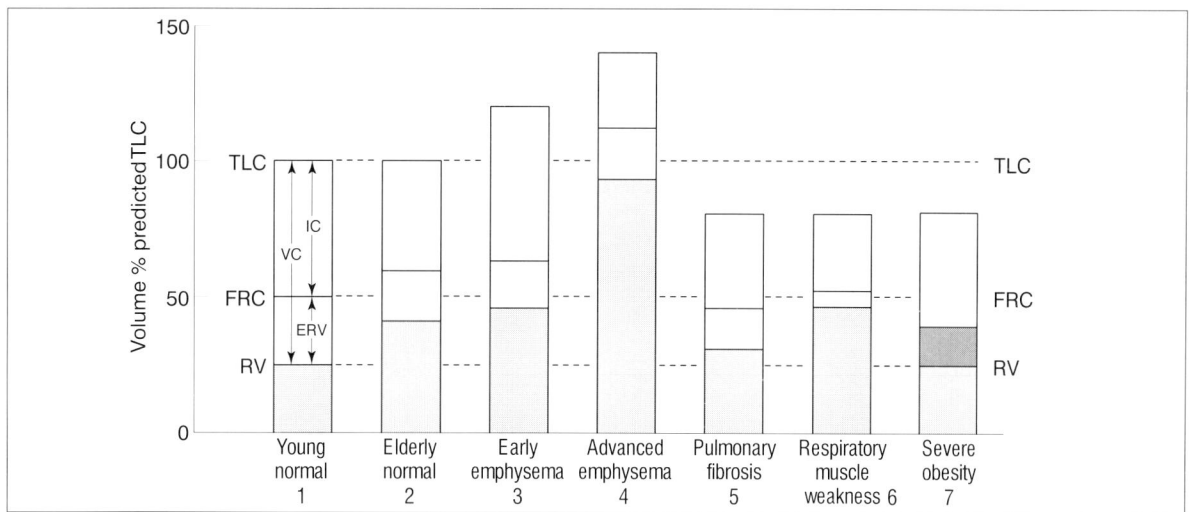

Volume expressed as % predicted TLC; hatched area represents RV, height of each column TLC and the difference (RV to TLC) VC; horizontal lines indicate FRC (FRC – RV = ERV). Note: (2) with aging in healthy subjects RV and FRC increase and VC falls but TLC is unchanged; (3) the pattern described as early emphysema, with an increased VC, is rarely seen; (4) in advanced emphysema the proportionate increases in RV and FRC are usually much greater than the increase in TLC; VC is usually reduced in patients with symptomatic airway obstruction; (5) intrapulmonary and (6) extrapulmonary restriction are similar apart from a tendency for RV to increase in the latter; (7) severe obesity shows a reduction in ERV

(with or without a low FEV_1/VC). This picture can result from a balance of opposing influences, e.g. with pulmonary fibrosis tending to shrink the lungs and airway obstruction tending to produce hyperinflation. In such a situation the net effect on TLC may be deceptively little and tests of lung mechanics may underestimate the severity of the lung destruction. A clue to such combined pathology may be given by a dramatically reduced CO transfer factor as this is likely to be impaired by both disease processes. Obese patients have a reduction in FRC and a small ERV, so that they are breathing close to their residual volume. Their closing volume exceeds their ERV, and airway closure will be present in the tidal breathing range, giving rise to arterial hypoxemia. In gross obesity, TLC is also reduced.

- A large TLC occurs in severe emphysema, especially with 'giant' bullae.
- A small TLC has multiple causes:
  loss of aerated lung units
  diffuse fibrosis
  pleural disease
  respiratory muscle weakness
  gross abdominal enlargement and obesity.
- RV is raised in all causes of diffuse intrapulmonary airflow obstruction, and to a lesser extent in pulmonary vascular congestion and expiratory muscle weakness.
- Expiratory reserve volume (ERV) is reduced in severe obesity.

References

1 Rahn H, Otis AB, Chadwick LE, Fenn WO. The pressure-volume diagram of the thorax and lung. *Am J Physiol* 1946; **146**: 161–78.

2. Gibson GJ & Pride NB. The assessment of lung elasticity. *Br J Dis Chest* 1976; **70**: 143–84.
3. Pride NB & Milic-Emili J. Lung mechanics. In: Calverley P & Pride NB (eds) *Chronic obstructive pulmonary disease*. London: Chapman and Hall 1995: 135–60.
4. Zapletal A, Paul T & Samanek M. Pulmonary elasticity in children and adolescents. *J Appl Physiol* 1976; **40**: 953–61.
5. Gibson GJ, Pride NB, Davis J, Schroter RC. Exponential description of the static pressure-volume curve of normal and diseased lungs. *Am Rev Respir Dis* 1979; **120**: 799–811.
6. Meneely GR & Kaltreider NL. The volume of lung determined by helium dilution. *J Clin Invest* 1949; **28**: 129–39.
7. DuBois AB, Botelho SY & Comroe JH. A new method for measuring airway resistance in man using a body plethysmograph. *J Clin Invest* 1956; **35**: 327–32.
8. Mead J. Volume displacement body plethysmograph for respiratory measurements in human subjects. *J Appl Physiol* 1960; **15**: 736–40.
9. Barnhard HJ, Pierce JA, Joyce JW, Bates JH. Roentgenographic determination of total lung capacity. *Am J Med* 1960; **28**: 51–60.
10. Rodenstein DO & Stanescu DC. Reassessment of lung volume and measurement by helium dilution and by body plethysmography in chronic airflow obstruction. *Am Rev Respir Dis* 1982; **126**: 1040–4.
11. Leith DE & Mead J. Mechanism determining residual volume of the lungs in normal subjects. *J Appl Physiol* 1967; **23**: 221–7.
12. Michels A, Decoster K, Derde L, Vleurinck C, van de Wocstijne KP. Influence of posture on lung volumes and impedance of respiratory system in healthy smokers and non-smokers. *J Appl Physiol* 1991; **71**: 294–9.
13. Pride NB. Physiology. In: Clark TJH, Godfrey S & Lee T H (eds) *Asthma,* 3rd edn. London: Chapman and Hall 1992: 14–72.

4 Respiratory Muscles
J Moxham

- **INTRODUCTION**
  Normal function
  Disease
  Load/capacity balance
  Clinical assessment

- **ASSESSMENT OF RESPIRATORY MUSCLE STRENGTH**
  Simple tests
  Vital capacity, lung volumes, and transfer factor
  Blood gases
  Maximum mouth pressures
  Sniff nasal pressures
  Advantages and disadvantages of simple tests
  More invasive, volitional tests
  Sniff esophageal pressure
  Assessment of diaphragm strength
  Advantages and disadvantages of sniff Pes and sniff Pdi
  Expiratory muscle strength
  Advantages and disadvantages of PEmax and cough Pga
  Non-volitional tests: phrenic nerve stimulation
  Transcutaneous electrical stimulation
  Magnetic stimulation
  Twitch mouth pressure
  Reliability of phrenic nerve stimulation
  Advantages and disadvantages of electrical and magnetic phrenic nerve stimulation
  Sequential assessment of respiratory muscle strength

- **ASSESSMENT OF RESPIRATORY MUSCLE ENDURANCE**
  Sustained hyperventilation
  Sustained pressure development
  Clinical applications

- **ASSESSMENT OF RESPIRATORY MUSCLE FATIGUE**
  Methods of studying muscle fatigue
  Electromyography (EMG)
  Maximal relaxation rate
  Response to nerve stimulation
  Clinical relevance

INTRODUCTION

Normal function

The respiratory muscles perform the crucial function of sustaining ventilation. The major inspiratory muscle is the diaphragm which has left and right domes, each innervated by a phrenic nerve which originates in the cervical spinal cord and tracks down through the neck to the thoracic cavity where it runs over the pericardium before branching through the ipsilateral dome. Contraction of the diaphragm has two actions, (a) lowering the dome like a piston, and (b) elevating and expanding the lower rib cage. The latter action depends on the 'zone of apposition,' where the diaphragm lies apposed to the internal surface of the ribs. Both actions enlarge the lungs; this is accompanied by a reduction in pleural pressure and expansion of the rib cage, and increase in abdominal pressure and outward movement of the abdomen. Other important inspiratory muscles are the scalenes and sternomastoid muscles in the neck which elevate the upper rib cage, and the external intercostal and parasternal intercostal muscles.

The most important expiratory muscles are the muscles of the abdominal wall, whose contraction raises abdominal pressure which is transmitted across the diaphragm to produce a positive intrathoracic pressure. Internal intercostals have some expiratory action and in circumstances where the shoulder girdle is fixed, contraction of pectoral muscles can aid expiration.

At rest, the role of the inspiratory muscles, particularly the diaphragm, is dominant, while expiration is largely passive. During exercise, other inspiratory muscles are recruited and the expiratory muscles play an important role in reducing FRC and aiding the action of the diaphragm. Expiratory muscles provide the effector mechanism of cough.

The force produced by the inspiratory muscles is greatest at small lung volumes; that of the expiratory muscles is greatest at large lung volumes. With hyperinflation, not only is the diaphragm shortened, but the zone of apposition is reduced so that the inspiratory action on the lower rib cage is reduced.

Disease

Severe weakness leads to breathlessness and ventilatory failure. It is therefore entirely appropriate that the pulmonary function laboratory is able to assess the strength of the respiratory muscles. The referring clinician wishes to know the answer to the following questions:

- Are the respiratory muscles weak?
- If there is weakness, how severe is this?
- Is the extent of weakness clinically important?
- Which of the respiratory muscles are most affected?
- Is weakness improving or deteriorating?

These are important clinical questions and the laboratory should be capable of answering them.

Load/capacity balance

The clinical significance of respiratory muscle weakness will depend, not only on the severity of the weakness, but also on the load imposed on the ventilatory system (Figure 4.1). Thus, when the function of the lung is entirely normal, severe respiratory muscle weakness is required before breathlessness or ventilatory failure develops. However, if respiratory disease, for example airways obstruction or pulmonary fibrosis, increases the load on the ventilatory system moderate weakness will then contribute to symptoms.

Figure 4.1 Balance between capacity of respiratory muscles and load

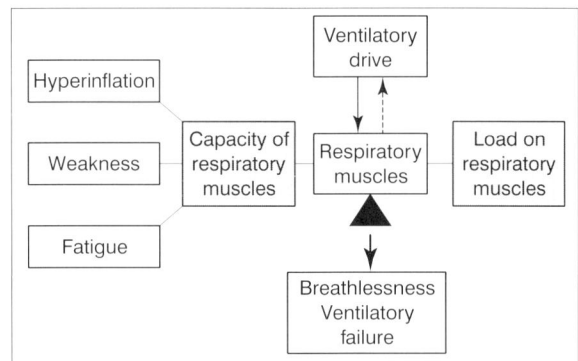

The pulmonary function laboratory can help in assessing both the reduction in ventilatory capacity due to respiratory muscle dysfunction and the increase in ventilatory load due to respiratory disease. The measurement of the dynamic compliance of the respiratory system is particularly important in assessing ventilatory load.

Clinical assessment

Prior to referral to the pulmonary function laboratory the clinician will have gained valuable information about possible respiratory muscle weakness from the history, examination, and imaging techniques.

Causes There are many causes of respiratory muscle weakness:

Neurogenic
  Motor neurone disease
  Polyneuropathy (e.g. Guillain-Barré syndrome)
  Surgical trauma of phrenic nerves
  Neuralgic amyotrophy
  Poliomyelitis
  Multiple sclerosis
  Traumatic tetraplegia
  Acute porphyria

Neuromuscular junction
  Myasthenia gravis
  Eaton-Lambert syndrome

Muscular
  Muscular atrophy (particularly resulting from poor nutrition)
  Muscular dystrophy
  Inflammatory myopathies
  Myotonic dystrophy
  Systemic lupus erythematosus
  Acid maltase deficiency
  Thyroid myopathy
  Biochemical abnormalities (e.g. acidosis, hypophosphatemia)
  Steroid therapy

Patients with known generalized neuromuscular disease, usually affecting limb or bulbar function, are likely to have respiratory muscle weakness, affecting in most cases both the inspiratory and expiratory muscles. Specific lesions of the phrenic nerves, developing either spontaneously or following cardiothoracic surgery, cause unilateral or bilateral diaphragm weakness without affecting other respiratory muscles. Muscles may be weakened not only by specific dystrophies but by inflammation, loss of bulk in severe disease, generalized metabolic disorders and systemic corticosteroid treatment. In severe airways obstruction with hyperinflation, inspiratory muscle function may be reduced by muscle shortening even though there is no intrinsic abnormality of the muscles.

Symptoms Severe respiratory muscle weakness causes breathlessness but moderate weakness may cause few problems unless there is an additional load on the ventilatory system due, for example, to infection. Patients with neuromuscular disease are often capable of little exercise, and breathlessness may therefore be a late development. Severe weakness causes nocturnal hypoventilation which disrupts sleep and causes morning headache, daytime sleepiness, and impaired intellectual function. Patients with severe diaphragm weakness have typical symptoms of orthopnea and breathlessness when standing or sitting in water.[1] Weakness of bulbar muscles and muscles of expiration impair cough and predispose to aspiration and chest infection.

Physical examination Examination may reveal the physical signs of neuromuscular disease, for example wasting and fasciculation. Wasting of the accessory muscles in the neck is easier to appreciate than wasting of the intercostal muscles. With severe weakness poor expansion of the thorax will be apparent. Severe diaphragm weakness causes abdominal paradoxical movement,[1] best seen when supine, when the abdomen moves inwards during inspiration because of the upward motion of the weakened diaphragm.

Imaging With diaphragm weakness one or both hemidiaphragms may be elevated on chest X-ray. With severe global respiratory muscle weakness the lung volumes appear small on chest X-ray but this can be easily misinterpreted as inadequate effort rather than a result of severe weakness. Screening of diaphragm movement during a sniff maneuver demonstrates paradoxical upward movement of the paralyzed diaphragm. Diaphragm movement during respiration can also be assessed by ultrasound. When there is severe bilateral weakness or paralysis, patients may increase tidal volume by contracting abdominal muscles during expiration, thereby reducing end-expiratory lung volume. At the onset of inspiration the abdominal muscles relax, abdominal pressure falls, and the diaphragm descends. When the diaphragm is screened it can appear to move normally during early inspiration despite severe weakness or paralysis.

ASSESSMENT OF RESPIRATORY MUSCLE STRENGTH

A range of tests, of varying complexity and invasiveness, are available to assess respiratory muscle strength. All laboratories should be able to undertake simple tests whereas more complex measurements will be undertaken in specialist centers.

Simple tests

Vital capacity, lung volumes, and diffusing capacity (transfer factor)

Weakness of the inspiratory muscles reduces inspiratory capacity, and weakness of expiratory muscles reduces expiratory capacity, and therefore global respiratory muscle weakness reduces vital capacity (VC) (Figure 4.2).

Figure 4.2 Effect of respiratory muscle weakness on lung volumes

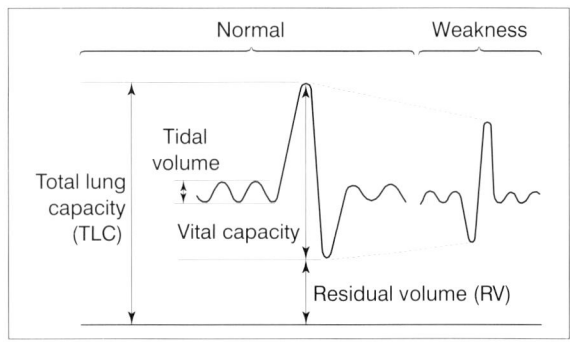

Figure 4.3 ΔVC as index of bilateral diaphragm weakness

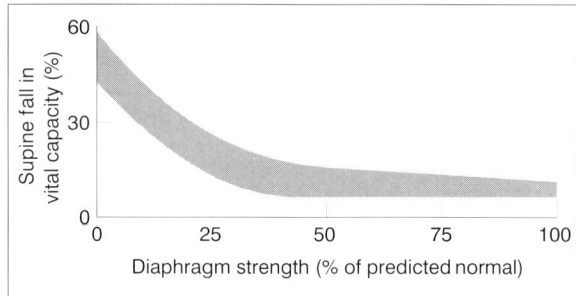

Relationship between percentage fall in vital capacity on adopting the supine posture and diaphragm strength (assessed by measuring transdiaphragmatic pressure during maximum sniffs). Fall in vital capacity is seldom substantial until strength is reduced to 30% of normal.

The simplicity of the VC maneuver makes it ideal for repeated measurements as, for example, in the monitoring of Guillain-Barré syndrome or muscular dystrophy. With substantial diaphragm weakness the VC is reduced and falls further when the patient is supine (Figure 4.3); in normal subjects the supine fall is less than 10% of the sitting values.[2]

Because relatively small pressures are necessary to fully inflate the lung, mild/moderate weakness does not cause a fall in VC. In chronic respiratory muscle weakness (for example following poliomyelitis), reductions in the compliance of the lung and chest wall and sometimes atelectasis result in greater reductions in VC for a given level of weakness. Important shortcomings of VC are the volitional nature of the maneuver and that it is non-specific, being reduced by a wide range of respiratory disor-

Lung function in six patients with severe isolated diaphragm weakness

n = 6	FEV$_1$/VC ratio	VC % pred (seated)	VC % fall (seated to supine)	TLC % pred	RV % pred	D$_{LCO}$ % pred	K$_{CO}$ % pred
mean	0.81	48	37	67	104	65	128
highest	1.00	69	55	83	139	78	167
lowest	0.76	36	30	54	83	44	101

Comment In these six cases, VC is reduced to half normal seated and falls by one third when supine, TLC is consistently reduced, RV is sometimes above normal (up to 139%); the diffusing capacity (D$_{LCO}$) is reduced to two thirds of normal but K$_{CO}$ is increased (up to 167%). The increased K$_{CO}$ is important because it helps distinguish muscle weakness from other intrapulmonary disorders associated with a small TLC (for example pulmonary fibrosis) [see also Chapter 17]). From Laroche et al,[3] with permission.

ders including airways obstruction, pulmonary fibrosis, and obesity.

Notwithstanding limitations, VC remains a remarkably useful simple measurement for the assessment of respiratory muscle weakness. Furthermore, a normal supine VC excludes clinically significant weakness.

Blood gases

Respiratory muscle weakness leads to hypoxemia, mainly due to ventilation/perfusion mismatch, and eventually ventilatory failure (*global* hypoventilation) which leads to hypoxemia and hypercapnia. When the function of the lung is relatively normal hypercapnia does not occur until there is profound weakness, with strength reduced to approximately one quarter of normal.[4] Hypercapnia will occur sooner if there are additional loads on the system, such as an intercurrent infection. Commonly, hypercapnia first develops during sleep. During wakefulness the reduced capacity of the ventilatory system in relation to the demands placed upon it can be sustained by increased respiratory drive but during sleep, when respiratory drive falls, the reduction in ventilation leads to hypercapnia. Hypoventilation is particularly severe during rapid eye movement (REM) sleep. An elevated morning bicarbonate and base excess are early indications of nocturnal hypercapnia. Overnight oximetry traces are useful in assessing hypoxemia. With severe weakness repeated episodes of nocturnal hypoventilation impair ventilatory control and result in established daytime hypercapnia. At this stage treatment with nocturnal non-invasive ventilatory support can reverse ventilatory failure (see Chapter 13). Such treatment can, in carefully selected patients, substantially improve the quality of life. However progressive respiratory muscle weakness eventually leads to irreversible persistent ventilatory failure. Weakness affecting the muscles of the upper airway can be important, predisposing to obstructive sleep apnea. It is of clinical importance to identify such weakness, since apnea can be treated by nocturnal continuous positive airway pressure (CPAP) therapy.

Maximum mouth pressures

When routine lung function tests suggest the possibility of respiratory muscle weakness it then becomes important to measure specifically the strength of the inspiratory and expiratory muscles.

Method

Conventionally respiratory muscle strength is most commonly assessed by measuring maximum static expiratory and inspiratory mouth pressures.[5] These pressures vary with lung volume (see Chapter 3). Maximum expiratory pressure (P$_E$max) is measured during a maximum expiratory effort at TLC, against a closed airway; maximum expiratory pressure generated at the mouth is recorded. Maximum inspiratory pressure (P$_I$max) is measured at the mouth during a maximum inspiratory effort against a closed airway at either RV or FRC. The measurement of P$_I$max and P$_E$max is quick, non-invasive, and normal values, albeit with a wide range, have been established. Simple, portable mouth pressure meters are available. (Fig. 4.4).

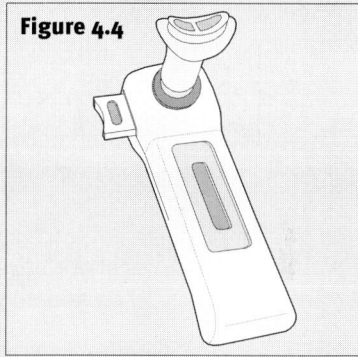

Figure 4.4

Some laboratories use a flanged mouthpiece similar to that used when performing other lung function tests, whereas others use a tube mouthpiece that is pressed against the face around the mouth. Normal subjects generate larger P$_I$max and P$_E$max with a tube mouthpiece, but most patients do best with the flanged mouthpiece.[6] Men can generate larger pressures than women and there is some decline with age. Despite the availability of published normal values it is usually preferable for each pulmonary function laboratory to establish its own normal ranges for P$_I$max and P$_E$max. A P$_I$max of –80 cmH$_2$O or a P$_E$max of +80 cmH$_2$O excludes important weakness of the inspiratory or expiratory muscles. Such a result is therefore of great value.

Reliability and clinical application Problems can arise with the interpretation of low values. Many individuals find the maneuver difficult and this, in part, explains the wide range of normal values. There is also a wide natural variation in muscle strength between individuals. Some patients only achieve very low values despite not having real weakness of their respiratory muscles. Even when highly motivated, some patients with neuromuscular disease causing weakness of the facial muscles and hands have difficulty in performing the P$_I$max or P$_E$max maneuver satisfactorily.

Reference values There are several studies of P$_I$max and P$_E$max in healthy males and females, including those > 60 years.[5,7,8] The best known studies in young and middle-aged subjects are quoted in the paper of Enright et al[8] (references 3–7 in their article). Smaller pressures are generated with conventional flanged mouthpieces than circular tube mouthpieces (c. 60% for P$_E$max and 80% for P$_I$max),[6] but flanged mouthpieces are what most laboratories use. With flanged mouthpieces, the lower limit of normal for P$_I$max is < −70 cmH$_2$O in men and < −35 cmH$_2$O in women (< −40 cmH$_2$O and < −25 cmH$_2$O in those > 65 years); for P$_{E\,max}$, the lower limit of normal is > 90 cmH$_2$O in men and > 50 cmH$_2$O in women (but not significantly different in elderly subjects).[8]

Clinical applications As a result of difficulties with performing the maneuver, approximately half of patients judged to be weak by P$_I$max have normal respiratory muscle strength when assessed by alternative methods. Notwithstanding the difficulties of the maneuver, in patients who are adept at mouth pressure measurements the technique is an excellent simple way of assessing respiratory muscle strength and is particularly useful for sequential measurements. Studies of maximum respiratory pressures confirm that hypercapnia only develops when respiratory muscle strength is considerably reduced[4] (Figure 4.5). In most patients with generalized neuromuscular disease there is a broadly similar reduction in P$_I$max and P$_E$max, although occasional patients have disproportionate diaphragm weakness affecting P$_I$max but not P$_E$max. Hyperinflation associated with severe airways obstruction impairs inspiratory mus-

Figure 4.5 Hypercapnia in patients with myopathy

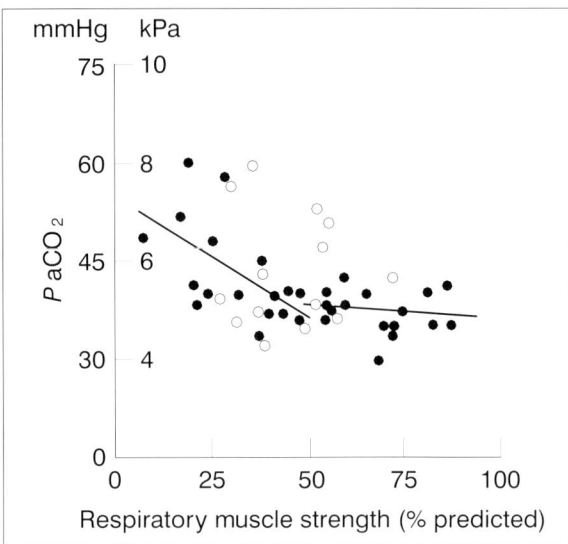

Relationship between arterial carbon dioxide pressure (PaCO$_2$) and respiratory muscle strength in 33 patients with uncomplicated myopathy (●, regression line) and 14 patients with myopathy plus chronic lung disease (○). Respiratory muscle strength expressed as the sum of static P$_I$max and P$_E$max, expressed as a percentage of predicted value and divided by two. Hypercapnia is unusual unless strength is reduced to approximately 30% of normal. [From Braun NMT et al[4], Thorax 1983; 38:616–23, with permission].

cle performance although most studies suggest that P$_I$max remains normal when the increased lung volume is allowed for; hyperinflation does not affect the expiratory muscles. For subjects who have difficulty with the P$_I$max maneuver (which is also used for assessing Pdi), pressure generation is often greater during a rapid inspiratory sniff.

Sniff nasal pressure (sniff Pna)

Method

Normal individuals and patients are familiar with the sniff maneuver. During a rapid maximum effort at FRC negative sniff pressures are generated within the thorax in a reproducible manner. During sniffing the aperture of the nasal passages narrows, producing a high resistance to flow, and volume change within the thorax is relatively small, approximately 500 ml. If a plug is inserted into one nostril with a pressure catheter passed through the plug so that its distal end is within the nose opening, sniffing through the other nostril with the mouth closed generates a negative pressure in the posterior nasopharynx that is similar to esophageal pressure. This pressure (sniff Pna) (Figure 4.6) is therefore a good measure of global inspiratory muscle strength. Normal values for sniff Pna have been described, and a sniff Pna more negative than 60 cmH$_2$O excludes significant inspiratory muscle weakness.[9]

Figure 4.6 Pressures generated during a rapid inspiratory sniff

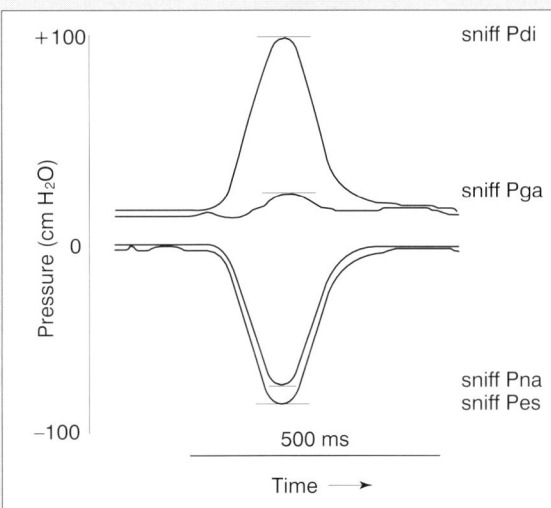

Pressure recorded at the nasal opening in an occluded nostril (see text). When sniff Pdi or Pes is measured the sniff is usually performed through both nostrils. The mouth should be closed during sniffs. Sniff Pdi or Pes is measured as change from the preceding baseline pressure and is usually performed at FRC.

Reliability The measurement is particularly useful in patients who have difficulty in performing the P$_I$max maneuver. A disadvantage of sniff Pna is that in patients with airways obstruction such as COPD the transmission of the negative intrathoracic pressure to the nose is dampened so that sniff Pna is less negative and underestimates inspiratory muscle strength. Nevertheless sniff Pna has considerable potential for the non-invasive measurement of inspiratory muscle strength and represents an important advance in our capacity to assess simply the respiratory muscles in the laboratory.

Advantages and disadvantages of simple tests

Vital capacity
- Simple, available, but non-specific.
- Rather insensitive, but normal supine VC excludes important respiratory muscle weakness.

Maximum effort mouth pressures
- Good for sequential measurements in 'trained' patients.
- Underperformance common.
- Good pressures exclude significant respiratory muscle weakness.

Sniff nasal pressure
- Applicable to most patients.
- Problems with transmission of intrathoracic pressure in COPD; sniff maneuver sometimes difficult with bulbar disease.

More invasive, volitional tests

After completing simple tests to assess respiratory muscle function, the answer to the basic question 'Is there true weakness of the respiratory muscles?' sometimes remains unanswered. In some patients, although weakness seems likely on the basis of the screening tests, a more specific and quantitative assessment is required. Furthermore, it may be clinically helpful to try to partition any weakness between the diaphragm and the other inspiratory muscles. In these circumstances it is necessary to position esophageal and gastric balloon catheters. A gastric balloon catheter can also be used to assess expiratory muscle strength.

Sniff esophageal pressure

Method

Maximum sniff esophageal pressure (sniff Pes) is the best available measurement of global inspiratory muscle strength.[10] The placement of an esophageal balloon is invasive but in practice is well tolerated by the vast majority of patients. Almost all patients find the sniff maneuver easy to perform. The maximum sniff efforts are made through an unoccluded nose with the mouth shut, and efforts are made from FRC. Sniff efforts are performed every 1–2 minutes and can be repeated without tiring. Patients achieve maximum efforts rapidly and there is little learning effect. The normal range of sniff esophageal pressure is narrower than that for Pimax and the test is therefore more useful for detecting weakness. A substantial number of patients who are judged to be weak on the Pimax test have normal strength when assessed by sniff Pes. A sniff Pes more negative than 80 cmH$_2$O in men and 70 cmH$_2$O in women excludes significant inspiratory muscle weakness.

Dynamic compliance and other measures of load
In addition, measurement of the esophageal pressure swings during resting ventilation and during exercise provides valuable information on the load imposed on the ventilatory system. If change in volume during breathing is measured using a spirometer or integrated pneumotachograph, dynamic compliance can be calculated (see Chapter 2 p. 32 and Chapter 3). These measurements, which can be amplified to include work, total lung resistance, and intrinsic PEEP (see Chapter 12), greatly facilitate understanding the clinical significance of any documented respiratory muscle weakness because they give information on the balance between load and capacity (Figure 4.1).

Sniff Pna can provide equally useful information as sniff Pes without the need for an esophageal balloon but there are some patients, e.g. those with COPD, in whom sniff Pna is less reliable than sniff Pes.

Assessment of diaphragm strength

To assess diaphragm strength specifically, it is necessary to measure changes in transdiaphragmatic pressure (Pdi), expressed as the difference between esophageal and gastric pressure. Note that while Pimax and sniff Pes are reported as negative (subatmospheric) pressures, Pdi is positive during a maximum inspiratory effort (Figure 4.6). Experimental work in animals confirms that transdiaphragmatic pressure is a good reflection of diaphragm muscle tension.

Sniff transdiaphragmatic pressure (sniff Pdi)
Historically, Pdi has been measured during a maximum static inspiratory effort at FRC against a closed airway. This maneuver is identical to, and has all the disadvantages of, the Pimax maneuver. With this technique the results of transdiaphragmatic pressure are variable and the normal range is very wide. Sniff Pdi has a narrower normal range and more reproducible results. Sniff Pdi shares the advantages of sniff Pes discussed above and is therefore the measurement of choice for the assessment of diaphragm strength.[11]

Sniff Pdi is greater than 100 cmH$_2$O in normal males and greater than 70 cmH$_2$O in females. The technique allows the accurate assessment of diaphragm weakness and is particularly valuable for sequential assessment. From the measurement of sniff Pdi in a large number of patients with varying degrees of diaphragm weakness it is now clear that orthopnea, paradoxical abdominal motion, and supine fall in VC only develop when sniff Pdi is less than 30 cmH$_2$O or approximately 25% of normal strength[1] (Figure 4.3).

Advantages and disadvantages of sniff Pes and sniff Pdi

- Most patients can perform the sniff maneuver.
- No problems with pressure transmission.
- Invasive technique.
- Rely on maximum voluntary efforts.

Expiratory muscle strength

The strength of the expiratory muscles, principally the abdominal and internal intercostal muscles, is measured by recording PEmax (see above). As with Pimax, some patients find the maneuver difficult to perform and the range of normal values is wide, so whereas a high PEmax reliably excludes expiratory muscle weakness a low value can frequently be difficult to interpret. Better techniques are needed for assessing expiratory muscle strength, which is particularly reduced in advanced neuromuscular disease and in tetraplegia, leading to an ineffective cough.

Cough gastric pressures Patients find cough to be a natural maneuver and can produce maximal expiratory pressures with little training. Although the measurement requires passing a gastric balloon catheter the values produced are often higher than for P$_E$max. Many patients with low P$_E$max values have normal expiratory muscle strength as judged by cough gastric pressures. The use of cough gastric pressure is relatively recent and requires further evaluation but it appears likely to be a useful additional test.

Advantages and disadvantages of P$_E$max and cough Pga

- Advantage of the P$_E$max maneuver is that it is non-invasive and widely available.
- Disadvantage of P$_E$max is that some patients do not perform the maneuver maximally; interpretation of low values can be difficult.
- Advantage of the cough Pga maneuver is that coughing is a natural maneuver that most patients perform maximally.
- Disadvantage of cough Pga is necessity of a gastric balloon catheter.
- Correct approach is to measure P$_E$max and, if the result is low, to measure cough Pga.

Non-volitional tests: phrenic nerve stimulation

Until recently, stimulation of the phrenic nerve has been achieved electrically; this is a highly skilled technique which has been little used clinically. The recent development of magnetic stimulation has greatly increased the possibility of making non-volitional tests of inspiratory muscle strength, such as Pdi in response to a simple twitch, in the clinical setting and may even be applied in the Intensive Care Unit.

Transcutaneous electrical stimulation

Using surface electrodes the phrenic nerves can be electrically stimulated in the neck close to the posterior border of sternomastoid at the level of the hyoid cartilage. Supramaximal stimulation is possible and therefore maximal twitch Pdi responses can be measured, as can the electromyograph (EMG) response. The diaphragm EMG can be measured from an esophageal electrode but is usually recorded from surface electrodes placed in the seventh interspace in the anterior axillary line. In normal subjects and patients the phrenic nerve conduction time is less than 9.5 ms (Figure 4.7).

The size of the EMG action potential can be used to assess that stimulation is supramaximal. Each phrenic nerve can be stimulated separately and so it is possible to assess the two sides individually. However, the technique has numerous disadvantages. Electrical stimulation is uncomfortable for the subject, precluding stimulation at frequencies much greater than 1 Hz. It can frequently be difficult to achieve a satisfactory stimulation position, therefore supramaximal activation is not always possible and variability in twitch Pdi substantial. In practice, whereas a high twitch response excludes hemidiaphragm weakness, a low response is often difficult to interpret with certainty. The reported normal values for bilateral electrical twitch Pdi at FRC are wide (8.8–33 cmH$_2$O), presumably reflecting the difficulty of bilateral supramaximal stimulation. However, because it is frequently possible to achieve some response, the technique remains valuable for confirming that diaphragm function is present and for measuring the phrenic nerve conduction time. This may be useful in assessing the prognosis when there is unilateral or bilateral diaphragm weakness, as for example after damage to the phrenic nerve during cardiothoracic surgery.

Figure 4.7 Surface electromyogram of diaphragm after ipsilateral stimulation of phrenic nerve

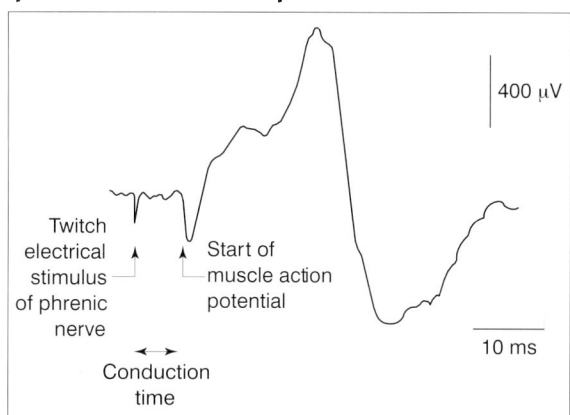

Normal phrenic nerve conduction time is < 9.5 ms. The size of the muscle action potential can be used to assess maximality of the applied twitch. (Reproduced with permission from Oxford University Press and Laroche CM, Moxham J & Green M. Respiratory muscle weakness and fatigue. Quart J Med 1989; **71**: *373–97)*

Magnetic stimulation[12]

Methods
Magnetic stimulation is substantially less uncomfortable than electrical stimulation and requires less precise positioning.

Magnetic stimulation of the phrenic nerves by posterior stimulation of phrenic nerve roots
Supramaximal bilateral phrenic nerve stimulation can be achieved using a circular magnetic coil placed over the cervical phrenic nerve roots. The neck of the subject is flexed and the magnet is pressed against the skin with its center over the level of C6 or C7 spinous processes.

Figure 4.8

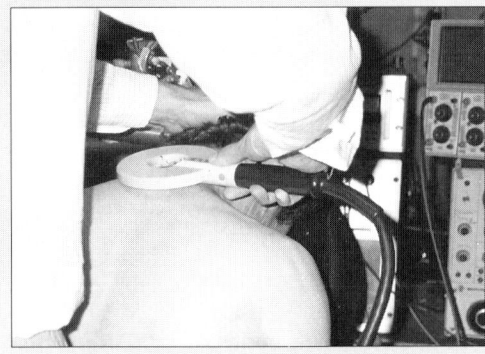

Figure 4.9

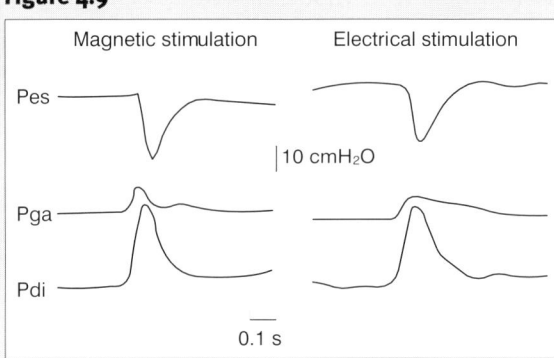

With cervical stimulation the twitch Pdi at FRC is similar to that elicited by bilateral electrical stimulation although the amplitude is slightly larger. This is due to a more negative twitch Pes.[13]

This increased esophageal component is due to stimulation of the muscles of the upper thorax rendering the rib cage slightly stiffer and thereby allowing the diaphragm contraction to generate a more negative Pes. In clinical practice this slight non-specificity of cervical magnetic stimulation does not importantly reduce the clinical value of the technique for the assessment of diaphragm strength.

Anterior magnetic stimulation of the phrenic nerves
Smaller, twin, magnetic coils can be used to stimulate the individual phrenic nerves anteriorly in the neck;[14] with anterior magnetic stimulation it is easy to achieve supramaximal stimulation rapidly and reproducibly. Using such coils on each side, supramaximal stimulation can be easily achieved and the response obtained is closely similar to that achieved by successful bilateral electrical stimulation. With unilateral anterior magnetic stimulation the twitch Pdi at FRC is approximately 10 cmH$_2$O and with bilateral stimulation 25 cmH$_2$O. Values of twitch Pdi are usually about 20–30% of those produced in a well-performed sniff Pdi or Pdimax maneuver. The normal range is relatively narrow and diaphragm weakness is likely when bilateral twitch Pdi is less than 19 cmH$_2$O.

Figure 4.10

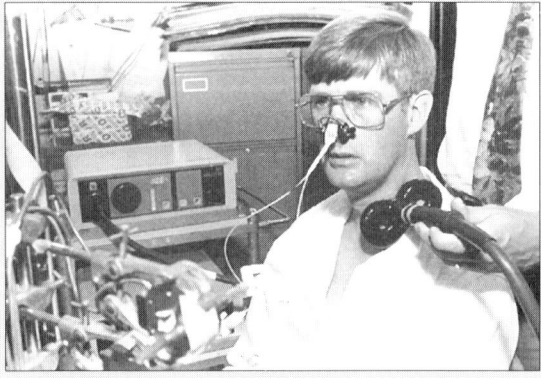

Twitch Pdi and Pes are measured from esophageal and gastric balloons passed pernasally.

Twitch mouth pressure

During a voluntary sniff maneuver the pressure in the pharynx usually closely reflects Pes (see above). Similarly, when the phrenic nerve is stimulated it is possible to use the pressure measured at the mouth (twitch Pmo)[15] as an indication of twitch Pes. To measure twitch Pmo the patient breathes on a mouthpiece which is occluded at FRC and the phrenic nerves are then magnetically stimulated. To make sure that the glottis remains open it is often best if the subject makes a small expiratory effort and the slight increase in mouth pressure triggers the stimulator (Figure 4.11).

Figure 4.11 Twitch mouth pressure with cervical magnetic stimulation in a normal subject

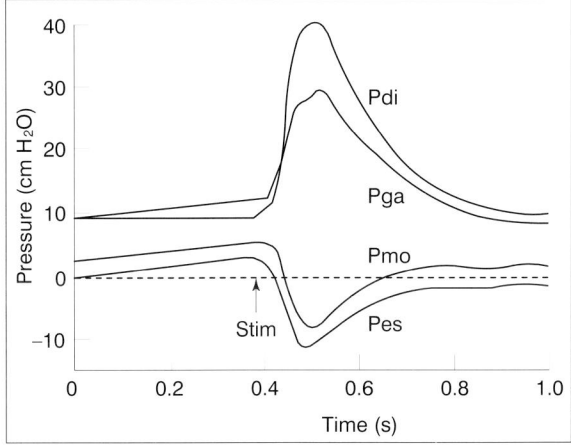

Twitch pressures are measured as the change from the pressure immediately before triggering. Twitch Pmo is currently under evaluation in the clinical setting.[16] As with sniff Pna, twitch Pmo may not reflect twitch Pes in the presence of airways obstruction, but may well prove to be an excellent non-volitional and non-invasive technique for assessing diaphragm strength and weakness in other situations.

Reliability of phrenic nerve stimulation The diaphragm has to be relaxed when nerve stimulation is applied. The preceding contraction history is important because twitch pressures are increased following the voluntary contraction of any skeletal muscle, the phenomenon known as twitch potentiation. For the diaphragm large voluntary efforts can increase twitch Pdi by 60%. It is important to assess the diaphragm after the patient has been breathing quietly for a period of 10–15 minutes. Twitch Pdi is affected by diaphragm length and therefore by lung volume. Stimulation should be at FRC; stimulation at 1.0 L above FRC reduces a normal twitch Pdi by about 5 cmH$_2$O. A disadvantage of magnetic stimulation is difficulty in recording the diaphragm EMG from surface electrodes because of stimulus artifact and excitation of other chest wall muscles.

Advantages and disadvantages of electrical and magnetic phrenic nerve stimulation

- Magnetic stimulation has many advantages, and few disadvantages, when compared with electrical stimulation.
- Magnetic stimulation is less uncomfortable for the subject, optimal positioning is quicker, and the twitch Pdi response is more reproducible because supramaximal stimulation is easier.
- The equipment for magnetic stimulation is expensive and not yet widely available.
- Cervical magnetic stimulation is also not completely specific for the diaphragm but bilateral anterior stimulation largely overcomes this problem.
- The recording of diaphragm EMG with magnetic stimulation is difficult, and electrical stimulation remains an important technique to study diaphragm EMG.

Sequential assessment of respiratory muscle strength

To decide whether or not the respiratory muscles are weak can be simple in some patients and difficult in others. The question can be answered with greatest efficiency and accuracy by proceeding from simple to more complicated tests.[17] If weakness is present, invasive tests are required to assess its severity. The specific assessment of diaphragm strength entails measuring Pdi.

Table 4.2 Schema for investigating the respiratory muscles

CLINICAL	
History and examination	Respiratory muscle involvement is likely in any patient with a neurological or muscle disorder
STANDARD SIMPLE TESTS	
Sitting and supine vital capacity (VC)	Normal supine VC excludes important respiratory muscle weakness
Lung function, including Kco	The combination of reduced TLC and normal or raised Kco in a patient with reduced lung volumes suggest respiratory muscle weakness
Arterial (or arterialized ear lobe) blood gas analysis	Hypoxemia due to weakness implies moderately severe disease: hypercapnia indicates severe weakness
PI and PEmax	PImax (at FRC or RV) more negative than 70–80 cmH$_2$O excludes important inspiratory muscle weakness. PEmax at TLC > 80 cm H$_2$O excludes important expiratory muscle weakness
SNIFF TESTS (at FRC)	
Non-invasive	
If PImax reduced, measure sniff nasal pressure	Sniff Pna more negative than 60 to 70 cm H$_2$O excludes important inspiratory muscle weakness
Esophageal balloon	
If sniff nasal pressure reduced (or if significant co existing lung disease) measure sniff esophageal pressure	Sniff Pes more negative than 70 to 80 cmH$_2$O excludes important inspiratory muscle weakness
Esophageal and gastric balloons	
If sniff Pes reduced and/or specific assessment is required of diaphragm weakness, measure transdiaphragmatic pressure	Sniff Pdi of 70 to 100 cm H$_2$O excludes important diaphragm weakness
NON-VOLITIONAL TESTS (at FRC)	
Esophageal and gastric balloons and phrenic nerve stimulation	
If sniff Pdi reduced (or in patients unable to perform voluntary maneuvers) stimulate phrenic nerves magnetically and measure Pdi	Twitch Pdi (unpotentiated) >10 cm H$_2$O (unilateral) or 20 cm H$_2$O (bilateral) excludes important diaphragm weakness

ASSESSMENT OF RESPIRATORY MUSCLE ENDURANCE

Tests of respiratory muscle endurance[18] are not as well developed or as widely applied as measurements of strength. They presuppose a determined and fully motivated subject. In practice many patients find endurance tests difficult and it is frequently impossible to distinguish whether impairment or inadequate effort is responsible for a poor performance. Most commonly, respiratory muscle endurance is assessed by the ability of subjects to sustain high levels of ventilation or respiratory pressures.

Sustained hyperventilation

Endurance can be investigated by asking subjects to ventilate maximally for prolonged periods, conventionally between 2 and 15 minutes.[18] During prolonged hyperventilation it is important to monitor the end-tidal CO_2 and maintain it at a normal level thereby avoiding hypocapnia. This is usually achieved by ventilation circuits that allow partial rebreathing plus the addition of extra CO_2. Sustained maximum voluntary ventilation represents substantial exercise and involves the vigorous recruitment of many muscles not commonly involved in ventilation.

The value of maximum voluntary ventilation (MVV) that can be sustained for a brief period of 12–15 s ('sprint MVV') cannot be sustained for longer periods. In normal subjects the level of ventilation rapidly falls during the first minute and thereafter approaches a plateau (Figure 4.12). In well-motivated normal subjects, plateau values for sustained MVV are about 70% of sprint MVV. In normal subjects sustained MVV leads to respiratory muscle fatigue with slowing of maximum relaxation rate (MRR) (see below) of both the inspiratory[19] and expiratory muscles and also a reduction in both twitch Pdi[20] and twitch Pga. In COPD the fall in maximum ventilation over the duration of the test is less than in normal subjects, and in some patients ventilation does not fall at all. This finding suggests that intrapulmonary mechanical factors rather than muscle strength per se limit sustained MVV in COPD. Furthermore, in COPD the diaphragm does not develop a reduction in twitch Pdi nor low frequency fatigue following sustained MVV.

A related approach is to assess the period for which varying percentages of sprint MVV can be sustained. In normal subjects the maximum sustainable ventilation ranges between 50 and 80% of sprint MVV. Alternatively, patients can be required to sustain a relatively low level of ventilation for 2 or 3 minutes and then the target level of ventilation is increased in a progressive step-wise fashion until ventilation cannot be sustained.[18]

Sustained pressure development

The endurance properties of the inspiratory muscles can be studied by asking individuals to breathe through an inspiratory resistance and thereby generate a large change in pressure with each breath. Conventionally the pressure generated within the mouthpiece is displayed in front of the subject and a target pressure is also set. The individual seeks to reach the target pressure with each breath for as long as possible. The larger the percentage of the maximum inspiratory pressure (Pimax) that has to be achieved, the shorter is the time for which the inspiratory resistive loading can be sustained.[21] If transdiaphragmatic pressure (Pdi) is measured, the endurance time for the diaphragm can be measured in an analogous fashion. The load on the diaphragm can be expressed as the tension (strictly pressure) time index (TTdi) which relates tidal pressure requirement to maximum pressure:

$$TTdi = \frac{\Delta Pdi_{(tidal)}}{Pdi_{(max)}} \cdot \frac{T_I}{T_{TOT}}$$

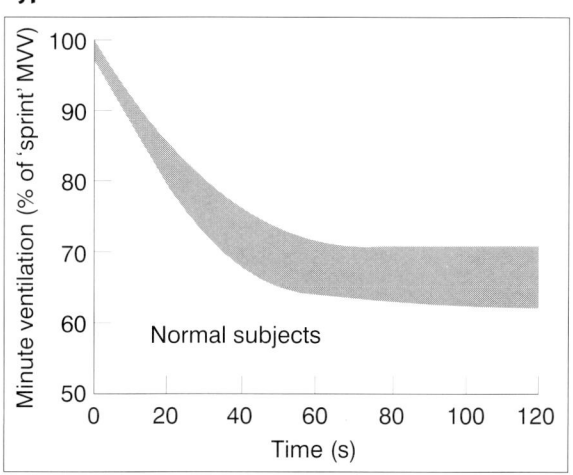

Figure 4.12 Decline in ventilation during voluntary hyperventilation

where T_I/T_{TOT} is the proportion of each breath spent on inspiration (duty cycle). When studied with *external* loads, a given Pdi (tidal) has to be sustained throughout inspiration; when used as an index of *internal* load during tidal breathing, peak tidal ΔPdi is used.

Great commitment by the subject is needed to achieve reproducible endurance times. In practice the results often tend to be variable, partly reflecting different levels of commitment between tests, and partly a learning effect whereby individuals spontaneously alter their pattern of breathing to minimize work and discomfort while still achieving the target pressures for as long as possible. These strategies can be thwarted by asking that individuals breathe at a particular respiratory rate and pattern, but this often makes the test more difficult and can also result in subjects stopping because of breathlessness.

Inspiratory threshold loading devices[18] have been developed to make the load imposed on the inspiratory muscles more reproducible. With these devices a valve or a weighted plunger does not permit airflow until a threshold pressure is reached. When this threshold is exceeded, the valve opens or the plunger is raised and there is then no resistance to airflow, although the threshold pressure has to be sustained. Inspiratory muscle endurance times are more reproducible when threshold loading devices are used.

Clinical applications

Sustained hyperventilation, inspiratory resistive loading, and threshold loaded breathing have all been used to assess the endurance of the inspiratory muscles and the impact of training programs. However these techniques are probably only useful in the hands of those performing such tests regularly and working with highly motivated normal subjects or patients.

Although these techniques are of potential interest in all patients with neuromuscular disease and muscle weakness, in practice they have been applied most to patients with COPD or asthma in whom the abnormality of the inspiratory muscles is usually functional due to the shortening imposed by hyperinflation and the load is greatly increased by increased airflow resistance, reduced dynamic compliance, and intrinsic PEEP. (Patients with advanced COPD may have some additional generalized muscle weakness due to poor nutrition and/or systemic corticosteroid treatment.) In COPD patients, exercise tests - either formally on cycle ergometer or treadmill or using 6 or 12 minute walk or shuttle walk tests (see Chapter 8) – provide useful, if indirect, information on respiratory muscle function and the ability to sustain increased ventilation and pressure requirements (see below).

Attempts have been made to improve respiratory muscle function by specific training programs; the available data suggest that, at best, such training is of marginal benefit.[22]

ASSESSMENT OF RESPIRATORY MUSCLE FATIGUE

When the ventilatory load on the respiratory system is excessive in relation to the ventilatory capacity patients develop breathlessness, reduced exercise tolerance, and eventually ventilatory failure. This 'task failure' might be due to fatigue of the respiratory muscles. Much research effort has been devoted in recent years to the study of respiratory muscle fatigue and its possible clinical importance.[23] Muscle fatigue can be investigated in many different ways.

Methods of studying muscle fatigue

Electromyography (EMG)

When skeletal muscle is excessively loaded there is a change in the high frequency component of the EMG signal from the muscle compared to the low frequency component, reducing the EMG high/low ratio. A fall in the EMG high/low ratio of the respiratory muscle has been observed in patients failing to wean from mechanical ventilation. Many other factors influence the high/low ratio, however, and it is not clear what relationship the ratio has to other indices of fatigue. This measurement has not been used extensively in clinical practice.

Maximal relaxation rate

When skeletal muscle is excessively loaded there is a progressive slowing of maximum contraction and relaxation rates. The slowing of maximum relaxation rate (MRR) is a predictable and relatively robust measurement. With rest, MRR rapidly returns to normal over approximately 10 minutes. The MRR of the respiratory muscles can be measured, usually from esophageal or transdiaphragmatic pressure wave forms during a sniff maneuver. When normal subjects undertake inspiratory resistive loading to exhaustion there is marked slowing of inspiratory muscle MRR.[24]

Response to nerve stimulation

Excessive muscle loading also leads to reduced peripheral muscle contractility. Following resistive loading there is a reduction in twitch Pdi and a shift to the right (less force at a given frequency of stimulation) of the frequency/force curve of the diaphragm.[25] Similar changes have also been documented for the sternomastoid muscle. These changes may last several hours and demonstrate that the respiratory muscles *can* develop low frequency fatigue following severe respiratory loading.

Clinical relevance

Chronic hypercapnia occurs in severe weakness associated with neuromuscular disease (Figure 4.5) and in severe COPD, where it is related to a combination of reduced Pimax and increased mechanical load. There has been much speculation about whether chronic hypercapnia indicates chronic respiratory muscle fatigue, and also whether fatigue develops in the acute crisis when the load is increased by infection or by other factors.

Using available techniques, how clinically relevant is respiratory muscle fatigue? The answer to this question remains uncertain but slowing of inspiratory muscle MRR develops in patients with severe COPD who exercise to extreme breathlessness (Figure 4.13). Non-invasive positive pressure ventilation, used to reduce the work of breathing in such patients, reduces the slowing of muscle relaxation rate, reduces breathlessness, and increases the distance that such patients can walk.[26] Similarly, in patients failing to wean from mechanical ventilation there is also a slowing of respiratory muscle MRR.[27] Slowing of MRR is a relatively early change in the fatiguing process but these observations do suggest that the inspiratory

Figure 4.13 Maximum relaxation rate of Pes before and after exercise

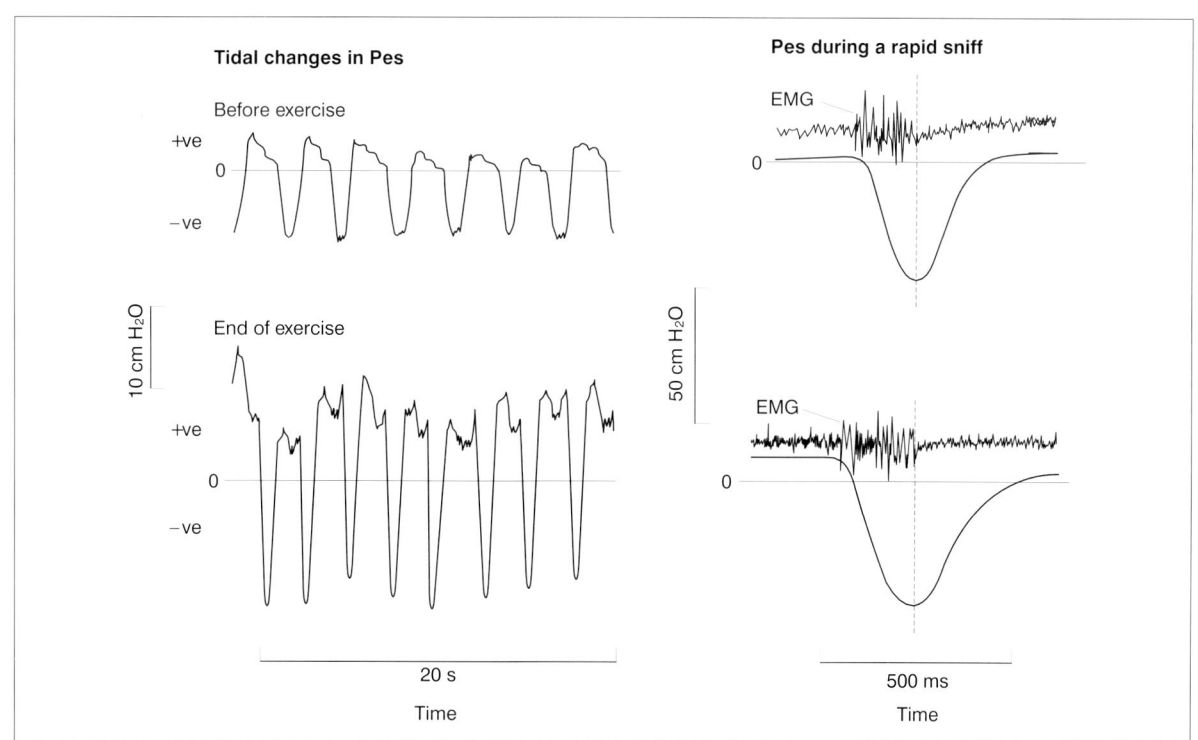

Changes before, and at the end of, exhaustive treadmill exercise in a patient with severe COPD. Left panels show the increase in tidal swings of Pes; right panels show the prolongation of relaxation of Pes during a rapid sniff. Surface EMG of the diaphragm indicates rapid termination of EMG activity when the most negative Pes is achieved.

muscles are excessively loaded and the fatiguing process has commenced. However, when COPD patients exercise to their limits it is not possible to demonstrate any reduction in twitch Pdi. This observation suggests that in some clinical situations, even though the respiratory muscles are hard pressed and the MRR slows, overt contractile failure probably does not occur. Contractile failure is avoided by a reduction in central drive. When low frequency fatigue is experimentally induced it is associated with muscle damage, and perhaps patients 'choose' task failure (even if this manifests itself as ventilatory failure) rather than inducing peripheral muscle damage and contractile failure. In this context it is of note that patients failing weaning trials develop rapid shallow breathing, and that similar breathing patterns are seen in many patients with acute ventilatory failure. Such breathing patterns reduce ventilatory work, albeit at the cost of hypoventilation and hypercapnia. Some patients in respiratory distress alternate predominantly diaphragmatic breathing with predominantly rib cage breathing, a strategy aimed perhaps at minimizing the load on particular respiratory muscles.

References

1. Mier A, Brophy C, Moxham J, Green M. Assessment of diaphragm weakness. *Am Rev Respir Dis* 1988; **137**: 877–83.
2. Allen SM, Hunt B & Green M. Fall in vital capacity with posture. *Brit J Dis Chest* 1995; **79**: 267–71.
3. Laroche CM, Carroll N, Moxham J, Green M. Clinical significance of severe isolated diaphragm weakness. *Am Rev Respir Dis* 1988; **138**: 862–6.
4. Braun NMT, Arora NS & Rochester DF. Respiratory muscle and pulmonary function in polymyositis and other proximal myopathies. *Thorax* 1983; **38**: 616–23.
5. Black LF & Hyatt RE. Maximal respiratory pressures: Normal values and relationships to age and sex. *Am Rev Respir Dis* 1969; **99**: 698–702.
6. Koulouris N, Mulvey DA, Laroche CM, Green M, Moxham J. Comparison of two different mouthpieces for the measurement of Pimax and PE max in normal and weak subjects. *Eur Respir J* 1988; **1**: 863–7.
7. Rochester DF & Arora NS. Respiratory muscle failure. *Med Clinics North Am* 1983; **67**: 573–97.
8. Enright PL, Kronmal RA, Manolio TA, Schenker MB, Hyatt RE. Respiratory muscle strength in the elderly: correlates and reference values. *Am J Respir Crit Care Med* 1994; **149**: 430–8.
9. Heritier F, Rahm F, Pasche P, Fitting J-W. Sniff nasal pressure. A non invasive assessment of inspiratory muscle strength. *Am J Respir Crit Care Med* 1994; **150**: 1678–83.
10. Laroche CM, Mier AK, Moxham J, Green M. The value of sniff esophageal pressure in the assessment of global inspiratory muscle strength. *Am Rev Respir Dis* 1988; **138**: 598–603.
11. Miller J, Moxham J & Green M. Sniff as a test of diaphragm function. *Clin Sci* 1985; **69**: 91–6
12. Similowski T, Fleury B, Launois S, Cathala HP, Bouche P, Derenne JP. Cervical magnetic stimulation: a new painless method for bilateral phrenic nerve stimulation in conscious humans. *J Appl Physiol* 1989; **67**: 1311–8.
13. Wragg S, Aquilina R, Moran J *et al.* Comparison of cervical magnetic stimulation and bilateral percutaneous electrical stimulation of the phrenic nerves in normal subjects. *Eur Respir J* 1994; **7**: 1788–92.
14. Mills GH, Kyroussis D, Hamnegard C-H, Wragg S, Moxham J, Green M. Unilateral magnetic stimulation of the phrenic nerve. *Thorax* 1995; **50**: 1162–72.
15. Hamnegard C-H, Wragg S, Kyroussis D, Mills G, Bake B, Green M, Moxham J. Mouth pressure in response to magnetic stimulation of the phrenic nerves. *Thorax* 1995; **50**: 620–4.
16. Hughes PD, Polkey MI, Kyroussis D, Hamnegard C-H, Moxham J, Green M. Measurement of sniff nasal and diaphragm twitch mouth pressure in patients. *Thorax* 1998; **53**: 96–100.
17. Polkey MI, Green M & Moxham J. Measurement of respiratory muscle strength. *Thorax* 1995; **50**: 1131–5.
18. Clanton TL. Respiratory muscle endurance in humans. In: Roussos Ch (ed) *The Thorax,* 2nd edn. New York: Marcel Dekker 1995: 1199–1230.
19. Mulvey DA, Koulouris NG, Elliott MW, Laroche CM, Moxham J, Green M. Inspiratory muscle relaxation rate after voluntary maximal isocapnic ventilation in humans. *J Appl Physiol* 1991; **70**: 2173–80.
20. Hamnegard C-H, Wragg S, Kyroussis D *et al.* Diaphragm fatigue following maximal ventilation in man. *Eur Respir J* 1996; **9**: 241–7.
21. Roussos C, Gross D & Macklem PT. Fatigue of inspiratory muscles and their synergistic behaviour. *J Appl Physiol* 1979; **46**: 897–904.
22. Smith K, Cook D, Guyatt GH, Madhavan J, Oxman AD. Respiratory muscle training in chronic airflow limitation: a meta-analysis. *Am Rev Respir Dis* 1992; **145**: 533–9.
23. Roussos C, Bellemare F & Moxham J. Respiratory muscle fatigue. In: Roussos Ch (ed) *The Thorax,* 2nd edn. New York: Marcel Dekker 1995: 1405–61.
24. Esau SA, Bellemare F, Grassino A, Permutt S, Roussos C, Pardy RL. Changes in relaxation rate with diaphragmatic fatigue in humans. *J Appl Physiol* 1983; **54**: 1353–60.
25. Moxham J, Morris AJR, Spiro SG, Edwards RHT, Green M. Contractile properties and fatigue of the diaphragm in man. *Thorax* 1981; **36**: 164–8.
26. Keilty SE, Ponte J, Fleming TA, Moxham J. Effect of inspiratory pressure support on exercise tolerance and breathlessness in patients with severe stable chronic obstructive pulmonary disease. *Thorax* 1994; **49**: 990–4.
27. Goldstone JC, Green M & Moxham J. Maximum relaxation rate of the diaphragm during weaning from mechanical ventilation. *Thorax* 1994; **49**: 54–60.

Section II
GAS EXCHANGE, CONTROL OF BREATHING, EXERCISE

5 Pulmonary Gas Exchange

J M B Hughes

- **INTRODUCTION**
  Oxygen transport overview

- **OXYGEN IN ARTERIAL BLOOD**
  Carriage of gases in blood
  Oxygen dissociation curve (ODC)
  Non-invasive measurements of arterial oxygenation
  PaO_2 from arterialized capillary blood
  Transcutaneous PaO_2 ($tcPO_2$)
  Pulse oximetry (SpO_2)
  Causes of hypoxemia
  Ventilation-perfusion mismatching: theory

- **GAS EXCHANGE IN DISEASED LUNGS**
  The three compartment model
  Dead space compartment
  Venous admixture compartment
  Quantitating gas exchange inefficiency for oxygen
  Deviation of PaO_2 from 'normal' values
  The ideal alveolar to arterial PO_2 gradient
  PaO_2/FiO_2 ratio
  Physiological shunt ($\dot{Q}s/\dot{Q}_T$ phys)
  Anatomic shunt ($\dot{Q}s/\dot{Q}_T$ anat)
  Responses to arterial hypoxemia
  Compensatory mechanisms
  FiO_2 increase
  Arterial PCO_2
  Clinical examples

- **MEASURING VENTILATION AND PERFUSION INHOMOGENEITY**
  Multiple inert gas elimination technique (MIGET)
  Distribution of ventilation (intraregional)
  Phase III and closing volume
  Inter-regional distributions of ventilation and perfusion
  Clinical applications

- **NITRIC OXIDE**
  Measurement of exhaled NO
  Therapeutic use of inhaled NO

INTRODUCTION

The majority of this chapter focuses on the assessment and interpretation of hypoxemia in the context of measurements of arterial oxygen tension (PaO_2) and arterial oxygen saturation (SaO_2). A brief review of techniques for measuring the distributions of ventilation ($\dot{V}_A$) and perfusion ($\dot{Q}$) follows, mismatching of these distributions being the most important clinical cause of arterial hypoxemia. First, gas exchange *as a whole* will be viewed, from the entry of oxygen into the lungs to its utilization by body tissues. Carbon dioxide travels in the reverse direction, but the principles are the same.

Oxygen transport overview

There are two means of transporting oxygen:

1. convection (bulk flow)
2. molecular diffusion coupled to chemical reaction with hemoglobin.

These two mechanisms operate in series between the mouth and the tissues. Convective flow requires an energy source to build up a head of pressure; in the steady state, fluids (gases or blood) flow downhill, down a pressure gradient. In a system of tubes (airways or blood vessels), the quantity of fluid passing through the system per unit time (the flow rate) is proportional to the overall pressure difference from one end to the other and the geometry of all the tubes in the system itself. The geometry is the reason for the pressure gradient itself, loss of pressure being caused by frictional resistance and the need to accelerate the fluid molecules at points of narrowing. For gas exchange, the energy for the convective flow of oxygen is provided by two pumps:

1. respiratory muscles, chiefly the diaphragm, for ventilation
2. the heart for blood flow.

The link between these two pumps is provided by **molecular diffusion** where molecules of a *particular* species move down *partial* pressure gradients by diffusive flux, in the absence of any externally applied energy. In **convective flow**, all molecules move together, e.g. oxygen, nitrogen, and carbon dioxide, driven by the *total* pressure (the blood pressure in the case of the circulation, and alveolar pressure for ven-

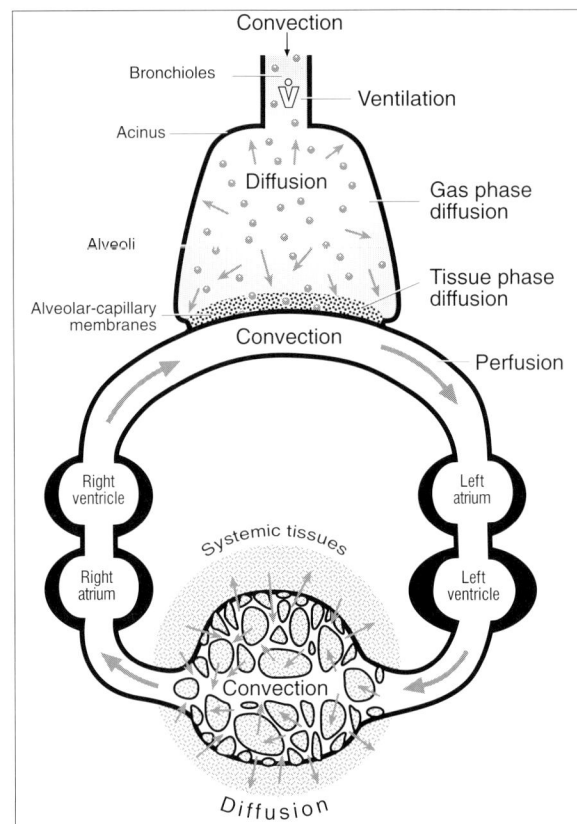

Figure 5.1 Oxygen transport from lung to tissues

Convection and diffusion operate in series. The acinus, distal to the terminal bronchioles, is the effective unit of gas exchange in normal lungs.

tilation). In diffusive flow, the movement of oxygen molecules in one direction, driven by a partial pressure difference, must be balanced (in a closed system) by an equal number of molecules of a different species (say carbon dioxide) moving in the other.

After crossing the red cell membrane by molecular diffusion, oxygen combines chemically with hemoglobin (Hb). This process is reversed in the body tissues, i.e. unbinding of O_2 from Hb and diffusion out of the red cell.

Note that *partial pressure* is equivalent to *concentration* only in gases in a gaseous medium or when physically dissolved in plasma or tissues, and only when the barometric pressure remains constant. The concentration of oxygen in air on the top of Mt Everest (21%) is the same as at sea level, but the barometric pressure, and therefore the partial pressure of oxygen, is less than a third of that at sea level.

The conventional view of pulmonary gas exchange focuses on convective flow of gas and blood (and the matching of one to the other throughout the lung), neglecting alveolar-capillary diffusion (in the gas and tissue phases) which is the link between them (Figure 5.1). Diffusion is not a limiting factor for gas exchange in normal lungs (though it may become so in diseased lungs and in normal subjects at altitude), because the anatomy of the gas exchanging units is so favorable to this mode of transport. The ultimate 'unit of gas exchange' is the acinus, which is the lung distal to a terminal bronchiole. There are about 50 000 acini, and each one contains about 5 000 alveolar sacs. Gas transport within an acinus is predominantly by molecular diffusion and not by convection.

OXYGEN IN ARTERIAL BLOOD

Carriage of gases in blood

The carrying capacity of blood for different gas species (O_2, CO_2, CO, etc.) varies widely, as shown in Figure 5.2; it is plotted as content (ml.L^{-1}) against partial pressure. Gases of clinical interest, such as oxygen, carbon dioxide, and carbon monoxide, form chemical bonds in blood mostly with hemoglobin. The relationship is curvilinear (S-shaped for oxygen) and is called a dissociation curve. The carrying capacity of blood for gas is the capacitance coefficient (β) which is the slope of the curve (Figure 5.2) at a particular PO_2 (in practice, over as narrow a range of PO_2 as possible). For the oxygen dissociation curve (ODC) β is highest in the 0–50 mmHg (0–6.7 kPa) range. β for oxygen represents its effective solubility in blood at a particular partial pressure. Gases which do not combine chemically, but which are just physically dissolved, have a linear relationship between concentration and pressure and so a single value for β; examples include anesthetic gases such as ether, nitrous oxide (N_2O), acetylene (used in research to measure cardiac output by rebreathing) and, of course, oxygen and CO in plasma.

The oxygen dissociation curve (ODC)

The ODC (Figure 5.3) for hemoglobin A has a sigmoid shape. The position of the curve is designated by the

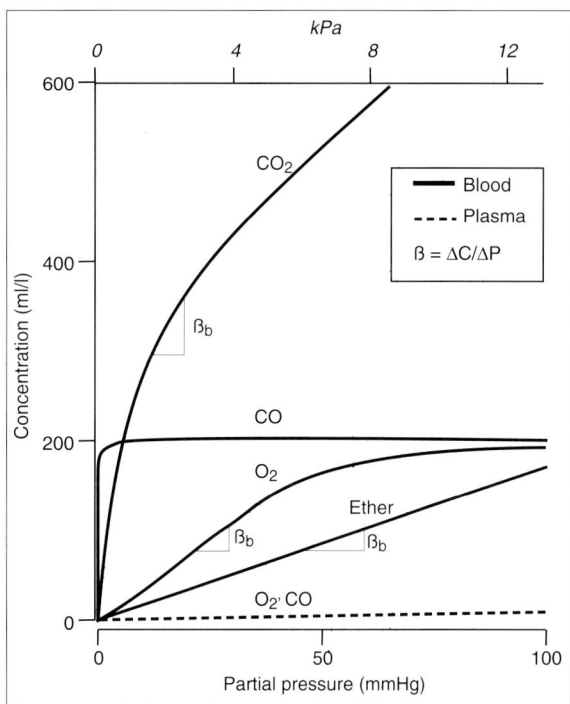

Figure 5.2 Concentration-pressure relationships for gases in blood

P_{50} which is defined as the PO_2 at 50% oxygen saturation (SO_2) or half maximum concentration. The normal value for P_{50} is 26–28 mmHg (3.5–3.7 kPa). A shift to the right (Figure 5.3) – raising P_{50} – occurs during exercise when there is tissue hypercapnia, acidosis, and hyperthermia, or with an increase in concentration of red cell 2:3 diphosphoglycerate (2:3 DPG), a glycolytic pathway intermediate. The higher P_{50} is beneficial on exercise because more oxygen is given up to the tissues; for a given PaO_2, the oxygen concentration or saturation is lower. The interaction of the ODC with carbon dioxide is called the Bohr effect. A shift to the left occurs with fetal hemoglobin, which has an exponential rather than sigmoid shape. The low P_{50} (about 19 mmHg [2.53 kPa]) of fetal blood means that in umbilical venous blood, where the PO_2 is only 30 mmHg [4.0 kPa], the hemoglobin saturation is 74% which is 16% higher than in maternal placental blood at the same PO_2. Oxygen will be given up to the tissues with some difficulty, but the fetus does not require to do much exercise!

The oxygen content of blood (ml.L^{-1}) is the sum of a small amount dissolved in plasma (about 1.5% of

Figure 5.3 Oxygen dissociation curve (ODC) for whole blood and plasma

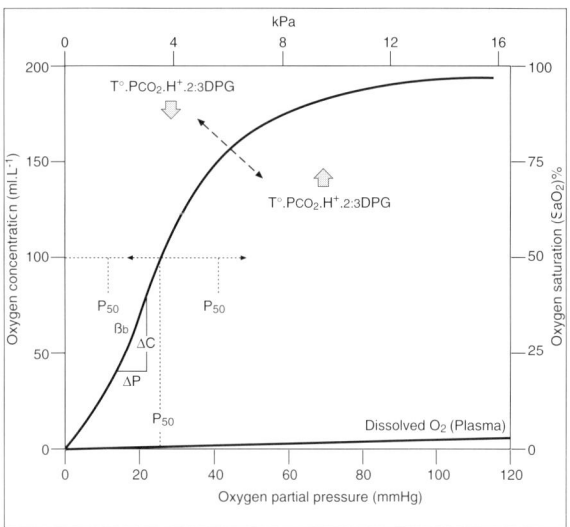

Table 5.1 Aide memoire for the oxygen dissociation curve

SaO_2 (%)	PaO_2 (mmHg)	PaO_2 (kPa)	Comments
97.5	100	13.3	Arterial blood
96	80	10.7	Lower limit for arterial blood
89	60	8.0	On the knee of the ODC. Moderate hypoxemia. (A convalescent patient qualifies for home oxygen therapy)
75	40	5.3	Severe hypoxemia. Needs O_2 therapy acutely. (Normal value for mixed venous blood at rest)
50	27	3.6	P_{50}. Mixed venous blood on moderate exercise

the total breathing air, and 8% of the total breathing 100% O_2) and that combined with hemoglobin:

$$O_2 \text{ content} = PO_2 \times \beta_p O_2 + SO_2 \times [Hb] \times 1.39$$

where $\beta_p O_2$ is the carrying capacity of plasma for oxygen (0.003 ml.dL^{-1} mmHg^{-1}), [Hb] is the hemoglobin concentration (g.dL^{-1}), and 1.39 ml.O_2.g^{-1} is the capacity of Hb for oxygen.

The oxygen content of blood is more often calculated from measurements of SO_2, PO_2 and [Hb], than actually measured. The modern pulse oximeter provides a non-invasive and reasonably accurate measurement of the saturation of arterial blood with oxygen (SaO_2), as a percent of the maximum saturation at PO2 >150 mmHg (20 kPa).

Non-invasive measurements of arterial oxygenation

From the ODC (Figure 5.3), the difference between a 'normal' PaO_2 (100 mmHg [13.3 kPa]) and a definitely 'abnormal' PaO_2 (60 mmHg [8.0 kPa]) is 40 mmHg [5.3 kPa], whereas the change of SaO_2 is only 8.5% (97.5–89%). Therefore, because of the shape of the ODC, PaO_2 is a more sensitive index of mild degrees of hypoxemia than SaO_2. Below 60 mmHg (8.0 kPa), SaO_2 becomes more sensitive. Measurements of PaO_2 have always been regarded as more 'definitive' and an advantage is that $PaCO_2$ and pH are measured at the same time. SaO_2 can also be calculated from PaO_2, assuming a standard ODC; this is more accurate than the converse – calculating PaO_2 from SaO_2 – because $PaCO_2$ and pH, which can shift the ODC (Figure 5.3), are not taken into account. The only argument against the frequent use of PaO_2 is that it is invasive, requiring arterial puncture. PaO_2 can be measured from a 'capillary' sample from the arterialized earlobe, which is discussed in the next section.

Typical values for arterial blood in a healthy subject, breathing air:

O_2 content = 100 [mmHg] × 0.003   +   0.975 × 14.5 × 1.39

            = [0.3 ml.dL^{-1} in plasma]   +   [19.65 ml.dL^{-1} combined with Hb]

            = 19.95 ml.dL^{-1} in whole blood, 98.5% being hemoglobin bound

Measurement of PaO_2 from arterialized capillary blood

The technique involves making a small cut in the periphery of the earlobe, after previous warming with vasodilator cream. Blood, which must be freely flowing, is collected in a capillary tube, as anaerobically as possible, and analyzed immediately. Blood from the earlobe is a mixture of blood from capillaries and venules, and it cannot have the same PO_2 as pure arterial blood because there is a gradient of PO_2 from 90–100 mmHg (12–13.3 kPa) at the arterial end of the capillary bed to 40 mmHg (5.3 kPa) at the venous end. Nevertheless, if the capillary bed is dilated sufficiently and blood flow increased 10–20 fold (without a change in $\dot{V}O_2$ – see Fick Equation),* the arteriovenous difference narrows so much that capillary and venous PO_2 approach arterial PO_2. The arteriovenous PO_2 difference is likely to be smaller and more favorable if PaO_2 and PvO_2 are on the steep part of the ODC (< 60 mmHg [8.0 kPa]). In fact, with good vasodilatation and, most importantly, good technique, there is convergence of arterial PO_2 and arterialized PO_2 at PaO_2 levels < 70 mmHg (9.3 kPa).[1] Arterialized values > 80 mmHg (10.7 kPa) underestimate PaO_2 by 4.4 ± 4.4 (SD) mmHg (0.59 kPa). The results on exercise are very similar to those at rest, the larger (a-v̄) PO_2 difference on exercise being offset perhaps by greater vasodilatation in the earlobe. Failure to arterialize the capillary blood sufficiently means that arterialized PO_2 will underestimate the true PO_2; in the opposite sense, poor collection with air contamination will raise arterialized PO_2 above arterial PO_2. Sometimes, the two errors may cancel each other.

Like measurements of SaO_2 using pulse oximetry, arterialized capillary PO_2 is least reliable in the higher PaO_2 range (> 70 mmHg [9.3 kPa]). An advantage over pulse oximetry is that measurements of PCO_2 and pH are obtained from the capillary sample, and these track arterial values even more closely than PO_2. It is suitable for use by non-medical staff, provided great care is taken over blood spillage and accidental skin pricks, especially when hepatitis B and human immunodeficiency virus (HIV) positive patients are studied.

*FICK EQUATION:
Gas transport = arteriovenous content difference × cardiac output
$\dot{V}O_2$ = [CaO_2 – CvO_2] × [$\dot{Q}$]

Transcutaneous measurements of PaO_2 ($tcPO_2$)

A Clark polarographic electrode placed on the skin measures the PO_2 in subdermal tissues. Like the measurement of arterialized PO_2 from the earlobe, the arteriovenous PO_2 difference must be virtually eliminated to obtain an accurate arterial estimate. This is achieved by heating the skin to 40–42°C. While the method works satisfactorily in neonates where the epidermis is very thin, substantial underestimates of PaO_2 may occur in adults (much greater than with arterialized earlobe samples) because of individual differences in the anatomy and physiology of the dermis and epidermis. Calibration against a simultaneous arterial sample is therefore needed. $tcPO_2$ may be able to follow trends in arterial PO_2 over time in adults, but a spot sample is not reliable.

The measurement of $PaCO_2$ with transcutaneous electrodes is well established as a reliable monitor of long-term trends, i.e. overnight in patients with nocturnal hypoventilation. The small arteriovenous difference for PCO_2 at rest is an advantage.

Pulse oximetry (SpO_2)

Pulse oximetry detects transmitted light at two wavelengths, corresponding to deoxygenated and oxygenated hemoglobin. The light emitters and detector face each other separated by tissue (finger or earlobe) 5–10 mm thick. The signal is the difference in absorbance between the peripheral systolic pulse wave and the sub-

Requirements for the accurate estimation of SaO2 with pulse oximetry

■ Adequate arterial pulsation	Use vasodilator cream
■ Minimal venous pulsation	Keep finger probe near heart level
■ [COHb] < 3%	Avoid smoking for 24 hours
■ Steady state	Wait a minimum of 5 minutes
■ Interference (but skin pigmentation OK)	Avoid nail polish, very bright lighting

sequent diastole – a difference of only 1–10% of the total light absorbance. Carboxyhemoglobin [COHb] (and methemoglobin) absorb light at the same wavelength as deoxyhemoglobin, so that HbO_2% is overestimated in the presence of COHb.

With these reservations, pulse oximetry is acceptably accurate at rest and on exercise when compared with simultaneous estimates of oxygen saturation from arterial blood samples.[2] In non-smokers (COHb < 3%), the differences at rest and on exercise were < 2%, with a trend for the finger probe to underestimate and the ear probe to overestimate true arterial saturations.

The pulse oximeter is so patient friendly and so user friendly (the machine calibrates itself in about one minute) that technique can become sloppy and the results unreliable. Better results will be obtained if readings are written down at one minute intervals on a proforma sheet (patients can do this for themselves) for ten minutes in order to confirm the reliability of the measurement. The strength of pulse oximetry is its ability to follow changes – from rest to exercise, from air to oxygen breathing, and for continuous overnight monitoring. It can also be used in places where arterial puncture is not feasible – in patients' homes, for example.

Laboratory and domiciliary uses of pulse oximetry (SpO_2)

- Assessment for home oxygen therapy:
    1. SpO_2 on air and on oxygen via nasal prongs at different flow rates
    2. SpO_2 at end of 'walk test' breathing air or oxygen (via portable cylinders).
- SpO_2 monitoring during progressive or steady state exercise testing.
- SpO_2 monitoring overnight for obstructive sleep apnea diagnosis.
- SpO_2 monitoring at home (done by the patient) during the day or overnight.
- Assessment of 'fitness to fly' (see Chapter 13) using 15% FiO_2.
- Substitute for arterial sampling in children or when serial observations are required.

Causes of hypoxemia (low PaO_2)

■ Low oxygen partial pressure (P_IO_2)	Altitude
■ Hypoventilation (low $\dot{V}_E$)	Respiratory center depression Neuromuscular diseases
■ Diffusion limitation ('alveolar-capillary block')	Exercising with low P_IO_2 or low D_{LO_2}
■ $\dot{V}_A/\dot{Q}$ mismatching	Any intrapulmonary disease
■ Anatomic right to left shunts	Pulmonary arteriovenous malformations Intracardiac shunts

$\dot{V}_A/\dot{Q}$ mismatching (see next section) accounts for the hypoxemia in the majority of cases. More than one mechanism may be operating at any one time. Effective hypoxemia also occurs when PaO_2 is normal but blood oxygen content (concentration) is low, such as in anemia, carbon monoxide poisoning, and methemoglobinemia.

Arterial hypoxemia is not serious in itself. As far as the bodys tissues are concerned, oxygen delivery is more important:

$$O_2 \text{ delivery} = \text{arterial oxygen content} \times \text{tissue blood flow}$$

Low tissue blood flow (in relation to the metabolic demand for oxygen [local $\dot{V}O_2$]) will cause tissue hypoxia irrespective of the arterial PO_2 or SaO_2.

Hypoventilation is defined as inadequate total minus dead space ventilation in relation to metabolic demand (oxygen uptake and carbon dioxide production). To maintain the respiratory quotient (RQ – usually 0.8 and which is imposed on the lung by tissue metabolism), P_ACO_2 must rise as P_AO_2 falls in a ratio of 0.8, i.e. approximately equally. The end result is a combination of hypoxemia and hypercapnia (low P_AO_2 and high P_ACO_2). Common causes of hypoventilation are the shallow breathing associated with respiratory depression or neuromuscular weakness; the low tidal volume means that a large proportion of the total ventilation is wasted ventilating the anatomic dead space. In the long term, hypoventilation may lead to retention of secretions, secondary atelectasis, $\dot{V}_A/\dot{Q}$ mismatching and further hypoxemia. The term *alveolar hypoventilation* is also used, referring to a situation where total minus dead space ventilation has not increased sufficiently to maintain $PaCO_2$ at normal levels (the $PaCO_2$ being high in the first place because of severe $\dot{V}_A/\dot{Q}$ mismatching [see section on Arterial PCO_2]).

Diffusion limitation is characterized by an alveolar-end-capillary oxygen tension difference in all or most lung units. Failure of oxygen equilibration between gas and blood is caused by a low $D_{LO_2}/[\dot{Q}_T.\beta_{O_2}]$ ratio – the ratio of the diffusive and perfusive conductances (see Figure 6.2). If the gas to blood gradient at the proximal (venous) end of the pulmonary capillary (alveolar to mixed venous PO_2) is nominally 100%, the end gradient (alveolar to end-capillary PO_2) will be 13% when $D_{LO_2}/\dot{Q}_T.\beta = 2.0$, and 37% when $D_{LO_2}/\dot{Q}_T.\beta = 1.0$. Normal values at rest are 4–6, falling on exercise to 2–3 because the increase of $\dot{Q}_T$ outstrips that of D_{LO_2}. β is higher when PaO_2 is low (because of the shape of the ODC), and substantial hypoxemia may occur when normal subjects exercise at extreme altitudes. In subjects with very low D_{LCO} (and thus low D_{LO_2}), and whose exercise capacity is not limited by severe airflow obstruction – typically patients with end-stage fibrosis or the hepatopulmonary syndrome (see Chapter 16) – the increase in $\dot{Q}_T$ far exceeds their very small increase in D_{LO_2}, and significant arterial oxygen desaturation occurs on mild to moderate exercise. This used to be called 'alveolar capillary block', and was later attributed to $\dot{V}_A/\dot{Q}$ mismatching. While $\dot{V}_A/\dot{Q}$ mismatch is the cause of the hypoxemia at rest, *diffusion limitation* is the reason for the further desaturation on exercise.

Ventilation-perfusion mismatching: theory

$\dot{V}_A/\dot{Q}$ mismatching is clinically the most common cause of arterial hypoxemia. As an extreme example, imagine the immediate effect of complete blockage by an embolus of the left main pulmonary artery, combined with complete obstruction by a tumor of the right main bronchus. Without ventilation, the blood flow (equivalent to the whole cardiac output) through the right lung would be unoxygenated (once the small oxygen stores in that lung had been exhausted), and would act as a 'physiological shunt'. The $\dot{V}_A/\dot{Q}$ ratio would be zero and the PO_2 and PCO_2 of the blood leaving the right lung would be the same as that entering it, i.e. of mixed venous composition (40 and 46 mmHg [5.3 and 6.0 kPa]) respectively. The other lung, with ventilation but no pulmonary blood flow, would act as 'physiological dead space' with a $\dot{V}_A/\dot{Q}$ ratio of infinity (∞) and an alveolar PO_2 and PCO_2 which would equal the inspired partial pressures (150 mmHg [20 kPa] and zero, respectively). Thus, there would be no gas exchange.

Figure 5.4 Oxygen-carbon dioxide diagram

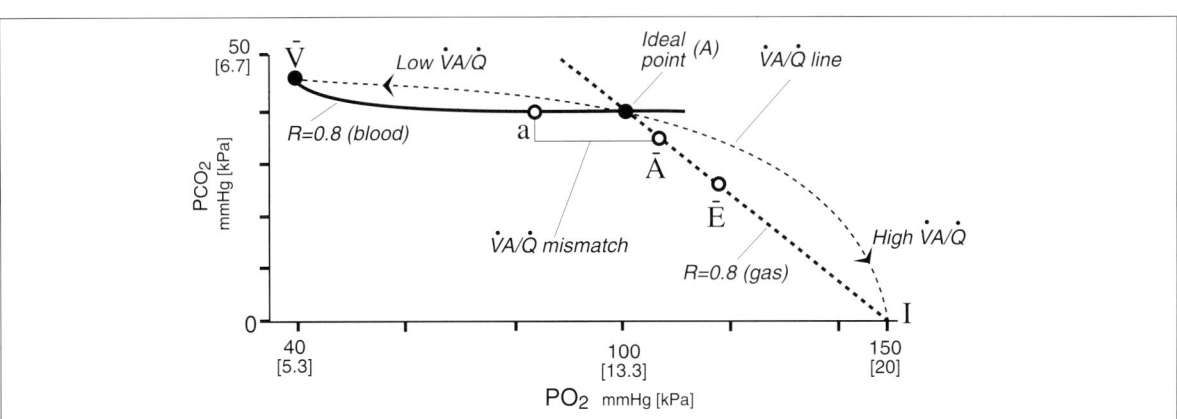

All possible combinations of alveolar PO_2 and PCO_2 for $\dot{V}_A/\dot{Q}$ ratios from zero to infinity for the given inspired (I) and mixed venous (v) compositions. Ideal point corresponds to $\dot{V}_A/\dot{Q}$ ratio of 0.86. With increasing $\dot{V}_A/\dot{Q}$ mismatch, arterial PO_2 falls along blood R line with an increasing 'ideal – a' PO_2 difference and alveolar PCO_2 moves down gas R line (total dead space fraction = [ideal – E] / [ideal – I]).

As $\dot{V}_A/\dot{Q}$ ratios increase from zero to infinity, so P_AO_2 increases from 40 to 150 mmHg (5.3 to 20 kPa) and P_ACO_2 decreases from 46 mmHg (6.0 kPa) to zero. For a resting subject, breathing air, Figure 5.4 shows every value of $\dot{V}_A/\dot{Q}$ from 0 to ∞ in terms of their alveolar PO_2 and PCO_2 values. At rest, if the lung were entirely uniform, with the total alveolar ventilation (say 4.3 L.min^{-1}) and pulmonary blood flow (say 5.0 L.min^{-1}) distributed evenly between all gas exchanging units, the $\dot{V}_A/\dot{Q}$ ratio would be 4.3/5.0, i.e. 0.86, which would mean that all alveoli would have a PO_2 of 100 mmHg (13.3 kPa) and a PCO_2 of 40 mmHg (5.3 kPa). This notion of a perfectly homogeneous lung is the basis of the 'ideal point' in Figure 5.4. The 'ideal point' represents a gold standard against which the efficiency of the *real lung* as a gas exchanger can be assessed. Gas exchanging units in real lungs have a spread of $\dot{V}_A/\dot{Q}$ values on either side of the 'ideal' value of 0.86. Blood coming from units with a $\dot{V}_A/\dot{Q} < 0.86$ will lower the oxygen content (and SaO_2) of the mixed arterial blood. With increasing $\dot{V}_A/\dot{Q}$ inhomogeneity PO_2 falls, following the line marked 'R = 0.8 (blood)' in Figure 5.4. The reason for this is that in the steady state the overall RQ of the body must be satisfied, so that:

$$[C\bar{v} - Ca]CO_2 / [Ca - C\bar{v}]O_2 = 0.8$$

This constrains CaO_2 and $CaCO_2$ (and PaO_2 and $PaCO_2$ derived from them) to certain combinations which fall along the so-called 'blood R' line (Figure 5.4).

GAS EXCHANGE IN DISEASED LUNGS

The three compartment model

In Figures 5.1 and 5.2 the lungs were considered as homogeneous gas exchange compartments *in series*. Diseased lungs are not uniform, consisting of many gas exchange units *in parallel* with different $\dot{V}_A/\dot{Q}$ ratios and different values for P_AO_2 and P_ACO_2 (Figure 5.4). Although diseased lungs contain units with a wide spectrum of function, it is simplifying and helpful to think in terms of only three compartments (Figure 5.5). Thus, we analyze the lung **as if** it consisted of an 'ideal' compartment where the $\dot{V}_A/\dot{Q}$ ratio is the same as that at the 'ideal point' (Figure 5.4), coupled with two other compartments representing the extreme ends of the spectrum, one with $\dot{V}_A/\dot{Q}$ ratio of zero (a non-ventilated shunt compartment) and one where $\dot{V}_A/\dot{Q} = ∞$ (an unperfused dead space compartment).

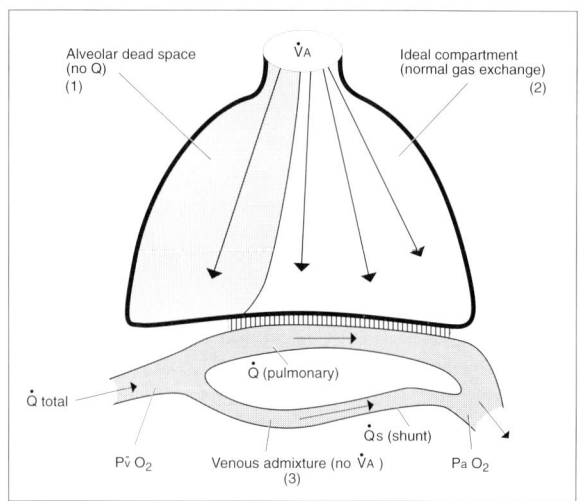

Figure 5.5 Parallel three compartment gas exchange

Alveolar ventilation ($\dot{V}_A$) – i.e. total ($\dot{V}_E$) minus anatomic dead space ventilation – is distributed to two compartments, one which is ventilated but unperfused (alveolar dead space or wasted ventilation), and one which is ventilated and perfused equally ('ideal' compartment, close to a 1:1 ratio). Blood flow is also distributed to a third compartment which is unventilated (shunt or wasted blood flow), and causes arterial hypoxemia. Note, this is an 'as if' model which, in conjunction with the O_2-CO_2 diagram, 'explains' the shift of arterial (a) and alveolar (A) PO_2 and PCO_2 away from the 'ideal' point in Figure 5.4.

Dead space compartment

Dead space refers to those parts of the respiratory system where there is little or no gas exchange because of a lack of pulmonary blood flow. There is an obligatory dead space extending from the mouth to the respiratory bronchioles (150–200 ml), the so-called *anatomic dead space*. There is, in addition, an 'alveolar' dead space which refers to gas exchanging units with reduced or absent blood flow, and $\dot{V}_A/\dot{Q}$ ratios higher than the 'ideal' of 0.86. The three compartment model of the lung (Figure 5.5) treats these units as an equivalent dead space by analyzing the difference between alveolar and mixed expired PCO_2 as if it were due to a combination of units with a normal P_ACO_2 and units with zero P_ACO_2 (no pulmonary blood flow and $\dot{V}_A/\dot{Q} = ∞$). Arterial PCO_2 is substituted for alveolar PCO_2. As mixed expired PCO_2 ($P\bar{E}CO_2$) includes anatomic dead space gas, the dead space is the sum of the alveolar and anatomic components and is called the 'physiological' dead space. It is expressed as a fraction of the tidal volume (V_D/V_T):

$$V_D/V_T \text{ [physiol]} = [P_A - P_{\bar{E}} / P_A - P_I] \, CO_2$$

or, since P_ICO_2 is zero and P_ACO_2 and P_aCO_2 are virtually identical in normal lungs:

$$[P_aCO_2 - P_{\bar{E}}CO_2] / P_aCO_2$$

V_D/V_T [physiol] at rest has a wide range (0.3–0.45)[3] and depends on the pattern of breathing. On exercise in normal subjects the ratio falls to < 0.2 (most of the V_D is anatomic) and values greater than 0.3 indicate abnormal alveolar dead space, i.e. high $\dot{V}_A/\dot{Q}$ units caused by maldistribution of pulmonary blood flow. Conceptually (Figure 5.4), think of the dead space as a shift of points $\bar{A}$ and $\bar{E}$ away from the **ideal point** (A) down the gas R line.

Venous admixture compartment

Venous admixture (also called physiological shunt [$\dot{Q}_S/\dot{Q}_T$]) is the converse of dead space. There is little or no gas exchange because of a lack of ventilation. Physiological shunt refers to units whose $\dot{V}_A/\dot{Q}$ ratio is less than the ideal ratio (Figure 5.4). These units have a low PO_2 and a low CaO_2. The arterial PO_2, with increasing amounts of shunt, moves away from the 'ideal' point along the (R= 0.8 [blood]) line (Figure 5.4). The physiological shunt is analyzed in **'as if'** terms – *as if* a certain amount of mixed venous blood had been added to arterial blood to produce the observed CaO_2. The normal physiological shunt (< 5%) includes a contribution (about 1%) from the extrapulmonary or obligatory shunt (see section on Anatomic Shunt).

$$\dot{Q}_S/\dot{Q}_T \text{ [phys]} = [C_A - Ca]O_2 / [C_A - C\bar{v}]O_2$$

where C_A is the oxygen content at the 'ideal' point (Figure 5.4). For clinical work, SaO_2 is usually substituted for CaO_2. The difficulty is that the measurement of $C\bar{v}O_2$ (mixed venous oxygen content) requires blood to be sampled from the pulmonary artery. In practice, [Ca – C$\bar{v}$]O_2 is assumed to be 50 ml.L^{-1} (or 25% SaO_2) which is reasonable for resting conditions. But, on exercise or in high or low cardiac output states, this assumption cannot be made. Breathing air, 'ideal' SaO_2 is taken to be 97.5%.

Because of the shape of the ODC, [$S_A - Sa$]O_2 is too small to be measured accurately until PaO_2 has decreased to ≤ 84 mmHg (11.2 kPa), i.e. until SaO_2 ≤ 95%. Although the physiological shunt is insensitive in detecting mild hypoxemia, it is a useful measure of gas exchange *efficiency* because it is independent of the shape of the oxygen dissociation curve.

Quantitating gas exchange inefficiency for oxygen

Deviation of PaO_2 from 'normal' values

What is a 'normal' PaO_2? Recent surveys have confined themselves to life-long non-smokers who have normal pulmonary function and whose PaO_2 is measured in the sitting position. PaO_2 rises by about 10 mmHg (1.3 kPa) in pregnancy[4] (and there is a corresponding fall in $PaCO_2$) but there are no other effects of gender. Remember that many people live at moderate altitudes. In Denver, USA, at height 1610 m (5280 feet), a normal PaO_2 would be 20–30 mmHg lower than at sea level. Because of the shape of the ODC, SaO_2 would still exceed 90%.

> **Four factors determining PaO_2 in healthy subjects at sea level:**
>
> - Age
> - Body mass index (BMI)
> - $PaCO_2$
> - Posture

PaO_2 on average declines by about 4 mmHg (0.53 kPa) per 10 years, from 100 mmHg (13.3 kPa) at age 20 years to 80 mmHg (10.7 kPa) at age 70 years. In a recent study of 194 healthy subjects (93 were women), aged between 40 and 90 years:[5]

$$PaO_2 \text{ (mmHg)} = 143.6 - 0.39.\text{age} - 0.56.\text{BMI} - 0.57.PaCO_2 \text{ [SEE 7.48]}$$

From this survey, the lower limits of normal (– 1.64 × SEE) encompassing 95% of a healthy population are shown in Table 5.2.

Some of the values in apparently healthy elderly subjects, seated, are quite low, especially if they are overweight and do not compensate by lowering $PaCO_2$.

Table 5.2 Lower limits of normal for PaO$_2$ in the sitting position[5]

Age (yr)	BMI# (kg.m^{-2})	PaCO2 ——— (mmHg	*PaO2 [kPa]) ———
40	25	35 [4.7]	82 [10.9]
40	34	40 [5.3]	74 [9.85]
75	25	35 [4.7]	68 [9.1]
75	34	40 [5.3]	60 [8.0]

\# Normal BMI is < 30
*For mean value, add 12.3 mmHg [1.6 kPa]

The decline in PaO$_2$ with age is caused by an increase in $\dot{V}_A/\dot{Q}$ inequality. Subjects > 75 years old do not show any further decline with age, nor any dependence on PaCO$_2$ or BMI, their mean ± SD for PaO$_2$ being 83.4 mmHg (11.1 kPa) ± 9.15 mmHg (1.2 kPa).

Arterial PO$_2$ is lower in the supine posture, compared to sitting, in those middle-aged and elderly subjects with a high closing volume[6] and in smokers (see Figure 5.7).

The ideal alveolar to arterial PO$_2$ gradient [A-aPO$_2$]

The [A-aPO$_2$] gradient is illustrated in Figure 5.4. In practice the 'ideal point' is used for P$_A$O$_2$ rather than the true mean alveolar ($\bar{A}$ in Figure 5.4) which is very difficult to measure without anatomic dead space contamination. The larger the gradient, the greater the $\dot{V}_A/\dot{Q}$ inhomogeneity. Although this index is used extensively in published papers on pulmonary gas exchange, its use in clinical practice has declined. The ideal P$_A$O$_2$ is calculated (from Figure 5.4) as:

$$P_AO_2 = P_IO_2 - [P_ACO_2/R] *$$

In the steady state the R of the lung ($\sim \dot{V}CO_2/\dot{V}O_2$) is assumed to be equal to the overall metabolic RQ usually close to 0.8 at rest in the steady state, fasting. The alveolar air equation adjusts PaO$_2$ to the value of alveolar PO$_2$. This is important because any change in minute ventilation which decreases or increases P$_A$CO$_2$ must cause an almost equal change in P$_A$O$_2$ in the opposite direction. With hyperventilation, P$_A$CO$_2$ (and PaCO$_2$) fall and P$_A$O$_2$ rises. PaO$_2$ may appear 'normal' just because P$_A$O$_2$ is high, but the calculated [A-aPO$_2$] will be greater than normal. Conversely, when P$_A$CO$_2$ rises (with hypoventilation, for example) P$_A$O$_2$ must fall and the reduction in PaO$_2$ which follows does not mean that gas exchanging efficiency has deteriorated. Unfortunately, the alveolar-arterial gradient (for an equivalent degree of venous admixture [physiological shunt]) is influenced by the shape of the ODC and is larger on the flat part of the curve (PO$_2$ > 75 mmHg [10 kPa]), as shown in Table 5.3.

Table 5.3 Effect of raising PaCO$_2$ and lowering F$_I$O$_2$ on PaO$_2$ and A-aPO$_2$

	F$_I$O$_2$	P$_A$O$_2$	PaCO$_2$ ——— (mm Hg	PaO$_2$ [kPa])	A-aPO$_2$ ———	$\dot{Q}_S/\dot{Q}_T$ (%)
A	0.14	60 [8]	32 [4.3]	56 [7.5]	4 [0.5]	9.0
B	0.21	60 [8]	72 [9.6]	56 [7.5]	4 [0.5]	9.0
C	0.21	100 [13.3]	40 [5.3]	86 [11.5]	14 [1.9]	9.0

The 'physiological' shunt has been kept constant at 9% of cardiac output in all examples (**A**, **B**, and **C**) as an indicator of a fixed amount of $\dot{V}_A/\dot{Q}$ mismatching. P$_A$O$_2$ and PaO$_2$ are lower in **A** because of a low inspired oxygen concentration and in **B** because of a high alveolar and arterial PCO$_2$. But the [A-aPO$_2$] gradient is independent of the level of PaCO$_2$. The alveolar-arterial oxygen tension gradient [A-aPO$_2$] is highly dependent on the position of P$_A$O$_2$ and PaO$_2$ on the ODC. [A-aPO$_2$] is higher in example **C** because the ODC is relatively flat at these PO$_2$s. $\dot{Q}_S/\dot{Q}_T$ is independent of the shape of the ODC and is a more reliable index of gas exchange efficiency when PaO$_2$ is reduced.

The A-aPO$_2$ widens with aging.[7] Since the fall of PaO$_2$ with age is trivial, the increase in A-aPO$_2$ tracks the fall in PaO$_2$. A-aPO$_2$ ranges from 6–10 mmHg (0.8–1.3 kPa) at age 20 years to 26–30 mmHg (3.5–4.0 kPa) at age 70.

PaO$_2$/F$_I$O$_2$ ratio

This empirical index of efficiency may be more useful in the Intensive Care Unit when inspired oxygen concentrations are changing. In the following example

*There is a small nitrogen correction, usually ignored clinically, equal to [PaCO$_2$ × F$_I$O$_2$ × (1–R)/R] which adds about 2 mmHg (0.27 kPa) to the calculated P$_A$O$_2$.

Table 5.4 Effect of increasing F_IO_2 on PaO_2 and indices of gas exchange efficiency

	F_IO_2	P_AO_2	PaO_2	A-aPO_2	PaO_2/F_IO_2	$\dot{Q}s/\dot{Q}_T$ (%)	SaO_2 (%)
			mm Hg [kPa]				
A	0.21	100 [13.3]	59 [7.9]	41 [5.4]	281 [38]	20	89
B	0.4	235 [31]	72 [9.6]	163 [21.4]	180 [24]	20	92
C	0.6	378 [30.4]	92 [12.3]	286 [38.1]	153 [20.5]	20	95
D	1.0	673 [90]	200 [26.7]	473 [63.3]	200 [26.7]	20	100

(Table 5.4), a change of inspired oxygen in the range 40–100%, at a constant $\dot{Q}s/\dot{Q}_T$, resulted in a threefold increase of the alveolar-arterial gradient [A-aPO_2] but no systematic change in the PaO_2/F_IO_2 ratio.

Physiological shunt ($\dot{Q}s/\dot{Q}_T$ phys)

Shunt (or venous admixture) has been discussed earlier. It is a very useful measure of the efficiency of arterial oxygenation which is independent of the shape of the oxygen dissociation curve. Shunt requires a measurement of pulmonary arterial oxygen content (or saturation); while it is reasonable to take a value for the [$SaO_2 - S\bar{v}O_2$] difference of 25% (or 50 ml.dL^{-1} O_2 content) in the steady state at rest, such assumptions are not warranted in sick patients.

Anatomic shunt ($\dot{Q}s/\dot{Q}t$ anat)

The 'physiological' shunt equation is used but the measurements are made while the subject is breathing 100% O_2 from a Douglas bag, with a nose clip and mouthpiece. An arterial sample is taken for PO_2, PCO_2 and [Hb] after at least 15 min breathing. The idea is to wash out the nitrogen from all gas-containing alveoli. Deep breaths are required at periodic intervals. By replacing nitrogen with oxygen, the P_AO_2 in all ventilated units (even with $\dot{V}_A/\dot{Q}$ as low as 0.001) will come to equal [Pb – PH_2O – P_ACO_2], i.e. 673 mmHg (90 kPa). This eliminates $\dot{V}_A/\dot{Q}$ inequality as a cause of any A-aPO_2 gradient. Ideal P_AO_2, although strictly 673 mmHg, is often taken as 650 mmHg (86.7 kPa) for clinical purposes. The A-aPO_2 and $\dot{Q}s/\dot{Q}_T$ on 100% oxygen represents $\dot{V}_A/\dot{Q}$ independent gas exchange inefficiency.

Perfusion of airless lobes or lobules too large to be oxygenated by diffusion from neighboring normal lung behaves like an 'anatomic' shunt.

Causes of an intrapulmonary anatomic shunt

- **Extrapulmonary:**
  R-L intracardiac shunt (including Thebesian veins)*
  Bronchial vein to pulmonary vein connections

- **Intrapulmonary:**
  Pulmonary arteriovenous malformations (PAVMs)
  Dilated capillaries in hepatopulmonary syndrome
  Lobar or lobular collapse or consolidation

The principal source of error in the measurement of the anatomic shunt is failure to eliminate nitrogen completely from slowly ventilated acinar units. The method is unreliable if there is moderate or severe airflow obstruction. Even in young normal subjects, PaO_2 rises on average to only 619 mmHg (82.5 kPa) – equivalent to a 3.2% shunt of the cardiac output; a further increase to 630 mmHg (84 kPa) occurs if deep breaths are taken[7] and finally to 658 mmHg (87.7 kPa) with the hyperventilation of exercise,[8] which is equivalent to 0.95% shunt. Thus, the true anatomic shunt is about 1% of cardiac output.

An alternative way of measuring the anatomic shunt is to inject radiolabeled albumin particles too large (> 15 μm) to pass through the normal pulmonary microvascular channels. In anatomic shunting, a measurable fraction of the injected dose reaches the systemic circulation, when it can be imaged quantitatively with a gamma camera looking at high flow organs such as the kidney and brain. In the case

---
* Coronary veins draining into the left atrium or ventricle

of PAVMs, there is a good correlation between the radioisotope and 100% oxygen methods.[9]

Responses to arterial hypoxemia

Compensatory mechanisms

The immediate response to hypoxemia is hyperventilation resulting from stimulation of the peripheral chemoreceptors in the carotid body (see Chapter 7). Hypercapnia and acidosis greatly increase the hypoxic ventilatory response. Hyperventilation is the most efficient way for the body to raise arterial PO_2. Hypoxic pulmonary vasoconstriction (diverting blood flow away from units with low PaO_2 and low $\dot{V}A/\dot{Q}$ ratios) and increasing the cardiac output are much less effective methods. The level of $PaCO_2$ is more 'ventilation dependent' than the level of PaO_2, so the ventilatory response to arterial hypoxemia usually leads to hypocapnia. The ventilatory response to a given PaO_2 (in absolute terms) may be reduced by abnormal lung or chest wall mechanical properties, particularly airflow obstruction (see Chapter 7).

Oxygen delivery to the tissues may be increased by raising cardiac output; the best example is pulmonary arteriovenous malformations (PAVMs – see Chapter 16). Alternatively, more red cells may be produced to increase the oxygen carrying capacity of blood (secondary polycythemia); this happens in some hypoxemic patients and in normal subjects on high altitude exposure. Thirdly, the oxygen dissociation curve may be shifted to the right to release oxygen to the tissues more easily, as occurs in some hemoglobinopathies where there is a failure to make sufficient hemoglobin. Compensatory mechanisms, or the lack of them, may explain in part why PaO_2 or exercise capacity may be higher or lower than predicted.

PaO_2 at rest is well preserved in mild to moderate emphysema, fibrosing alveolitis, and heart failure because of a high resting ventilation, but the stimulus to increase ventilation may arise from structures in the lung or chest wall as much as from arterial hypoxemia. $PaCO_2$ tends to be low. The hypoxemia of pneumonia and intrapulmonary shunts is not responsive to hyperventilation because blood is perfusing non-ventilated lung (see next section). Patients with neuromuscular disease cannot mount an effective ventilatory response to hypoxemia and hypercapnia, and the seriousness of their condition may be difficult to detect unless note is taken of their rapid and shallow pattern of breathing.

PaO_2 at rest better than expected	PaO_2 at rest worse than expected:
Emphysema	Asthma
Fibrosing alveolitis (CFA/IPF)	Pulmonary embolism
Heart failure	Pneumonia
	Intrapulmonary shunting
	Neuromuscular/chest wall restriction

FIO_2 increase

In an exacerbation of the disease, compensatory mechanisms may be overwhelmed, and patients present to hospital with a lower PaO_2 and an often higher $PaCO_2$ than usual. What increase in inspired oxygen levels needs to be given to raise SaO_2 to a reasonably normal level, say $\geq 95\%$? In simple terms, there are two scenarios:

1. The 'refractory hypoxemia' associated with severe pneumonia or the adult respiratory distress syndrome (ARDS), when high levels of FIO_2 are required.
2. Exacerbations of COPD or asthma when small increases of FIO_2 suffice; in COPD high levels of FIO_2 may be dangerous (see section on Arterial PCO_2).

In ARDS, the chest X-ray shows widespread pneumonic consolidation. These areas act as a shunt, being filled with inflammatory cells and edema fluid. They have no ventilation ($\dot{V}A/\dot{Q}$ ratio = zero) and the increase in FIO_2 will not be 'seen' by them. The non-pneumonic regions, for simplicity, may be considered normal or 'ideal', and their PaO_2 rises as FIO_2 is increased (see Table 5.4). The shunt regions, on the other hand, will reflect the composition of mixed venous blood. How does increasing the PaO_2 to normal lung raise PaO_2? There are three mechanisms:

1. The SaO_2 of the 'ideal' compartment will increase from 97.5% at PaO_2 100 mmHg [13.3 kPa] to 100% at PaO_2 200 mmHg [26.6 kPa].
2. For every 100 mmHg [13.3 kPa] increase in PaO_2, an extra 0.3 ml O_2 dL^{-1} blood will be dissolved in the

plasma of non-shunting blood. If arterial SO_2 is < 100%, this dissolved oxygen will combine with Hb.
3. The increase in the O_2 content of arterial blood stemming from (1) and (2) will, if cardiac output and oxygen consumption remain constant, increase $S\bar{v}O_2$ and the O_2 content of blood perfusing the shunt compartment.

In Table 5.4, with a shunt compartment of 20% ($\dot{V}_A/\dot{Q}$ ratio = zero), SaO_2 rose from 89 to 95% when FIO_2 was increased from air (0.21) to 0.6.

In the absence of shunt, when arterial hypoxemia is caused by units with low (< 0.1) but not zero $\dot{V}_A/\dot{Q}$ ratios, lower concentrations of FIO_2 suffice. The reason is that the nitrogen concentration in all ventilated units will fall as P_AO_2 rises (with very low $\dot{V}_A/\dot{Q}$ ratios the process may take some time). In three compartment model terms, this has the effect of reducing the venous admixture or physiological shunt. Taken to the extreme, when 100% O_2 is breathed and all alveolar nitrogen is washed out of all alveoli, the physiological shunt is eliminated and only the anatomic shunt remains (see preceding section, Anatomic Shunt). So, in Table 5.4, if the SaO_2 of 89% in **A** had been caused by a 20% *physiological* shunt (no zero $\dot{V}_A/\dot{Q}$ units), an FIO_2 of 0.35 (and not 0.6) would have been enough to raise SaO_2 to 95% because the '*effective*' physiological shunt would have fallen from 20% to 12.5%. In the absence of radiographic evidence of pneumonic consolidation, a relatively modest increase in FIO_2 is sufficient to improve arterial oxygen tension and content substantially, and 24% or 28% inspired oxygen is usually adequate.

Arterial PCO_2

The mechanisms leading to a rise of $PaCO_2$ are the same as those which lower PaO_2, except for altitude. Except for hypoventilation, the effects of gas exchange inefficiency are less noticeable on $PaCO_2$ than PaO_2. This is because the slope of the dissociation curve for carbon dioxide (Figure 5.3) is steeper and more linear than that for oxygen. Therefore, carbon dioxide transport is more *ventilation dependent*. $\dot{V}_A/\dot{Q}$ inhomogeneity raises $PaCO_2$ just as it lowers PaO_2. Nevertheless, hyperventilation which raises $\dot{V}_A/\dot{Q}$ ratios is more effective in lowering $PaCO_2$ than in raising PaO_2, because the plateau in the ODC limits further oxygen uptake at PO_2 > 90 mmHg (12 kPa). $\dot{V}_A/\dot{Q}$ mismatching in lung disease may be associated with a high, normal, or low $PaCO_2$, depending on the ventilatory responses to hypoxemia, hypercapnia, acidosis, and other influences (see Chapter 7).

The term '*alveolar hypoventilation*' should be reserved strictly for patients with a high $PaCO_2$ caused by low ventilation *[total minus dead space]* (respiratory center depression or neuromuscular/chest wall disease). Usually, breathing is fast and shallow and the ratio of anatomic dead space to tidal volume is abnormally high. *Alveolar hypoventilation* is used, loosely, to describe patients with hypercapnia resulting from $\dot{V}_A/\dot{Q}$ mismatch whose minute ventilation has not increased sufficiently to overcome their inefficiency of CO_2 transport. In the 'blue bloater' syndrome (COPD with hypercapnia, edema, polycythemia, and pulmonary hypertension), total ventilation is normal or high and not reduced. The term 'alveolar hypoventilation', applied to them, merely means a high $PaCO_2$. Nevertheless, they may also have true hypoventilation (see below).

Clinical examples

Patients with COPD and hypercapnia have a more rapid and a shallower pattern of breathing than COPD patients without hypercapnia (see Figure 7.6). In an exacerbation of their disease, PaO_2 falls and $PaCO_2$ rises further. Their very shallow breathing means that the [V_D anat + phys / V_T] ratio may exceed 0.6 (normal ≤ 0.4). Worsening hypercapnia is due to a combination of true hypoventilation and deterioration in $\dot{V}_A/\dot{Q}$ mismatching. The low V_T fails to clear the anatomic dead space effectively, and $PaCO_2$ rises. If uncontrolled oxygen is administered (FIO_2 > 0.35) to increase PaO_2, the hypoxic stimulus to the peripheral chemoreceptors is reduced and minute ventilation declines even more so that $PaCO_2$ may rise to very high levels (> 75 mmHg [10 kPa]). Another factor, though less important, is inhibition of pulmonary hypoxic vasoconstriction by the increased P_AO_2. This may increase local mismatching of ventilation and blood flow, and further compromise CO_2 elimination. Oxygen therapy for the hypercapnic COPD patient in an exacerbation should always be controlled, starting with 24% inspired oxygen and increasing to 28% (occasionally higher) only if $PaCO_2$ is stable.

Exacerbations of asthma and acute pulmonary embolism (PE) are associated with falls in $PaCO_2$. A normal or raised $PaCO_2$ in an attack of asthma is a serious sign, indicating (a) very severe $\dot{V}_A/\dot{Q}$ mismatching and (b) inability to increase $\dot{V}_E$ to compensate, which suggests that the respiratory muscles are stretched to their limit. Conversely, a normal $PaCO_2$ (and normal PaO_2) virtually rules out the diagnosis of *severe* PE. Pulmonary embolism should be considered if a hypercapnic COPD patient unexpectedly becomes more breathless and $PaCO_2$ is found to be lower than usual.

Extremely low values of $PaCO_2$ (< 25 mmHg [< 3.3 kPa]) may be found in the chronic hyperventilation syndrome. $PaCO_2$ < 15 mmHg (2.0 kPa) is usually a sign of a metabolic acidosis, e.g. uncontrolled Type I diabetes mellitus or acute renal failure.

MEASURING VENTILATION ($\dot{V}_A$) AND PERFUSION ($\dot{Q}$) INHOMOGENEITY

A major difficulty in assessing maldistribution of $\dot{V}_A$ and $\dot{Q}$ is the small volume (c. 0.06 ml) of each acinus (the effective unit of gas exchange) because it is beyond the resolving power of external imaging techniques using radionuclides and of direct sampling of gas with a flexible bronchoscope. Investigators have had to rely on measurements of the input and output functions of the lungs as a whole (all 50 000 acini), from which local $\dot{V}_A$ and $\dot{Q}$ distributions are derived using increasingly sophisticated mathematical and statistical analyses.

Multiple Inert Gas Elimination Technique (MIGET)

The MIGET approach, pioneered by Wagner, West, and colleagues,[10] measures the distribution of $\dot{V}_A/\dot{Q}$ in a 50 compartment model of the lung (Figure 5.6). This is a considerable advance, for research studies, over the three compartment model of Riley and Cournand. Six inert (non-reactive with Hb) gases with a wide range of solubilities (capacitance coefficients, β) are infused intravenously for 30 min, after which mixed venous, arterial and mixed expired samples are taken and analyzed by gas chromatography for the arterial retention [Pa/P$\bar{v}$] and alveolar excretion [PE/P$\bar{v}$ or PA/P$\bar{v}$] ratio of each gas (Figure 5.6, see facing page). The cardiac output (using inert gas concentrations and the Fick equation) and minute ventilation are also measured. Each tracer gas has a linear dissociation curve and a single value for β (Figure 5.3).

The key relationship is:

$$\text{Retention (R)} = Pa/P\bar{v} = \beta / [\beta + \dot{V}_A/\dot{Q}]$$

The relationship between Pa/P$\bar{v}$ β and $\dot{V}_A/\dot{Q}$ is shown in Figure 5.6 (**A** and **B**). There is a unique relationship between retention (Pa/P$\bar{v}$) and inert gas solubility (β) for each value of $\dot{V}_A/\dot{Q}$ (**A**). Pa/P$\bar{v}$ and PA/P$\bar{v}$ ratios for the six inert gases infused into the lung with moderate $\dot{V}_A/\dot{Q}$ inequality are shown in (**B**). Note the a-A gradients vary with the solubility of the inert gas and that the arterial values always lie above and the alveolar values below that for a homogeneous lung (h) with no $\dot{V}_A/\dot{Q}$ inequality. The a and A lines in **B** are unique for a particular $\dot{V}_A/\dot{Q}$ distribution. Plots of ventilation and blood flow versus $\dot{V}_A/\dot{Q}$ ratio (**C**) are derived as a best fit for the data in **B** on the basis of theory (**A**). In **C** the $\dot{V}_A/\dot{Q}$ distribution is fitted to 48 discrete values (compartments) plus one for shunt ($\dot{V}_A/\dot{Q} = 0$) and one for alveolar dead space ($\dot{V}_A/\dot{Q} = \infty$).

Though still an '*as if*' black box approach, MIGET is a more sophisticated analysis than the traditional three compartment model. Much information about $\dot{V}_A/\dot{Q}$ distributions in different respiratory conditions has been gained using the MIGET, together with insights into the pathological mechanisms involved. Several reviews are available.[11,12]

Distribution of ventilation (intraregional)

Maldistribution of ventilation, secondary to bronchial or bronchiolar narrowing or blockage, is the most common cause of $\dot{V}_A/\dot{Q}$ mismatching and arterial hypoxemia. In the three compartment model (Figure 5.5), maldistribution of ventilation is associated with shunt. Uneven ventilation is usually associated with airflow obstruction and slow gas mixing (long equilibration times for gases with wash-in or wash-out techniques).

Uneven ventilation may be inter-regional or intraregional, the latter referring to subsegmental regions beyond the resolution of radionuclide imaging techniques. The inter-regional differences seen on ventilation scans underestimate the amount of inhomogeneity found by other methods such as the single-breath nitrogen slope. Multi-breath nitrogen wash-out

Figure 5.6 MIGET technique

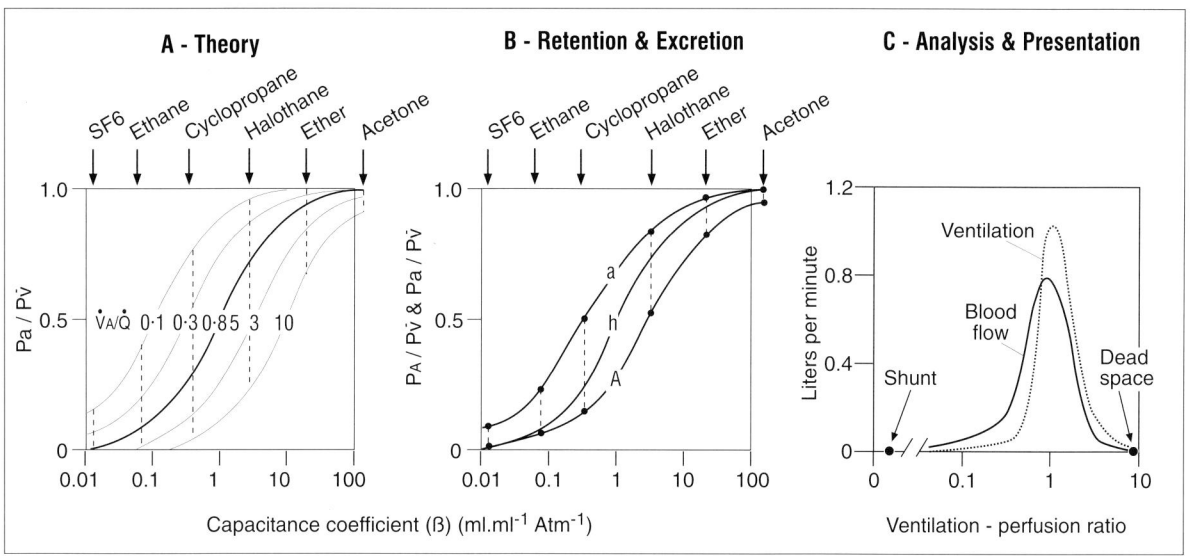

A. Each tracer gas (with its capacitance coefficient, β) has a unique Pa/Pv̄ value for a given V̇A/Q̇ ratio.

B. Values of arterial (a) retention (Pa/Pv̄) and alveolar (A) excretion (PA/Pv̄) for all six tracer gases in a lung with moderate V̇A/Q̇ dispersion (log SD 1.5 of a log normal V̇A/Q̇ distribution) compared to a theoretical homogeneous lung (h) with no V̇A/Q̇ dispersion.

C. Plot of ventilation and blood flow (smoothed) for 48 compartments (plus shunt and dead space) against V̇A/Q̇ as a best fit to explain data in **B** on basis of theory in **A**.

is the oldest and probably the most sensitive technique but it is time consuming to perform. Radiolabeled aerosols are easier to handle than radioactive gases, but they exaggerate inter-regional differences because of their poor diffusive mixing, and by impaction of the aerosol in the central airways in patients with airflow obstruction.

Techniques for showing maldistribution of ventilation

- Multi-breath nitrogen wash-out.
- Phase III and IV of single-breath nitrogen expiration.
- Radioactive gas and radiolabeled aerosol scans.
- Frequency dependence of compliance.
- Volume difference for TLC measurement between single-breath (e.g. during D_{LCO} measurement) and multi-breath or plethysmographic measurements.

Phase III and closing volume

Figure 5.7 shows the single-breath nitrogen expiration test, following a vital capacity inhalation of 100% oxygen. Four phases are apparent. In Phase I the anatomic dead space empties; Phase II is the transition in emptying from the bronchial and bronchiolar compartments to acinar/alveolar units. Phase III reflects alveolar emptying; a positive slope indicates uneven distribution of ventilation within and between lung regions. The abrupt change of slope at **A** and **B** marks the onset of Phase IV and reflects a change in the *inter-regional* pattern (between regions) of lung emptying. When the subject expires to residual volume prior to inhaling 100%O_2 the upper zone alveoli are more expanded than the lower and are less diluted with the subsequent single

Figure 5.7 Single-breath expired nitrogen concentration following 100% oxygen inspiration

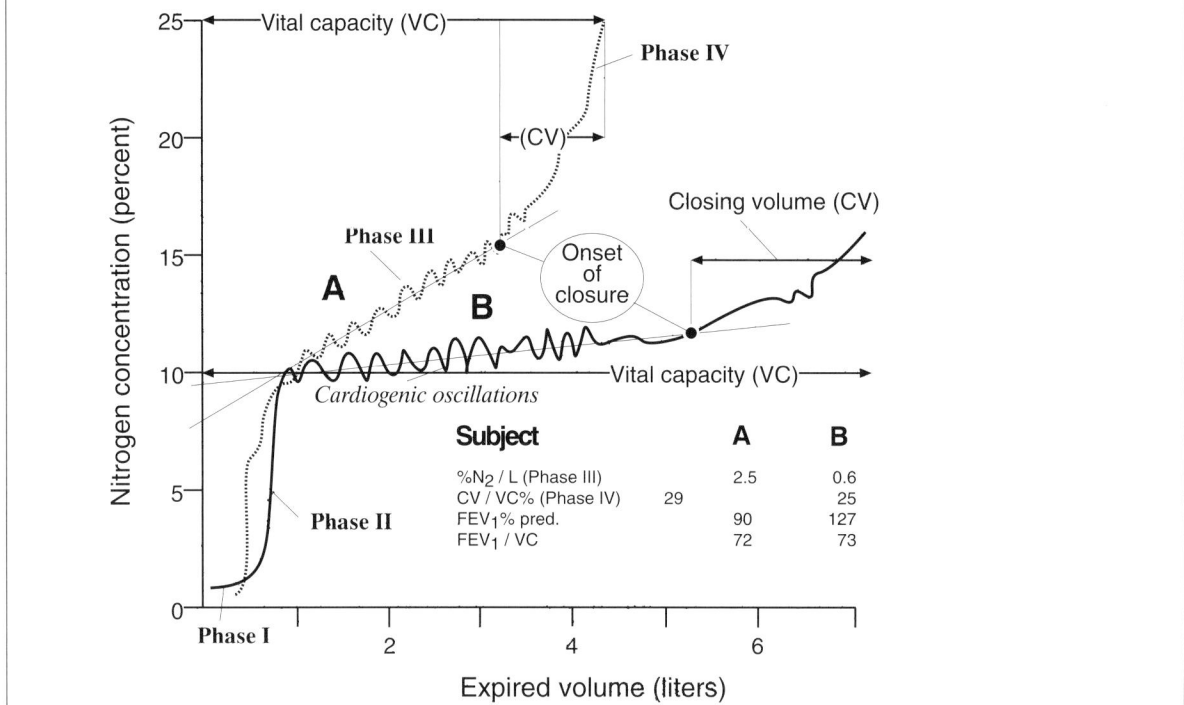

Two healthy middle-aged smokers. Greater Phase III slope (% N_2/L) in **A** indicates more uneven emptying. Abrupt change of slope at junction of Phase III and Phase IV indicates the lung volume at which some units in most dependent zones stop emptying (onset of airway closure). Subject **A** has more unevenness of ventilation distribution (larger Phase III slope) than subject **B** in spite of similar FEV_1/VC and closing volume/vital capacity (CV/VC) ratios. Subject **A** also had a lower PaO_2 (77 versus 100 mmHg [10.3 vs 13.3 kPa]).

breath of oxygen. The terminal rise in nitrogen concentration represents preferential emptying from the upper zones with their higher [N_2]. Phase IV is caused by functional closure of airways in the dependent parts of the lung where alveolar expansion and lung elastic recoil pressure at FRC are least. In Figure 7, the volume change from the onset of 'closure' to the end of expiration is designated closing volume. The closing capacity (CC) is the closing volume plus residual volume. If the closing volume exceeds the expiratory reserve volume, some airways will be closed during the tidal breathing cycle, and there will be some arterial hypoxemia.[6] This occurs with severe obesity. Closing volume increases with age, probably due to the declining elasticity of the lung parenchyma which exerts a distending pressure on the intrapulmonary airways.

Inter-regional distributions of ventilation and perfusion

Radioactive gas measurements (using xenon-133) in the 1960s showed systematic variations in alveolar expansion, ventilation and blood flow in the lung in a gravity-determined orientation, i.e. from non-dependent to dependent regions. The lung distorts (except at TLC) under the influence of its own weight. Non-dependent alveoli at FRC are expanded to 60% of their maximum compared to 40% of maximum for dependent alveoli.[13] Smaller alveoli (equivalent to the whole lung at a low volume) are on a more compliant part of the PV curve of the total lung (see Chapter 3) and their ΔVr^* will be greater for the same $\Delta Pplr$. Ventilatory

* r = function in a region

turnover ($\Delta V_r / FRC_r$) will also be greater because of the lower FRC_r. The dependent/non-dependent ventilation ratio ranges from 1.4 to 1.6 in the erect position and from 2.0 to 2.7 in the supine position.

There is a similar, though larger, increase in pulmonary blood flow from the top to the bottom of the lung, being 2:1 in the erect position and 2.9:1 in the supine position. This is due to the increase in pulmonary vascular pressures by 1.0 cmH$_2$O per cm distance, as outlined in Wests Zone I, II, III model.[14] The gravity gradient increases at lung volumes above FRC and virtually disappears at residual volume.[15] There are other influences on the distribution of pulmonary blood flow.[15]

Clinical applications

In the clinical setting, planar images (anterior, posterior, lateral, or oblique) of blood flow and ventilation are obtained from a gamma camera and interpretations are made by visual inspection. Three-dimensional images (single photon computer emission tomography, SPECT) are also available, but less often used. Perfusion distribution is measured after the injection, intravenously, of ^{99m}Tc-radiolabeled albumin particles (15–60 μm diameter) which become trapped in small pulmonary arteries in proportion to local blood flow. Less than 1% of the vascular cross-sectional area is blocked by the injection; the albumin particles are removed by macrophages within six hours. Ventilation is measured with radioactive gas inhalation (^{133}Xe or ^{81m}Kr) or with radioaerosols of conventional diameter (1–3 μm) or of very small particle size (Technegas™ – 0.01 μm diameter). The main application of $\dot{V}$ and $\dot{Q}$ scans lies in the confirmation or refutation of the diagnosis of pulmonary vascular obstruction due to pulmonary embolic disease. Segmental (usually multiple) defects in the perfusion scan in the presence of normal regional ventilation are diagnostic of pulmonary embolism. Destructive lung diseases cause 'matched' defects of ventilation and blood flow, usually in a subsegmental rather than a segmental distribution. A normal lung perfusion scan rules out pulmonary embolism. The other application of $\dot{V}$ and $\dot{Q}$ scans is in preoperative evaluation of the functional contributions of the lung to be resected versus that which will remain (see Chapter 15).

* ppb = parts per billion (10^{12}): ppm = parts per million

NITRIC OXIDE (NO)

Nitric oxide (previously 'endothelium-derived relaxing factor') is generated from L-arginine by the catalytic action of NO synthase (NOS), mostly in vascular endothelium. As its former name suggests, it relaxes vascular smooth muscle cells – by activating guanylate cyclase. NO is synthesized in other cells, including airway epithelium. NOS can be induced in inflammatory cells by cytokines and endotoxin; NO as an oxygen free radical can be toxic to bacteria (but bacteria may also produce NO!). High concentrations of NO are produced in the nose, especially in the paranasal sinuses. NO binds to hemoglobin with very high affinity (see Chapter 6 for measurements of diffusing capacity using NO) and nearly all NO produced in the periphery of the lung is quenched immediately by Hb. The source of NO in expired gas is thought to be mainly bronchial/bronchiolar with contributions from the upper respiratory tract, mainly nasal, directly or from dead space re-inspiration.

Measurement of exhaled NO

NO is measured by chemiluminescence, detection depending on a photochemical reaction between NO and ozone. The measurement must be carefully standardized because breathing history, breath-holding time, expiratory flow rate, and nasal contamination all affect the measurement. Expiration at a fixed flow rate against a small resistance (5–15 cmH$_2$O.L.s^{-1}) to obstruct the nose with the soft palate is recommended in the ERS Task Force Report.[16] NO in ambient air must be recorded. The normal expired plateau concentration of NO is 5–15 ppb.*

Factors affecting exhaled nitric oxide concentration[17]	
↑ NO	↓ NO
Asthma	Cigarette smoking
Bronchiectasis	Cystic fibrosis
Nasal disease	Autoimmune pulmonary hypertension
Upper respiratory tract infections	Corticosteroid therapy

Thus, exhaled NO may be a way of detecting airway inflammation and monitoring the response to treatment. Expired NO levels in COPD seem to be normal; this could help to distinguish COPD from asthma in ex-smokers.

Therapeutic use of inhaled NO

NO has been given by inhalation for its vasodilating properties. It is only a weak bronchodilator. The most dramatic effects have been in persistent pulmonary hypertension of the newborn where striking improvements in arterial oxygenation were achieved by inhaling 80 or 20 ppm,[18,19] presumably as a result of a fall in pulmonary artery pressure and in right to left shunt. Multicenter controlled trials are underway.

In adult ARDS, the results have been more variable, though oxygenation improves and pulmonary artery pressure decreases in two thirds of patients; but NO administration has not led to improvements in survival.[20] The theory is that inhaled NO will reduce pulmonary vascular resistance in ventilated units, diverting blood flow from unventilated units with 'pneumonic consolidation' which act as a shunt. NO also inhibits hypoxic pulmonary vasoconstriction; this may explain the failure of inhaled NO to improve oxygenation in patients with COPD[21] who have little or no shunt. In addition, Pap may not decrease if longstanding structural changes in the pulmonary vasculature have taken place.

Safety aspects associated with the administration of inhaled NO gas should not be neglected.[22]

References

1 Sauty A, Uldry C, Debetaz L-F, Leuenberger P, Fitting J-W. Differences in PO_2 and PCO_2 between arterial and arterialized ear lobe samples. *Eur Respir J* 1996; **9**: 186–9.

2 Powers SK, Dodd S, Freeman J, Ayers GD, Samson H, McNight T. Accuracy of pulse oximetry to estimate HbO_2 fraction of total Hb during exercise. *J Appl Physiol* 1989; **67**: 300–4.

3 Harris EA, Hunter ME, Seelye ER, Vedder M, Whitlock RML. Prediction of the physiological dead space in resting normal subjects. *Clin Sci Mol Med* 1973; **45**: 375–86.

4 Templeton A & Kelman GR. Maternal blood gases (PAO_2-PaO_2), physiological shunt and VD/VT in normal pregnant women. *Br J Anaesth* 1976; **48**: 1001–4.

5 Cerveri I, Zoia MC, Spagnolatti L, Berrayah L, Grassi M, Tinelli C. Reference values of arterial oxygen tension in the middle-aged and elderly. *Am J Respir Crit Care Med* 1995; **152**: 934–41.

6 Rea HH, Withy SJ, Seelye ER, Harris EA. The effects of posture in venous admixture and respiratory dead space in health. *Am Rev Respir Dis* 1977; **115**: 571–80.

7 Harris EA, Kenyon AM, Nisbet HD, Seelye ER, Whitlock RML. The normal alveolar-arterial oxygen tension gradient in man. *Clin Sci Mol Med* 1974; **46**: 89–104.

8 Harris EA, Seelye ER & Whitlock RML. Gas exchange during exercise in healthy people. II. Venous admixture. *Clin Sci Mol Med* 1976; **51**: 335–44.

9 Whyte MKB, Peters AM, Hughes JMB, Henderson BL, Bellingan GJ, Jackson JE, Chilvers ER. Quantification of right to left shunt at rest and during exercise in patients with pulmonary arteriovenous malformations. *Thorax* 1992; **47**: 790–6.

10 Wagner PD, Saltzman HA & West JB. Measurement of continuous distributions of ventilation-perfusion ratios: theory. *J Appl Physiol* 1974; **37**: 588–99.

11 Rodriguez-Roisin R (ed). Review Series: Contribution of multiple inert gas elimination technique to pulmonary medicine. *Thorax* 1994; **49**: 813–24, 924–32, 1027–33, 1169-74,1251–8. 1995; **50**: 85–91.

12 West JB & Wagner PD. Ventilation-perfusion relationships. In: Crystal RG, West JB et al (eds) *The Lung: Scientific Foundations*, 2nd edn. Philadelphia: Lippincott-Raven 1997: 1693–1709.

13 Milic-Emili J. Topographical inequality of ventilation. In: Crystal RG, West JB et al (eds) *The Lung: Scientific Foundations*, 2nd edn. Philadelphia: Lippincott-Raven 1997: 1415–23.

14 West JB, Dollery CT & Naimark A. Distribution of blood flow in isolated lung: relation to vascular and alveolar pressures. *J Appl Physiol* 1964; **19**: 713–24.

15 Hughes JMB. Distribution of pulmonary blood flow. In: Crystal RG, West JB et al (eds) *The Lung: Scientific Foundations*, 2nd edn. Philadelphia: Lippincott-Raven 1997: 1523–36.

16 Kharitonov S, Alving K & Barnes PJ. Exhaled and nasal nitric oxide measurements: recommendations. ERS Task Force Report. *Eur Respir J* 1997; **10**: 1683–93.

17 Barnes PJ & Kharitonov S. Exhaled nitric oxide: a new lung function test. *Thorax* 1996; **51**: 233–7.

18 Roberts JD, Polaner DM, Lang P, Zapol WM. Inhaled nitric oxide in persistent pulmonary hypertension of the new born. *Lancet* 1992; **340**: 818–9.

19 Kinsella JP, Neish SR, Shaffer E, Abman SH. Low dose inhalational nitric oxide in persistent pulmonary hypertension of the new born. *Lancet* 1992; **340**: 819–20.

20 Roissant R, Gerlach H, Schmidt-Ruhnke H, Pappert D, Lewandowski K, Stendel W, Falke K. Efficacy of inhaled nitric oxide in patients with severe ARDS. *Chest* 1995; **107**: 1107.

21 Barbera JA, Roger N, Roca J, Rovira I, Higenbottam TW, Rodriguez-Roisin R. Worsening of pulmonary gas exchange with nitric oxide inhalation in chronic obstructive pulmonary disease. *Lancet* 1996; **347**: 436–40.

22 Warren JB & Higenbottam T. Caution with use of NO. *Lancet* 1996; **348**: 629–30.

6 Diffusing Capacity (transfer factor) for Carbon Monoxide

J M B Hughes

- **BACKGROUND**
  What is the diffusing capacity?
  Clinical importance of the D_{LCO}
  Why use carbon monoxide to measure diffusion?
  Diffusion limitation versus perfusion limitation
- **THEORY AND PRACTICE**
  The single-breath D_{LCO} measurement
  Principles of measurement
  Resumé of single-breath D_{LCO} calculations and definitions
  Methodological key points
  Constant exhalation D_{LCO}
  Rebreathing D_{LCO}
- **COMPONENTS OF D_{LCO}**
  Membrane and reactive conductances of D_{LCO}
  Nitric oxide; D_{LNO}
- **D_{LCO} (T_{LCO}) IN HEALTHY SUBJECTS**
  Factors influencing the measurement of D_{LCO} (single-breath)
  Hemoglobin concentration
  Alveolar oxygen concentration
  Lung expansion
  Cardiac output
  Carbon monoxide back pressure
  Chronic cigarette smoking (not its acute effects)
  Normal values, units, reproducibility, quality control
  Calculation of alveolar volume (V_A)
- **CONCLUSIONS**
- **APPENDIX 6.I: WORKED OUT EXAMPLE OF D_{LCO} CALCULATION**

BACKGROUND

What is the diffusing capacity?

The diffusing capacity for carbon monoxide (D_{LCO}) – usually called the transfer factor (T_{LCO}) in Europe – measures the surface area of the lung available for gas exchange. The terms diffusing capacity (D_{LCO}) and transfer factor (T_{LCO}) are interchangeable; for convenience, the older term **diffusing capacity** will be used. D_{LCO} is actually the **diffusive conduc-**

tance, meaning 'ease of transfer' for CO molecules passing from alveolar gas to pulmonary capillary hemoglobin. Diffusive transfer of carbon monoxide involves two processes in series, illustrated schematically in Figure 6.1:

1. molecular diffusion across the alveolar and capillary membranes (membrane conductance)
2. chemical combination with hemoglobin [Hb] molecules (reactive conductance).

Molecular diffusion depends on the alveolar-capillary membrane surface area per unit thickness and the physical diffusivity of CO in tissue. The diffusivity (d) of a gas in a medium is proportional to [solubility.MW^{-2}] where MW^{-2} is the square root of its molecular weight.

The *reactive* process is related to the reaction rate of CO with [Hb] and the amount of [Hb] in the pulmonary microcirculation.

Clinical importance of the D_{LCO} (T_{LCO}) measurement

The D_{LCO} (T_{LCO}) is one of the key tests in the assessment of pulmonary function. It is a window on the pulmonary microcirculation. In cases of airflow obstruction, measurements of D_{LCO} help to distinguish asthma from bronchiectasis and to distinguish both from emphysema. In volume loss without airflow obstruction, the D_{LCO} (T_{LCO}) will tend to be preserved in extrapulmonary restriction, but it will be low in intrapulmonary alveolar and vascular disease.

Why use carbon monoxide to measure diffusion?

Diffusion limitation versus perfusion limitation

To understand intuitively the difference between perfusion and diffusion limitation for alveolar-capillary gas transfer, imagine an empty train arriving at a metro station. Gas molecules (passengers) are waiting on the platform. The capacity of the train is determined by the number of seats (hemoglobin [Hb] molecules or ml of blood). If there are very few doors, or if they are very narrow, the limiting process will be the *rate of entry* (~ diffusion) on to the train; increasing the frequency of trains (above a certain minimum) will not clear the platform faster. This is **diffusion limitation** which operates in the case of carbon monoxide. If the doors are wide and the train fills up rapidly and completely, increasing the frequency of trains (~ perfusion) will enable more pas-

Figure 6.1 Alveolar-capillary transfer of carbon monoxide

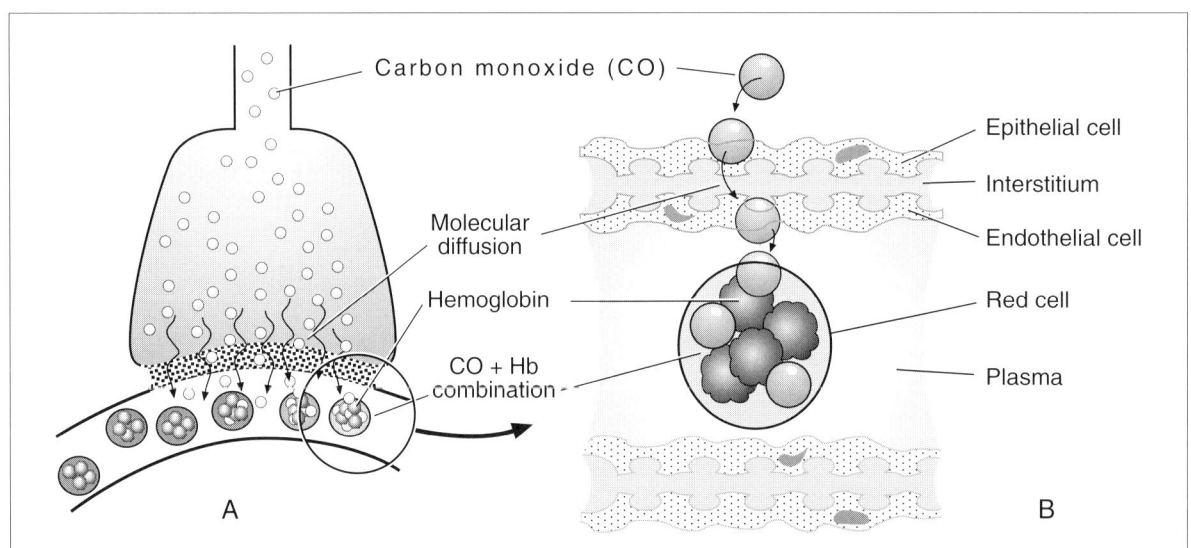

Schema of single alveolus (A) with enlargement (B) from inset of alveolar-capillary barrier for carbon monoxide. CO molecules cross the alveolar epithelium, interstitium, endothelial cell, plasma, and red cell membrane and interior by molecular diffusion (down a concentration gradient) before combining physicochemically with hemoglobin molecules in the red cells.

sengers to leave the station. This is **perfusion limitation**. The alveolar-capillary transfer of non Hb-reactive gases like acetylene is perfusion limited. Thus, acetylene (C_2H_2) and gases with similar properties (ether, freon-22, and nitrous oxide [N_2O]) are used to measure cardiac output with a rebreathing technique. Oxygen, of course, reacts with Hb but 200 times less strongly than CO. Its alveolar-capillary transfer is **perfusion and diffusion limited**; more correctly the efficiency of transfer is governed by the *ratio* of diffusion to perfusion.

In a more formal sense, the alveolar to end-capillary gas tension gradient for any gas (P_A-P_c') is determined by the ratio of diffusing capacity to perfusing capacity – the latter being pulmonary blood flow [~ cardiac output] times the capacity (β) of blood for a gas at a particular tension. Normalizing to the initial gradient (alveolar minus mixed venous [P_A–$P\bar{v}$]):

$$(P_A - P_c') / (P_A - P\bar{v}) = e^{-D_L/\beta\dot{Q}}$$

where β is capacity of blood for a particular gas, equivalent to a tangent to the slope of its dissociation curve, D_L is the diffusing capacity, and $\dot{Q}$ is pulmonary blood flow, $e^{-D_L/\beta\dot{Q}}$ is the exponential term governing the rate at which P_c approaches P_A, starting from $P\bar{v}$ (Figure 6.2).

For perfusion limited gases like acetylene $D_L/\beta\dot{Q}$ is > 10, alveolar-end–capillary equilibration is almost instantaneous, and the greater the blood flow the more gas will be transferred. For carbon monoxide, which is highly reactive with Hb, the very high value for β forces the $D_L/\beta\dot{Q}$ ratio down to < 0.01. During the whole capillary transit time, alveolar-capillary equilibration is negligible and plasma P_{CO} remains close to zero (assuming no prior exposure). The initial tension gradient (P_{ACO}-$P\bar{v}_{CO}$) operates continuously; CO molecules are driven into blood by the diffusion gradient and are immediately mopped up by hemoglobin molecules, acting as a huge sink. The Hb capacity for CO is so great that increasing the 'flow' of Hb will not increase CO uptake.

Oxygen reacts with Hb much less strongly than CO. $D_L/\beta\dot{Q}$ for oxygen varies from about 4–6 at rest to about 1.0 on exercise. Transfer is mostly perfusion dependent at rest (the alveolar-end–capillary gradient is very small) but becomes more diffusion dependent on heavy exercise, especially if inspired oxygen tension is low (as at altitude). The diffusing capacity for oxygen equals $D_{LCO} \times 1.2$.[1]

- Both perfusion and diffusion are rate limiting steps in the alveolar-capillary transfer of oxygen (and CO_2).
- CO transfer, because of its high affinity for hemoglobin, is diffusion-limited only.
- CO is the appropriate gas to measure the diffusing capacity.
- Alveolar-capillary CO transfer involves two processes in series:
  1. molecular diffusion
  2. combination with Hb.

Figure 6.2 Diffusion-perfusion relationships at the alveolar level

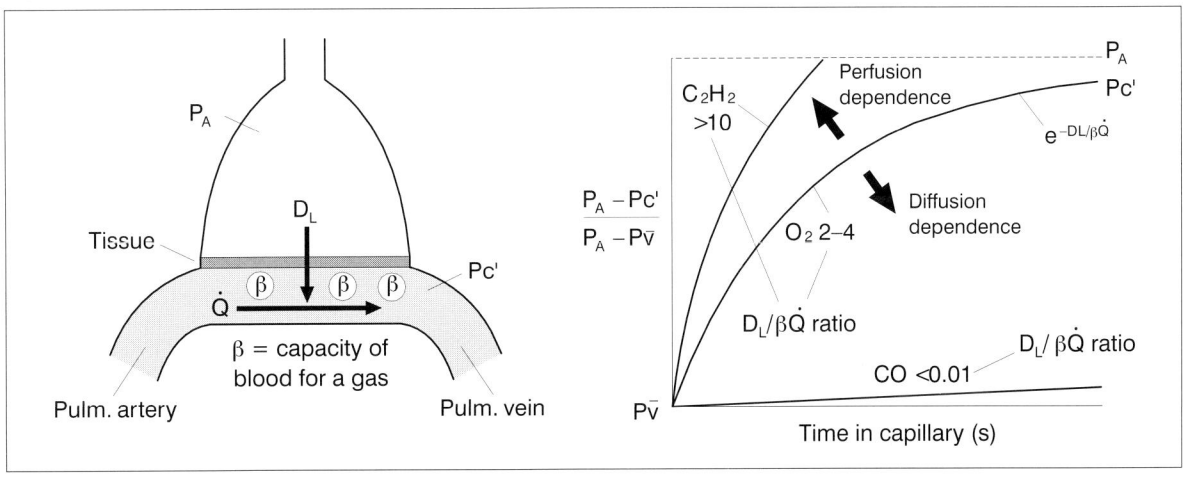

THEORY AND PRACTICE

The single-breath D_{LCO} (T_{LCO}) measurement

The single-breath D_{LCO} (T_{LCO}) is usually measured under specific conditions:

- at rest
- breath-holding at full inspiration
- corrected to a standard Hb concentration.

Higher values of D_{LCO} would be found on exercise, and lower values at lung volumes below TLC or with anemia. D_{LCO} represents the *potential* for gas exchange. It is not equivalent to the steady state arterial oxygen tension (PaO_2). For example, PaO_2 is often low in asthma but D_{LCO} is usually normal. Conversely, PaO_2 is often well maintained in emphysema or fibrosis in spite of a low D_{LCO}. PaO_2 at rest is mostly dependent on ventilation-perfusion matching, but the full inspiration to total lung capacity (in the measurement of D_{LCO}) is designed to minimize maldistribution of ventilation and $\dot{V}_A/\dot{Q}$.

- D_{LCO} (T_{LCO}) reflects the surface area available for gas exchange under resting conditions and at full inflation.
- The units of CO transfer are those of conductance (1/resistance) or quantity transferred per unit time and per unit driving pressure.
- D_{LCO} (T_{LCO}) is a measure of alveolar-capillary integrity and, as such, a window on the pulmonary microcirculation.

Principles of measurement

The single-breath diffusing capacity (D_{LCO} *[single-breath]*) was introduced as a clinical test by Ogilvie et al.[2] The principles are similar to those underlying the rebreathing technique (D_{LCO} *[rebreathing]*). The basic idea is best appreciated by a thorough understanding of the rebreathing method for D_{LCO} (see later), which should be read in conjunction with this section. The techniques for performing both measurements are outlined below.

Figure 6.3

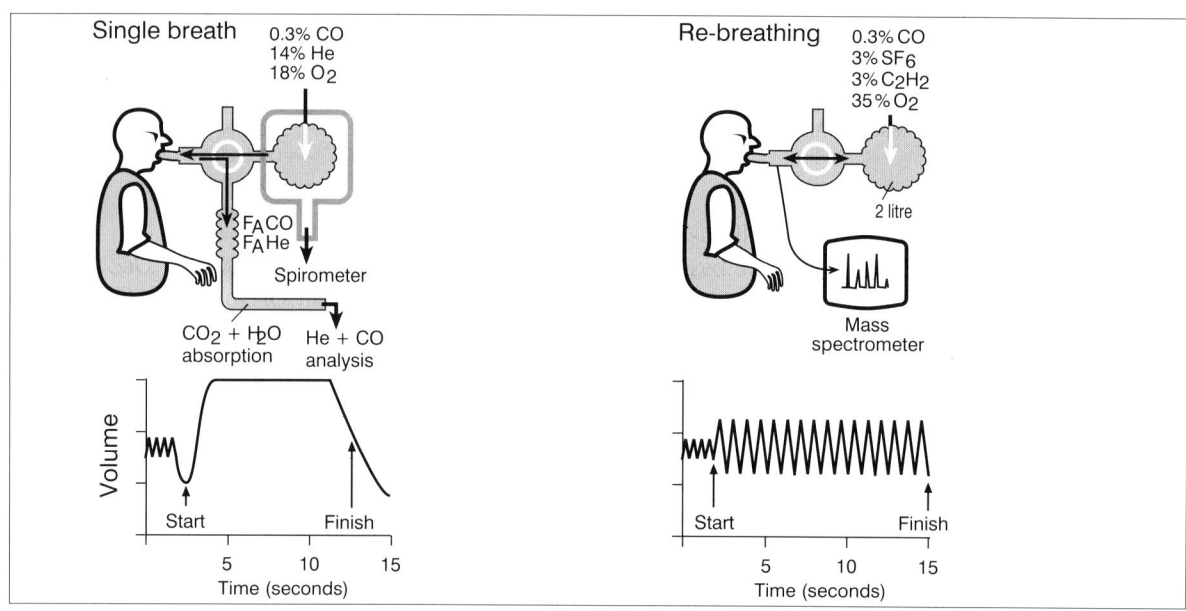

Single breath

*A **rapid** inspiratory vital capacity (from RV to TLC) is taken from a reservoir bag. The breath is held (automatically, against a closed shutter) for approximately 10 seconds at maximal inspiration, before a **rapid** and complete exhalation is made. The first 750 ml are discarded as contaminated with anatomic dead space gas, the next 500 ml are collected in a bag as an alveolar sample for analysis of CO and He.*

Rebreathing

The subject (either at FRC or RV) is switched into a bag of known volume and gas composition. The bag is filled and emptied every 1–2 seconds for 10–15 seconds while gas concentrations are sampled continuously. (see Figure 6.5a).

Figure 6.4 Single-breath D_{LCO}: gas concentrations versus time

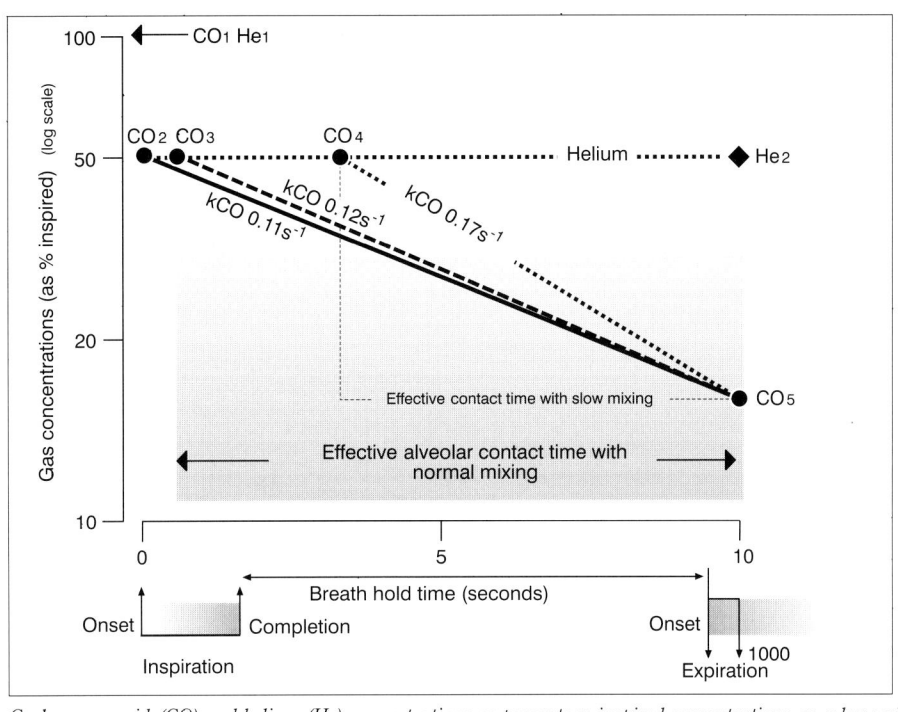

Carbon monoxide(CO) and helium (He) concentrations as percentage inspired concentrations on a log scale.

Unlike D_{LCO} (*rebreathing*) where there is continuous sampling of the CO and reference gas concentrations (Figure 6.5), only a single sample is usually obtained at the end of 10 s breath-holding in D_{LCO} (*single-breath*).

In outline, the calculations from Figure 6.4 proceed as follows:

Derivation of initial alveolar carbon monoxide concentration (CO_2) Knowing the dilution of the reference gas (helium) (He_2/He_1) the assumption is made that gas dilution is essentially instantaneous with the onset of inspiration (in normal lungs, this is a reasonable supposition, see Figure 6.5a) so that the alveolar concentration of CO at point CO_2 (before significant alveolar-capillary transfer has taken place) would have been the same as the expired helium value at point He_2. Thus, the initial alveolar CO concentration at time zero (CO_2) equals the inspired concentration (CO_1) times the helium dilution factor (He_1/He_2).

Derivation of alveolar contact time for CO The alveolar contact time has an important influence on the value of kCO. In Figure 6.4, the inspiratory vital capacity took 1.7 s to complete. There are several proposals[3] for the calculation of the 'effective' alveolar contact time and the choice is rather arbitrary. We favor the Jones and Meade[4] approach in which the contact time starts after one third of the inspired volume has been completed [CO_3] and ends when half the expired sample (usually taken between 750 and 1250 ml expired) has been collected.

Calculation of rate constant for alveolar-capillary CO transfer, or kCO Joining the CO concentrations, on the semi-log plot (Figure 6.4), at CO_2 and CO_5 gives a slope which, when divided by the 'alveolar contact time', equals the rate constant for CO uptake, or kCO. In this example, the concentration ratio CO_2/CO_5 = 50/16.7 = 3 and $\log_e$ of 3 = 1.1: the 'contact' time (CO_2 to CO_5) = 10 s so kCO = 1.1/10 = 0.11 sec^{-1}.

Effect of 'alveolar contact time' on carbon monoxide rate constant (kCO) If the inspiration is rapid, and the breath hold is about 10 seconds, the effect of a Jones-Meade correction is small (shift of CO_2 to CO_3 in Figure 6.4) and the kCO shifts by only 9% (1.1/9.4 = 0.117 s^{-1}). With a very slow inspiration (lasting 4–5 s) or, equally, very slow mixing (due to airflow obstruction) between inspired and residual gas, the effective alveolar contact time for CO might be as short as 6.4 s (CO4 to CO5 in Figure 6.4), giving a 'real' kCO of 0.17 s^{-1} (1.1/6.4) instead of 0.12 s^{-1} as conventionally measured by curve CO3/CO5. Thus, in the presence of a slow inspiration or slow mixing, the conventional calculation of contact time (CO3 to CO5) could conceal a much shorter 'real' contact time (CO4 to CO5) leading to a 32% underestimation of 'true' kCO.

Derivation of CO volume of distribution (referred to as 'alveolar volume' or [V_A])
By simple gas dilution principles, and assuming that gas mixing is rapid which, in the absence of airflow obstruction it is – see SF$_6$ curve in Figure 6.5, the volume of distribution of CO is

$$V_A = \text{inspired volume} \times (\text{He}_1/\text{He}_2)$$

The ratio (He2/He1) should be proportional to [1– RV/TLC = c.0.3] since the inspired volume should equal [TLC–RV], i.e. about 0.7. Note in Figure 6.4 (only an example) that (He2/He1) is low (0.5) implying an RV/TLC ratio of 50%.

See Appendix for details of conversion of volume to STPD conditions and the subtraction of dead space.

In D$_{LCO}$ (*single-breath*) the volume of distribution is the effective *alveolar* volume during breath-holding, but in D$_{LCO}$ (*rebreathing*, see later) the volume of distribution is the volume of the lungs when switched into the rebreathing bag plus the volume of the bag itself.

Constant exhalation D$_L$CO

A constant exhalation technique for D$_{LCO}$ has been introduced[5] which contains elements of D$_{LCO}$ (*rebreathing*) and D$_{LCO}$ (*single-breath*). The breathing maneuver is similar to D$_{LCO}$ (*single-breath*) except that the subject, after reaching maximal inspiration, exhales slowly and continuously against a fixed resistance at approximately 0.5 L.s^{-1}. CO is analyzed at a rate of 31 samples per second by a rapidly responding infra-red CO sensor. Because CO and the reference gas (CH$_4$ in this instance) are monitored continuously, the analysis is akin to D$_{LCO}$ (*rebreathing*) (Figure 6.5). D$_{LCO}$ with constant exhalation was identical to D$_{LCO}$ (*single-breath*) in 100 consecutive patients.[5] Alveolar volume (V$_A$) was less than V$_A$ (*single-breath*), because breath-holding at full inflation promotes better gas mixing; kCO is correspondingly higher.

Calculation of D$_L$co from data shown in Figure 6.4

$$D_{LCO} = \frac{[\text{kCO} \times \text{volume of distribution}]}{\text{barometric pressure}}$$

Intuitively, from Figures 6.3 and 6.4, if the volume of distribution was 4000 ml and supposing the lungs contained 100% carbon monoxide,* the quantity of CO diffusing across the alveolar-capillary surface would be **4000 ml × 0.12** s^{-1} or **4000 × 0.12 × 60** min^{-1} i.e. **28 800** ml.min^{-1}. Since the diffusing capacity is a conductance, i.e. flux per unit pressure, and the partial pressure of carbon monoxide (if lung gas were 100% CO) equals barometric pressure (Pb) (minus water vapor pressure) (P$_{H_2O}$) (**713 mmHg** or **95 kPa**), D$_{LCO}$ would be:

$$\frac{28\ 800}{713} = 40.4\ \text{ml.min}^{-1}\ \text{mmHg}^{-1}$$

or

$$\frac{28\ 800}{(22.4 \times 95)} = 13.5\ \text{mmol.min}^{-1}\ \text{kPa}^{-1}$$

- D$_{LCO}$ is the multiple of kCO and V_A divided by Pb.
- kCO is the equivalent of D$_{LCO}$/V$_A$ (K$_{CO}$).
- kCO and V_A are the **primary** measurements.
- A low D$_{LCO}$ is caused by a low K$_{CO}$ or a low V_A or both.

The crucial point to grasp is that the D$_{LCO}$ is the product of the rate constant for alveolar CO uptake (kCO) times the volume of distribution (V$_A$) divided by the effective barometric pressure. V$_A$ and kCO are the primary measurements from which D$_{LCO}$ is *derived*. Therefore, when D$_{LCO}$ is subsequently divided by V$_A$ to derive 'diffusing capacity per unit volume' (D$_L$/V$_A$), we are, except for the units, returning full circle to the rate constant kCO. The expression D$_L$/V$_A$ does not actually contain any volume information. Nevertheless, whether it is called D$_L$/V$_A$ or K$_{CO}$, it is a very useful index of the 'efficiency of alveolar CO uptake' or the 'diffusing capacity per alveolus'.

See Appendix 6.I (page 106) for a sample calculation.

---

* remember that CO can be a very toxic gas at lung concentrations > 0.3%

Resumé of single-breath D_{LCO} calculations and definitions

A. Using traditional nomenclature (ml and mmHg)

1. $[kCO(\text{min}^{-1}) \times V_A' (\text{ml})] / P_b - P_{H_2O} (\text{mmHg}) = D_{LCO}$ ml.min^{-1} mmHg^{-1}

2. $D_{LCO}/V_A = K_{CO}$ ml.min^{-1} mmHg^{-1} L^{-1}

   note V_A' (ml[STPD]) has become V_A (L[BTPS]) by multiplying by a BTPS factor/1000 which for P_b 760 mmHg is 0.0012 (see *Worked out example* in Appendix 6.I).

3. It follows that the rate constant kCO (min^{-1}) converts to K_{CO} (or D_{LCO}/V_A) only by dividing by the constant factors $(V_A'/V_A) \times (P_b - P_{H_2O})$, i.e. $0.0012 \times 713 = 0.856$ (for P_b 760 mmHg).

B. Using SI units (mmol and kPa)

1. kCO (min^{-1}) remains unchanged
   V_A' (ml STPD)/22.4 = V_A mmol
   P_b (mmHg)/7.5 = P_b (kPa)
   $P_b - P_{H_2O}$ = 101.3 − 6.3 = 95 kPa

   D_{LCO} = mmol.min^{-1} kPa^{-1} (conversion factor from traditional = 7.5/22.4 = .335)

2. $D_{LCO}/V_A = K_{CO}$ (mmol.min^{-1} kPa^{-1} L^{-1})

   V_A (mmol) converts to V_A (L.BTPS) by $22.4 \times 0.0012 = 0.0269$

3. kCO converts to K_{CO} by dividing by the factor

   $0.0269 \times 95 = 2.55$ (for P_b 101.3 kPa)

Methodological key points

- After prior explanation, guide the subject through the maneuver.
- Complete exhalation to residual volume first.
- Rapid and full inspiration to total lung capacity.
- Rapid exhalation after breath-hold.
- If first two D_{LCO}s do not agree to within 5%, do a third measurement.
- Apply the correction for [Hb].
- Check recent (last 8 hours) cigarette consumption. Measure carboxyhemoglobin fraction or alveolar P_{CO} if unexpectedly low values are found.

Rebreathing D_{LCO}

Measurement of D_{LCO} with a rebreathing technique is becoming more popular with the introduction of respiratory mass spectrometers sensitive enough to detect the stable isotope of carbon monoxide ($C^{18}O$) with a good signal-noise ratio. In fact, the rebreathing method serves as a good explanation of the theory of the single-breath D_{LCO}.

The basic idea is to measure the rate of uptake of carbon monoxide in a known lung volume and in a defined time period (see Figure 6.3 for details of the technique).

The concentration falls (relative to the inspired concentration) (see Figure 6.5a) for two reasons:

(a) dilution in the CO-free residual lung gas volume
(b) diffusion of CO across the alveolar capillary membranes.

Gas dilution is monitored with a reference gas which is inert and insoluble; helium is generally employed in the single-breath method (methane [CH_4] is also used) and sulfur hexafluoride (SF_6) is a convenient gas for the mass spectrometer (Figure 6.3, right) in the rebreathing method. The quantity of these gases which crosses the alveolar-capillary membranes by diffusion is negligible compared to carbon monoxide.

Figure 6.5a SF$_6$ and rescaled C^{18}O rebreathing curves

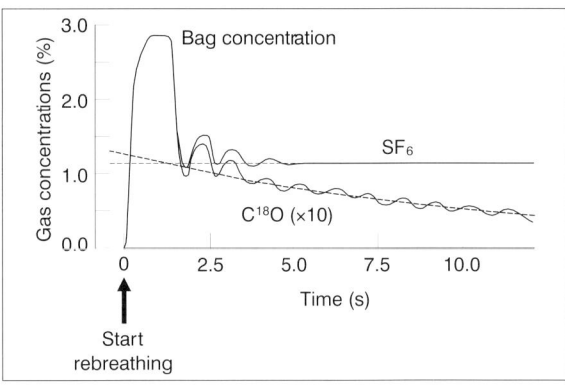

Peak concentrations (2.8% for SF$_6$) are those in the rebreathing bag initially. Note bag C^{18}O concentration was 0.28%.

Note the following points in Figure 6.5a:

1. The SF$_6$ curve reaches a steady level or equilibrium at 4.5 s after the onset of inspiration. From this moment C^{18}O is in contact with all ventilated alveoli. As this is a normal subject, gas mixing occurs very rapidly and is actually virtually complete by the second exhalation.
2. The C^{18}O concentration time curve departs from the SF$_6$ curve from the first exhalation and the divergence increases after gas mixing is completed, the subsequent concentration changes of CO being entirely caused by alveolar-capillary diffusion.

Figure 6.5b C^{18}O/SF$_6$ ratios during the rebreathing maneuver

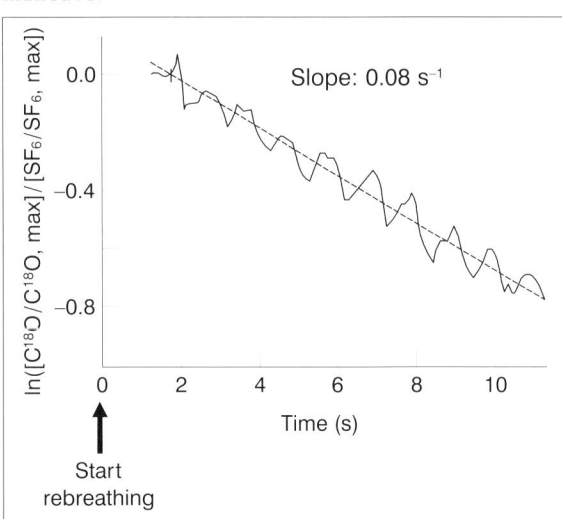

Figure 6.5b shows a semi-log plot of the C^{18}O/SF$_6$ ratio (both gases expressed as a fraction of their inspired, i.e. maximum, concentration). This slope equals the dilution-independent rate of alveolar uptake of carbon monoxide, designated kCO when k stands for the rate constant (see also Figure 6.4). In approximately 10 seconds (from 0 to 10 seconds on the time axis) the ln [C^{18}O/SF$_6$] has fallen from 0 to –0.8 which is a change of 0.08 s^{-1}. Thus CO is disappearing from alveolar gas at a constant rate of 8% per second.

COMPONENTS OF D$_{LCO}$

Membrane and reactive conductances of D$_{LCO}$

Roughton and Forster's paper[6] was a landmark in our understanding of D$_{LCO}$. They proposed that D$_{LCO}$ consisted of two conductances in series: the molecular diffusion component (from alveolar epithelium up to the interior of the red cell) called the membrane conductance (D$_M$), and the reactive conductance (θ.Qc) where θ is the rate of reaction of a gas with hemoglobin and Qc is the volume of blood in the capillaries. The inverse of these conductances (1/D$_M$ and 1/θ.Qc) represent resistances in series which can be added to give the Roughton-Forster equation:

$$\frac{1}{D_{LCO}} = \frac{1}{D_M} + \frac{1}{\theta.Qc}$$

At P$_A$O$_2$ >100 mmHg, 1/θ CO is directly proportional to PO$_2$ because of competition between O$_2$ and CO for hemoglobin. Therefore, by measuring D$_{LCO}$ (*single-breath*) with different oxygen concentrations in the reservoir bag (with or without pre-oxygenating the subject with 100% oxygen breathing), the Roughton-Forster equation can be solved (Figure 6.6). It is assumed that changing alveolar PO$_2$ does not alter pulmonary hemodynamics or cardiac output and by itself alter D$_{LCO}$. This assumption is reasonable in the case of normal subjects, but might not hold in the presence of lung disease and regional alveolar hypoxia.

Figure 6.6b shows single estimations of D$_{LCO}$ (*single-breath*) at four levels of P$_A$O$_2$.[7] This was achieved by pre-oxygenating the subject for 15 minutes (with 21, 39, 59 or 88% inspired O$_2$) before inhaling the standard CO mixture (in 18% oxygen). Note that the increase in

D_{LCO} with an increase in V_A (3.3 L at low versus 8.0 L at the high volume) is caused by an increase in membrane conductance, i.e. alveolar-capillary membrane surface area/thickness, rather than an increase in capillary volume. It is more usual to use low (18%) and high (85–90%) oxygen in CO mixtures, obtained commercially. Two points are obtained at each level (no pre-oxygenation is employed) and a straight line is drawn between the mean value of each pair of measurements. The oxygen concentration of the alveolar sample is measured by putting an oxygen analyzer in series with the CO and helium analyzers. Details of the procedure and calculations are given by Cotes.[8]

In most disease states, the reduction in D_{LCO} is accompanied by a fall in both D_M and Q_c and no extra information is gained, except in heart failure where D_M only is reduced.[9] In normal subjects, the increase in cardiac output on exercise is accompanied by linear increases in D_M and Q_c, by 30% and 60% respectively as cardiac output increases threefold (from 5 to 15 L.min^{-1}).[10]

The ratio $[1/D_{MCO} / 1/D_{LCO}]$ (rebreathing technique) is 0.63[10] and with the single-breath method 0.5.[9] This implies that 50–63% of the resistance to alveolar-capillary transfer resides in the membranes, leaving 37–50% in the combination with hemoglobin. The ratio remains 0.6 on exercise ($\dot{Q} = 15$ L.min^{-1}).[10] On the other hand, recent work using inhaled nitric oxide (NO) (see below), where D_{LNO} acts as a surrogate for D_M,[11,12] suggests that only 25% of the total resistance to CO transfer is in the membrane component, not 50–60%.

[θCO] which is the D_{LCO} of a drop of blood (or more correctly of a ml of hemoglobin in solution), is influenced by the density of hemoglobin binding sites, i.e. the blood hematocrit, as well as by alveolar PO_2. It is variations in θ which determine the relationship between [Hb] and D_{LCO} (Figure 6.6) and also enable us to calculate D_M and Q_c.

Nitric oxide: (D_{LNO})

Nitric oxide (NO) has an extremely high affinity for hemoglobin, θNO exceeding θCO by more than tenfold. The diffusing capacity for NO has been measured following inhalation of 0.004% NO gas.[11,12] The breath-hold time has to be reduced to 5 s or less because of the rapid disappearance of NO from alveolar gas. When D_{LCO} and D_{LNO} are measured simultaneously, $D_{LCO}/D_{LNO} = 0.23$.[11] D_{LNO} was unchanged when P_AO_2 was increased, suggesting that the resistance to alveolar-capillary transfer for this gas resides mostly in D_M. This was supported by a 34% fall in

Figure 6.6 Graphical solution of the Roughton-Forster equation

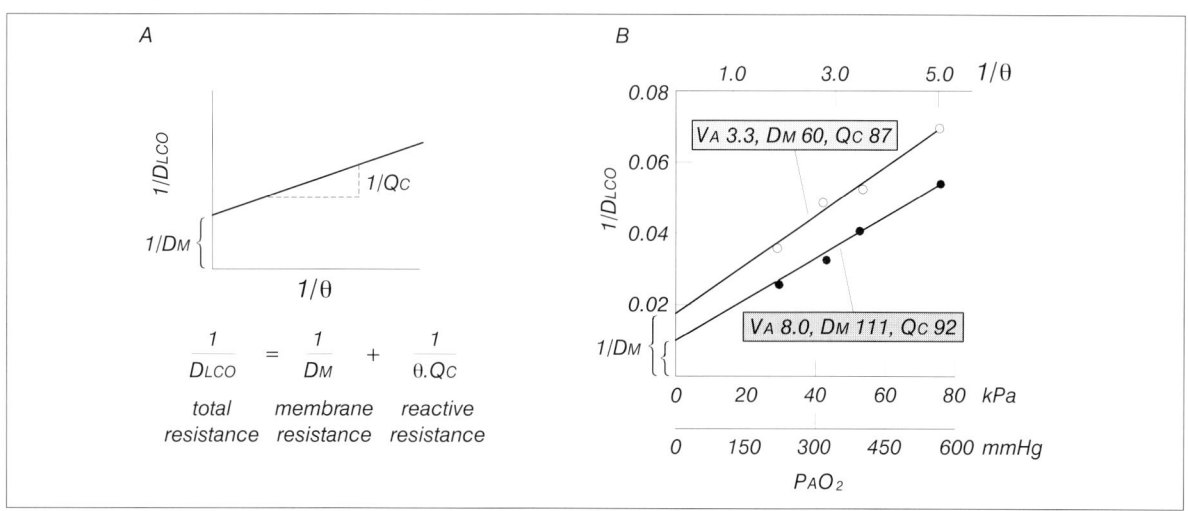

Panel (B) plots $1/D_{LCO}$ against alveolar PO_2. D_{LCO} was measured at four different inspired oxygen concentrations giving four different values of P_AO_2 and corresponding values of $1/θ$. Measurements made with a normal subject breath-holding at a high (8.0 L) or low (3.3 L) alveolar volume (V_A). Note increase in membrane conductance (D_M) at higher lung volume (87 to 111) but no change in microvascular volume (Q_c).

Traditional units shown for D_M (ml.min^{-1} mmHg^{-1}) and $1/D_{LCO}$ and $1/D_M$ (mmHg.ml^{-1} min). Units of $1/θ$ are [mmHg.L.ml^{-1} min] × 10^{-3}

D_{LNO} with a 3 L reduction in lung volume compared to 7% for D_{LCO}. To the extent that D_{LNO} measures D_M, the Roughton-Forster equation can be solved with a simultaneous $D_{LNO} - D_{LCO}$ measurement:

$$1/Qc = \theta CO\ [1/D_{LCO} - 2/D_{LNO}]*$$

The D_{LCO}/D_{LNO} ratio of 0.23 implies that 75% of the diffusive resistance resides in the reactive (θQc) component rather than in the membrane. Clinically, the sensitivity of D_{LCO} to diseases involving the pulmonary circulation alone, to increases in pulmonary blood volume (with exercise), to pulmonary hemorrhage, and to changes of hematocrit all point to θQc as the main rate limiting step for alveolar-capillary CO transfer.

There are no measurements of D_{LCO}/D_{LNO} ratio in different disease states.

D_{LCO} (T_{LCO}) IN HEALTHY SUBJECTS

Factors influencing the measurement of D_{LCO} (single-breath)

Hemoglobin concentration

θ in the Roughton-Forster equation (the rate of uptake of CO in blood) is a function of the oxygen tension (see Figure 6.6) and of the number of Hb binding sites for CO per ml blood.

θ is influenced by:

- alveolar PO_2
- hemoglobin concentration or hematocrit.

Cotes et al[13] proposed a [Hb] correction to D_{LCO} based on the Roughton-Forster equation, assuming a D_M/Vc ratio of 0.7 and a reference [Hb] of 14.5 g dL^{-1}.

D_{LCO} (corr)=D_{LCO} (obs). (10.2+[Hb])/1.7×[Hb].

Measurements before and after blood transfusion[14] have confirmed the accuracy of this correction. It is good practice to apply this correction to all measurements but particularly when patients with non-respiratory disease are studied. At [Hb] 7 g.dL^{-1} there is a 30% reduction in D_{LCO} (and K_{CO}) relative to [Hb] 14.5 g.dL^{-1} i.e. 4% reduction per g [Hb] fall – Figure 6.7, panel **D**. If severe anemia was accompanied by a rise

---

* 2/D_{LNO} occurs because D_M ~ diffusivity ~ [solubility.MW^{-2}] and NO solubility is twice that for CO.

> **Key points from the Roughton-Forster equation**
>
> - The membrane conductance (D_M) is in series with the hemoglobin-binding conductance (θQc).
> - D_M, but not Qc, increases as V_A increases.
> - $1/\theta$ is linearly related to alveolar PO_2 and inversely proportional to hematocrit.
> - D_{LNO} is largely a measure of D_M ($\theta NO \gg \theta CO$).
> - D_{LCO}/D_{LNO} ratio (0.23) suggests only 20–25% of overall diffusion resistance lies in the membrane.

in cardiac output, the Cotes equation might over-correct (see D_{LCO} versus $\dot{Q}$ in Figure 6.7, panel **B**).

Alveolar oxygen concentration

θ for CO is also inversely related to alveolar PO_2 (Figure 6.6) due to competition between oxygen and CO for binding sites on the Hb molecule. In everyday practice, variations in P_AO_2 between subjects can be ignored. The 17–18% oxygen concentration in the inspired reservoir for D_{LCO} (*single-breath*) has been chosen, so that P_AO_2 will remain around its normal value (105 mmHg/14 kPa) irrespective of the volume inspired, but North American practice is to have 21% oxygen in the reservoir. At altitude, e.g. Denver, Colorado, P_AO_2 may be 30 mmHg less, and a correction factor for the higher value of θ has been proposed.[15] Fuller discussion of this subject can be found in Crapo and Gardner[3] (p 1302).

Lung expansion

D_{LCO} (*single-breath*) is relatively independent of the lung volume at which the measurement is made with only a 3–4% decrease per 10% reduction in V_A (Figure 6.7, panel **A**). On the contrary K_{CO} (or D_{LCO}/V_A) increases exponentially as V_A declines (Figure 6.7, panel **C**) which explains the relative stability of D_{LCO} versus V_A. It is as if the gas exchanging part of the lung distal to the terminal bronchioles, the acini, were inflating and deflating like a concertina or a corrugated bellows, i.e. with a constant surface area so that the surface/volume ratio (analogous to K_{CO}) increases exponentially as volume declines.

Cardiac output

Increases in pulmonary blood flow are accompanied by increases in pulmonary arterial and venous pressures and by an increased pulmonary blood volume due to distension and recruitment of vessels, especially in the pulmonary microcirculation. This leads to the percentage increases in D_{LCO} shown in Figure 6.7 panel **B** (K_{CO} behaves similarly). In absolute terms, D_{LCO} (*rebreathing*) is 8.6 ml.min^{-1} mmHg^{-1} (or 2.9 mmol.min^{-1} kPa) *less* than D_{LCO} (*single-breath*) at $\dot{Q}$ = 5.0 L.min^{-1} but the gap narrows progressively as cardiac output increases.

Carbon monoxide back pressure

Ten successive measurements of D_{LCO} in a normal subject (equivalent to smoking several cigarettes acutely) raise alveolar CO to 0.004%. This concentration, which acts as a back pressure for alveolar-capillary transfer (raising $P\bar{v}_{CO}$), would have to be subtracted from the alveolar CO concentrations CO3 and CO5 (Figure 6.5), equivalent to a 2.7% and 8% fall in them and a 5% reduction in the slope (kCO) and in D_{LCO} and K_{CO}. At 0.004% plasma CO, the carboxyhemoglobin level will be about 10%. This is equivalent to reducing [Hb] by 10% and will reduce D_{LCO} by a further 5%. Thus, the maximum underestimation due to acute cigarette smoking or multiple tests will be 10%. Provided that subjects are asked about recent cigarette smoking and that the number of single-breath tests does not exceed five, a correction for CO back pressure is not required. See ATS recommendations[3] for further discussion of this point.

Chronic smoking (not its acute effects)

It is well known that a reduction in K_{CO} (D_{LCO}/V_A) correlates well with the extent of emphysema inferred in life from computed tomography or assessed directly by morphometry from lung sections. The K_{CO} is also reduced in asymptomatic middle-aged smokers with normal FEV_1.[16] Interestingly, ten years later there was no further fall in their K_{CO} in comparison to the age-

Figure 6.7 Lung expansion, cardiac output, and anaemia as determinants of single breath D$_{LCO}$ in normal subjects

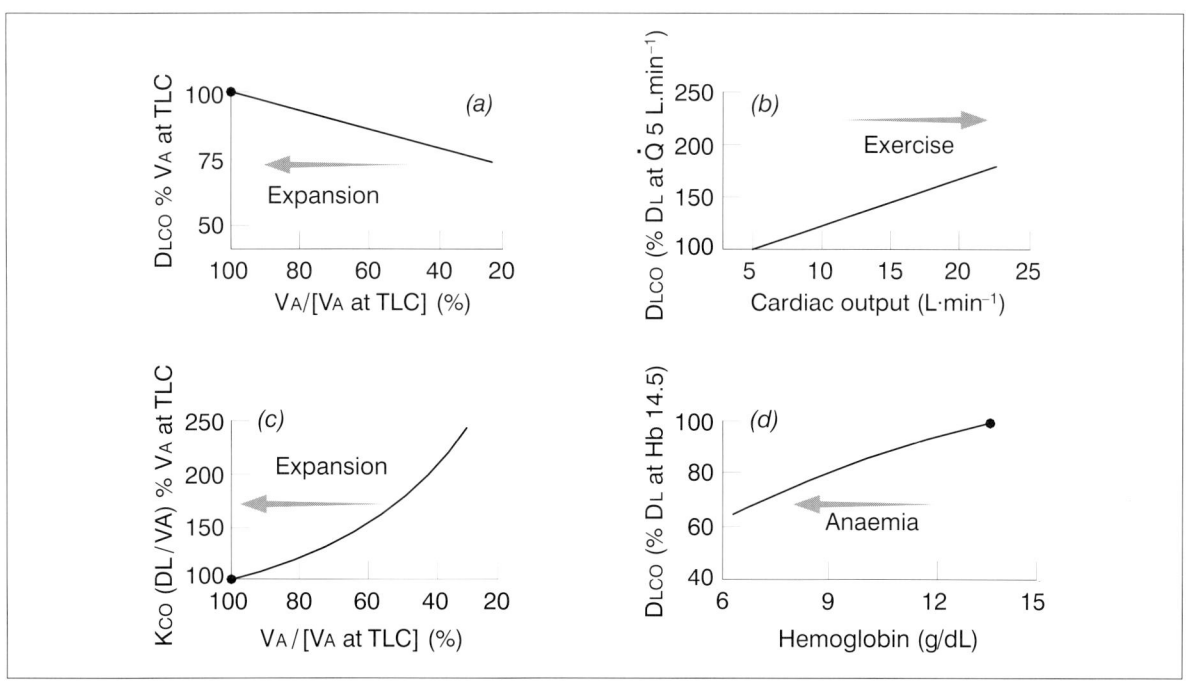

In panels (a) and (c), D_{LCO} and K_{CO} have been measured at lung volumes less than full inspiration, V_A being expressed as a percentage of the V_A at TLC. Panel (b) plots the increase in D_{LCO} in response to rises in cardiac output produced by steady state exercise (K_{CO} would behave similarly). Panel (d) charts the effect of chronic anemia.

related fall in non-smokers even though their FEV_1 declined per year at double the rate for never smokers. Those smokers, followed serially, who quit smoking in the first two years of the ten year follow-up showed an *improvement* in Kco in comparison to the age-related fall in non-smokers, (5% in absolute terms), whereas *never smokers* showed a 9% decline in absolute terms.[16] Therefore, the reduction in Kco in smokers who quit can be reversed.

Normal values, units, reproducibility, quality control

It is unfortunate that there is no agreement between North America and Europe over nomenclature and units, with *diffusing capacity* (D_{LCO}) in ml.min^{-1} mmHg^{-1} in use on one side of the Atlantic and *transfer factor* (T_{LCO}) in mmol.min^{-1} kPa^{-1} on the other side. The ratio D_{LCO}/T_{LCO} with their different units is 3:1 or $D_{LCO} \times 0.333 = T_{LCO}$.

Reference values are discussed in Chapter 19. For more information, consult the ERS[17] and ATS[3] recommendation statements. Kco (D_{LCO}/V_A), which is directly related to the rate constant for alveolar-capillary transfer (or gas-exchange 'efficiency'), should, in my opinion, be independent of sex and height and dependent only on age, but only one study[18] has shown this.

There are no ethnic differences for D_{LCO}. Since subjects of African and Asian origin tend to have lung volumes which are smaller for their height (by 10–15%), their Kco (D_{LCO}/V_A) will be higher.

With good technique, measurements of D_{LCO} and Kco (D_{LCO}/V_A) are reproducible to the extent that duplicate measurements are generally within 5% of each other. If duplicates lie outside this limit, the reason for the discrepancy should be sought. The question of quality control is addressed in the ATS[3], ERS[17] and BTS[19] recommendation documents.

Calculation of alveolar volume (V_A)

The basic D_{LCO} equation ($[V_A \times kCO]/Pb$) gives an estimate of CO uptake in the well ventilated part of the lung, i.e. V_A. In airflow obstruction, the V_A measured from helium dilution during a 10 second breath-hold may quite considerably underestimate the true lung gas volume at full inflation (TLC). In this case, the D_{LCO} calculated from V_A is a lower boundary value since gas exchange surface lies hidden in the poorly ventilated volume component (TLC–V_A). ($[TLC \times kCO]/Pb$) would give an upper boundary for D_{LCO}.[19] Although TLC was used as the 'alveolar volume' in the original clinical description of D_{LCO} by Ogilvie et al,[2] the use of TLC has not found favor subsequently, partly because the poorly ventilated units probably have a much lower than average kCO. Any solution represents a compromise since there is no absolutely correct way to weight kCO for the volume of distribution when kCO itself is unevenly distributed, as it is in the diseased lung.

An important practical point is that a separate measurement of absolute lung volume (i.e. TLC) is not required if V_A is derived from a single breath helium dilation, and this modification saves time which can be spent on other tasks.

CONCLUSIONS

1. The single-breath diffusing capacity D_{LCO} is one of the most widely used tests in pulmonary function assessment.

2. D_{LCO} (single-breath) is the multiple of the alveolar volume (V_A) and the rate constant for alveolar-capillary transfer (kCO), the latter being equivalent to Kco or D_{LCO}/V_A.

3. V_A reflects the number of contributing units and Kco represents the diffusing capacity per alveolus or the 'alveolar efficiency'.

4. D_{LCO} and Kco can detect microvascular damage in the absence of alveolar disease.

5. Low D_{LCO} supports the diagnosis of emphysema, fibrosis, or pulmonary vascular disease.

References

1. Meyer M, Scheid P, Riedl G, Wagner H-J, Piiper J. Pulmonary diffusing capacities for O_2 and CO measured by a rebreathing technique. *J Appl Physiol* 1981; **51**: 1643–50.

2. Ogilvie CM, Forster RE, Blakemore WS, Morton JW. A standardized breath holding technique for the clinical measurement of the diffusing capacity of the lung for carbon monoxide. *J Clin Invest* 1957; **36**: 1–17.

3. American Thoracic Society. Single breath carbon monoxide diffusing capacity (transfer factor), recommendations for a

standard technique – 1995 update. *Am Rev Respir Dis* 1995; **52**: 2185–98.

4   Jones RS & Meade FA. A theoretical and experimental analysis of anomalies in the estimation of pulmonary diffusing capacity by the single breath method. *Q J Exp Physiol* 1961; **46**: 131–43.

5   Wilson AF, Hearne J, Brenner M, Alfonso R. Measurement of transfer factor during constant exhalation. *Thorax* 1994; **49**: 1121–6.

6   Roughton FJW & Forster RE. Relative importance of diffusion and chemical reaction in determining rate of exchange of gases in the human lung. *J Appl Physiol* 1957; **11**: 290–302.

7   Lipscomb DJ, Patel K & Hughes JMB. Interpretation of increases in the transfer coefficient for carbon monoxide (T_{LCO}/V_A or K_{CO}). *Thorax* 1978; **33**: 728–33.

8   Cotes JE. *Lung Function; Assessment and Application in Medicine,* 5th edn. Oxford: Blackwell Scientific Publications 1993: 17.

9   Puri S, Baker BL, Oakley CM, Hughes JMB, Cleland JGF. Increased alveolar capillary membrane resistance to gas transfer in congestive heart failure. *Br Heart J* 1994; **72**: 140–4.

10 Hsia CCW, McBrayer DG & Ramanathan M. Reference values of pulmonary diffusing capacity during exercise by a rebreathing technique. *Am J Respir Crit Care Med* 1995; **152**: 658–65.

11 Guenard H, Varenne N & Vaida P. Determination of lung capillary blood volume and membrane diffusing capacity by measurement of NO and CO transfer. *Respir Physiol* 1987; **70**: 113–20.

12 Borland CDR & Higenbottam TW. A simultaneous single breath measurement of pulmonary diffusing capacity with nitric oxide and carbon monoxide. *Eur Resp J* 1989; **2**: 56–63.

13 Cotes JE, Dabbs JM, Elwood PC, Hall AM, McDonald A, Saunders MJ. Iron-deficiency anaemia: its effect on transfer factor for the lung (diffusing capacity) and ventilation and cardiac frequency during sub-maximal exercise. *Clin Sci* 1972; **42**: 325–35.

14 Clark EH, Woods RL & Hughes JMB. Effect of blood transfusion on the carbon monoxide transfer factor of the lung in man. *Clin Sci Molecul Med* 1978; **54**: 627–31.

15 Kanner RE & Crapo RO. The relationship between alveolar oxygen tension and the single-breath carbon monoxide diffusing capacity. *Am Rev Respir Dis* 1986; **133**: 676.

16 Watson A, Joyce H, Hopper L, Pride NB. Influence of smoking habits on change in carbon monoxide transfer factor over 10 years in middle aged men. *Thorax* 1993; **48**: 119–24.

17 Cotes JE, Chinn DJ, Quanjer PH, Roca J, Yernault J-C. Standardization of the measurement of transfer factor (diffusing capacity). *Eur Respir J* 1993; **6**(suppl 16): 41–52.

18 Bradley J, Bye C, Hayden SP, Hughes DTD. Normal values of transfer factor and transfer coefficient in healthy males and females. *Respir* 1979; **38**: 221–26.

19 BTS and ARTP recommendations. Guidelines for the measurement of respiratory function. *Respir Med* 1994; **88**: 165–94.

APPENDIX 6.1

Worked out example of the calculation of D_{LCO} (*single-breath*)

Data

1. Barometric pressure: 765 mmHg or 102 kPa
2. Room temperature: 23°C or 296°K
3. V_I [inspired volume (from reservoir bag at ATPD[a])] = 2700 ml
4. F_{ICO} = 0.3%
5. F_{IHe} = 10%
6. F_{ECO} = 0.05%
7. F_{EHe} = 5.26%
8. Alveolar contact time (Jones-Meade) = 10 s (t)
9. V_D (instrumental [50 ml] and anatomic dead space [150 ml]) = 200 ml (ATPD)

Calculations

A. Alveolar volume (V_A) = $[V_I - V_D] \times [F_{IHe}/F_{EHe}]$
= $[(2700 - 200) \times 0.94^b] \times [10/(5.26 \times 0.95^c)]$
= 4703 ml (STPD)[a]
= $4703/22.4^d$ = 210 mmol

B. kCO = $\log_e [(F_{ICO} \times F_{EHe} / F_{IHe})/F_{ECO}]/t$
= $\log_e [(0.3 \times 5.26 \times 0.95/10)/0.05]/t$
= $\log_e [0.15/0.05]^e/(10/60)$ min^{-1}
= $1 \times 60/10$ = 6 min^{-1}

C. D_{LCO} = $(V_A \times kCO)/Pb-PH_2O$
= $[4703 \times 6]/(765-47)$
= 39.3 ml.min^{-1} mmHg^{-1}
= $[210 \times 6]/(102-6)$
= 13.1 mmol.min^{-1} kPa^{-1}

D. V_A (.BTPS^l) = $4703 \times 1.2^f/1000$ = 5.64

E. D_{LCO}/V_A = 39.3/5.64
= 6.96 ml.min^{-1} mmHg^{-1} L^{-1}
= 13.1/5.64
= 2.32 mmol.min^{-1} kPa^{-1} L^{-1}

Notes

a. ATPD = ambient temperature and pressure, dry (from a cylinder)
   BTPS = body temperature (37°C or 310°K) and pressure (Pb) saturated with water vapor ($-P_{H_2O}$)
   STPD = standard temperature (0°C or 273°K) and pressure (760 mmHg/101 kPa), dry
b. 0.94 converts ATPD to STPD [(765/760) × (273/293)]
c. 0.95 corrects F_{EHe} for prior absorption of 5% CO_2
d. 22.4 converts ml to millimolar (for most gases)
e. $\log_e$ (napierian or natural logarithms): $\log_e 3 = 1$
f. 1.2 converts STPD to BTPS [(765/765-47) × (310/273)]

7 Control of Breathing
P M A Calverley

- **INTRODUCTION**
- **VENTILATORY CONTROL IN HEALTH**
- **ASSESSING VENTILATORY CONTROL**
  Measuring the output
  Minute ventilation and breathing pattern
  Additional measurements
  Chemosensitivity: responses to hypoxia and hypercapnia
  Arterial PCO_2 at rest
  Responses to increasing CO_2 and hypoxia
  (Practical aspects of testing
  Mechanical loading
  Types of load
  Practical aspects
  Breathing patterns
  Breath-holding time
- **VENTILATORY CONTROL IN DISEASE**
  Problems of interpretation
  Impaired gas mixing
  Mechanical inequalities
  Changes in respiratory muscles
  Mechanical loading
  Specific diseases
  Primary disorders of ventilatory control
  Abnormalities of ventilatory control due to altered respiratory mechanics
- **CONCLUSION**

INTRODUCTION

The maintenance of constant blood gas tensions, widely regarded as the primary function of the respiratory system, requires a sophisticated feedback mechanism capable of rapidly modifying ventilation to meet sudden changes in metabolic demands. Understanding how this is done has fascinated respiratory physiologists for decades. Theories about the control of breathing have influenced how treatments have been prescribed, e.g. low flow oxygen in the treatment of exacerbations of obstructive lung disease. In practice it is easier to infer the nature of the control problem from measurements of lung function such as changes in respiratory mechanics (FEV_1) and gas exchange (blood gas tensions) than from direct tests of the control of ventilation, which are complex, often cumbersome, and largely restricted to academic investigators. Testing ventilatory control is useful in the assessment of drug safety, particularly that of hypnotics, and in those infrequent patients with primary neurological diseases which produce unexplained hypoventilation. Nonetheless some understanding of ventilatory control is needed if the functioning of the lungs is to be viewed as a whole. This chapter reviews the control of ventilation in health, the conventional ways in which it is assessed and, finally, some practical examples of how the studies have improved our understanding of disease.

VENTILATORY CONTROL IN HEALTH

Most data about the neurophysiology of respiration are derived from very un-physiological studies in anesthetized animals. The neural mechanisms that operate here are still best regarded as a 'black box' whose internal wiring is difficult to interpret (this has been reviewed in detail elsewhere).[1] A simplified scheme of the overall control of ventilation is given in Figure 7.1.

The central feature in this scheme is the respiratory pattern generator, a complex oscillatory neural network lying in the dorsal medulla that dictates the basic rhythm of breathing. Mechanical and chemical inputs arising from changes in chest wall movement or blood gas tensions provide a feedback mechanism to the brain stem which modifies the intensity and timing of the respiratory neural output. This has a number of practical consequences:

- If the rib cage and diaphragm cannot produce adequate ventilation then mechanoreceptors in the joints and intercostal muscles provide positive feedback to increase the respiratory center output, changing both the timing and amplitude of nervous pulses in the phrenic nerves.

- If ventilation is insufficient and arterial oxygen tension falls, the peripheral chemoreceptors – receptors at the junction of the external and common carotid arteries which supply blood to the brain – will increase their discharge rate, but only when the PaO_2 is less than 60 mmHg (8.0 kPa).

- If $PaCO_2$ rises, the peripheral chemoreceptors increase their firing rate, especially if there is coexisting hypoxia.

- The main response to rising CO_2 is in the central medullary chemoreceptors which respond to changes in the CSF pH.

- Peripheral chemoreceptors can be removed surgically without ill effect and account for approximately 15% of resting ventilation.[2]

Nevertheless, this combination of chemical and mechanical feedback does not fully explain how we breathe. Breathing can be modified by direct control from the cerebral cortex, e.g. during speech, and differs when we sleep. The deeper the sleep the more regular and automatic breathing becomes. During sleep the response to changes in blood gas tensions or mechanical loading is less than during wakefulness. During rapid eye movement (REM) sleep breathing becomes irregular but remains shallow. There is dispute about how easy it is to arouse from this stage of sleep.

Studies of breathing during sleep have emphasized the need for coordinated respiratory activity of the upper airway and respiratory muscles. Activation of the genioglossus, pharyngeal and laryngeal mus-

Figure 7.1 Feedback control of ventilation

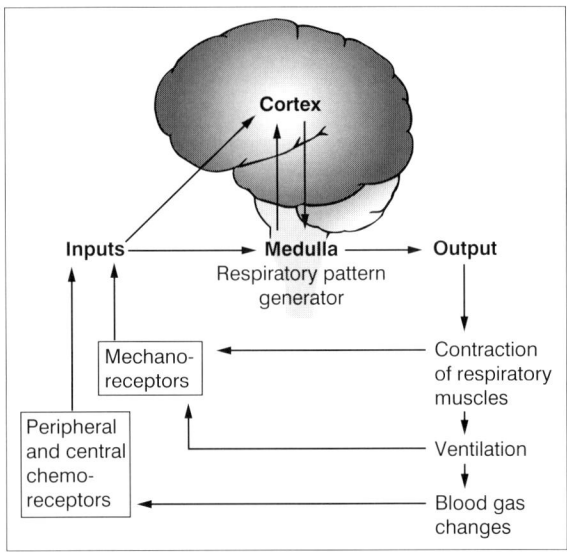

cles is necessary to prevent upper airway collapse with each inspiration and to ensure that the larynx is fully open. Moreover the influence of the degree of wakefulness on ventilatory control emphasizes the role of the cerebral cortex and respiratory perception in determining the breathing pattern of healthy humans.[3]

The best example of integrated cardiorespiratory control is during exercise where metabolic and ventilatory demands are closely matched. The precise mechanisms are still debated but in the *early* stages of exercise neural rather than chemical influences probably predominate.

> **Minute ventilation is influenced by:**
> - chemical and mechanical factors
> - sleep
> - talking, singing, anxiety, and other cortical inputs.

ASSESSING VENTILATORY CONTROL

There is no simple single number which explains how breathing is controlled. The investigator either opens the 'closed loop' of physiological control, e.g. by adding CO_2 to the inspired gas, or measures the breathing pattern under resting or challenge conditions and compares this with the pattern seen in normal subjects in similar situations. Both approaches assume that a quick test lasting from a few minutes to half an hour gives information that explains how ventilation is controlled over much longer periods. This is not the case, of course, and longer exposures to abnormal gas mixtures or mechanical loads produce different and sometimes opposite effects from those seen during acute testing. Thus, most tests of ventilatory control give insight into the immediate responses to changes in breathing conditions but are unreliable guides to longer term breathing pattern.

Finally we must be cautious about over-interpreting results obtained from studies of anesthetized animals where the effects of the higher centers are eliminated.

The testing of ventilatory control has gone through several phases. In the 1950s and 1960s attention focused on abnormalities of blood gas tensions, and investigators studied the response to raised CO_2 and lowered oxygen tensions. In the 1970s control in the face of the added respiratory loads associated with respiratory disease became important, while studies of the effect of diaphragm fatigue became popular during the 1980s when longer term exposures to abnormal gas mixtures were also first investigated. Simple tests such as studies of breathing pattern have now become more popular. Some laboratories still use the breath-holding time (BHT) as a crude assessment of deranged respiratory control.

With the exception of BHT all other tests relate an external stimulatory input (e.g. loading, changed inspired gases) to measures that directly or indirectly reflect respiratory center output. The most common of these is minute ventilation (the volume of air breathed in a minute) but important changes in respiratory timing can also occur during mechanical loading.

Ideally, the results of testing should be compared to a normal range of values but more often individuals are studied before and after interventions, for example with drugs. This approach is used because the reported ranges are very wide even for tests such as the response to CO_2 (see Table 7.1), while with some stimuli, such as resistive loading, no normal range has been reported. Thus most conclusions about ventilatory control are qualitative, telling us that something has happened but not necessarily by how much. The most frequently performed tests assess chemoresponsiveness.

Measuring the output

Minute ventilation and breathing pattern

Measurement of tidal ventilation Ventilation has traditionally been measured using a spirometer, by integrating flow at the mouth, or by measuring the volume of gas expired into a Douglas bag or gas meter over a defined period. Such techniques are impractical for prolonged monitoring and, in addition, the application of a nose clip and mouthpiece alters the pattern of resting breathing (Figure 7.2). These disadvantages are avoided by monitoring *external movements* of the chest wall, i.e. rib cage and abdomen, using devices such as pairs of magnetometers which measure displacement in a single dimen-

Figure 7.2 Patterns of breathing in normal resting subjects

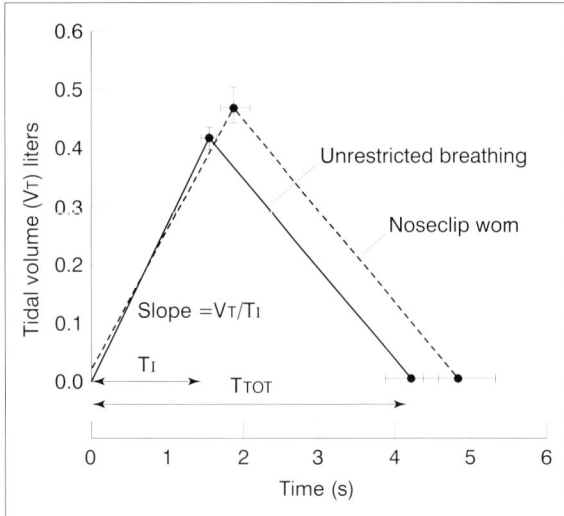

Data recorded during unrestricted breathing (solid line) and with nose clip in place (dashed line) using a respiratory inductance plethysmograph. Error bars are SEM. (data from Maxwell et al,[5]).

Analysis of breathing pattern Breathing patterns can be characterized simply by the tidal volume (V_T) and the frequency of breathing per minute (f).

$$\text{Minute ventilation } (\dot{V}_E) \text{ [L.min}^{-1}\text{]} = V_T \cdot f$$

Additionally, the total breath time (T_{TOT}) in seconds (which equals 60/f) can be subdivided into mean inspiratory (T_I) and expiratory (T_E) times. When V_T is divided by T_I the resulting term (V_T/T_I) reflects the mean inspiratory flow (L.s^{-1}) while the T_I/T_{TOT} ratio, often called the duty cycle, is the proportion of each breath spent on inspiration.

In this analysis:

$$\dot{V}_E = V_T/T_I \cdot T_I/T_{TOT}$$

Both approaches reduce the breath-by-breath variation to an average tidal volume and breath duration (or frequency). Each approach has value and offers complementary insights into the way breathing is controlled beyond simply measuring total minute ventilation.

A schematic tidal spirogram during unrestricted breathing in healthy subjects is shown in Figure 7.2. Measurements of volume and T_I, T_E and T_{TOT} were made using Respitrace™ belts.[5] Breathing without nose clip or mouthpiece is shown by the solid lines. When a nose clip was attached (dashed lines) V_T, T_I and T_{TOT} increased but minute ventilation was unchanged. When breathing is measured with a mouthpiece and apparatus such as a valve box or pneumotachograph, 'dead space' is added and the total ventilation usually increases.

Additional measurements

When there are mechanical abnormalities in the respiratory system (respiratory muscles, chest wall, or lungs) or an external mechanical load is applied, the ventilation produced by a given neural output is reduced. To allow for this, in addition to using ventilation (either in L.min^{-1} or expressed in relation to maximum ventilatory capacity) other measurements of neural output have been used.

Mouth occlusion pressure (pressure recorded 100 ms after the onset of inspiration against a closed airway – $P_{0.1}$) was devised to overcome the underestimation of ventilatory drive under loaded conditions since theoretically there should be no pressure loss due to changes in chest wall shape or variations in the speed

sion or the respiratory inductance plethysmograph (Respitrace™), which uses belts to measure change in cross-sectional areas of the two compartments of the chest wall. Konno and Mead[4] showed how the tidal motion of the lungs and chest wall could be measured by summing the volume displacements of the rib cage and abdomen to obtain tidal volume. Calibration is in two stages. First, the subject performs an 'isovolume maneuver' in which, with glottis closed, he gently shifts volume back and forth between rib cage and abdomen while the motion of each part is monitored. The relation between the two signals allows calibration in terms of the *relative* volume change of the two compartments. *Absolute* calibration is then achieved by comparison of the electrically summed signal with volume recorded by a spirometer or by integration of airflow at the mouth. It is important to appreciate that the calibration coefficients (i.e. relation between displacement and volume) vary and are very sensitive to changes in posture. Consequently accurate calibration of a signal recorded for a prolonged period, e.g. overnight, is not usually possible although breathing pattern and phase differences between rib cage and abdomen can still be reliably measured.

of contraction of the inspiratory muscles.[6] Direct comparisons in animal studies have confirmed that the $P_{0.1}$ is broadly representative of the phrenic neurogram. However, some muscle shortening does occur even when the airways are occluded, and abdominal wall muscle activation can modify the $P_{0.1}$ recorded. $P_{0.1}$ can be measured from a fast running paper trace speeded up just before manual occlusion during expiration or, more commonly, by computer controlled systems. In one frequently used system a helium-filled balloon is inflated in the inspiratory line and rapidly deflated approximately 150 ms after inspiratory effort begins. This should not be noticeable at low to moderate levels of inspiratory effort. Useful data have been collected using this method in patients, but delays in pressure transmission from the pleural space to the mouth, distortion of the chest wall and prior activation of the abdominal muscles during expiration all limit the ability of mouth pressure accurately to reflect phrenic neural traffic in many lung diseases, particularly COPD.

Other pressure measurements are sometimes recorded, including tidal pleural and transdiaphragmatic pressures (see Chapter 4). These tests involve swallowing esophageal and gastric balloons and are more uncomfortable for the subject. A non-invasive but less accurate alternative is the ratio of $P_{0.1}$ to mean inspiratory flow (VT/TI) through the preceding breath which is a measure of respiratory impedance, i.e. how much pressure is developed for a given amount of flow.

An even more direct recording is the measurement of the electrical activity of the crural diaphragm, usually expressed as arbitrary units of integrated EMG signal. This indicates activation of the diaphragm for each breath but is harder to quantify and involves swallowing an even more uncomfortable catheter. It can give information about the onset of inspiratory muscle fatigue but there are problems with signal sampling, ECG artifact, and patient discomfort, and currently the technique is used only in research laboratories.

Chemosensitivity: responses to hypoxia and hypercapnia

Arterial PCO_2 at rest

The response to increasing CO_2 or reducing O_2 and the interaction between the two stimuli has been

Assessment of CNS respiratory output

- Minute ventilation (and its subdivisions) from spirometer, pneumotachograph or chest/abdominal wall movements (e.g. Respitrace™).
- Mouth occlusion pressure ($P_{0.1}$).
- Pleural (esophageal) pressure or transdiaphragmatic pressure change.
- EMG of diaphragm.

worked out in great detail in normal subjects. At rest, alveolar ventilation is adjusted very precisely to maintain arterial PCO_2 close to 40 mmHg (5.3 kPa). The relation between alveolar ventilation ($\dot{V}_A$) and alveolar (arterial) PCO_2 at a given level of metabolic CO_2 production ($\dot{V}CO_2$) is curvilinear as given by the steady state equation:

$$PaCO_2 = \frac{\dot{V}CO_2}{\dot{V}_A} \cdot k \quad \text{where } k \text{ is a constant}$$

For CO_2 excretion it is the alveolar ventilation (total minus dead space ventilation) which is important, but usually only total ventilation ($\dot{V}_E$) is measured. The smaller the tidal volume the lower the $\dot{V}_A/\dot{V}_E$ ratio.

Responses to increasing CO_2 and hypoxia

When carbon dioxide is inhaled, there is a linear relationship between the rise in arterial CO_2 and the increase in ventilation, the slope of this relationship or 'gain' being a measure of the sensitivity of the control system (Figure 7.3a). Data are expressed as a linear regression with a correlation coefficient that usually exceeds 0.9.

Hypoxia is a less potent stimulus to ventilation until arterial PO_2 falls below 60 mmHg (8.0 kPa). There is a curvilinear relationship (Figure 7.3b) which can be expressed in terms of a shape constant A, but it is easier to transform this into a plot between SaO_2 and ventilation which is linear and can be presented in a similar but inverse fashion to the CO_2 response (Figure 7.3c). This relationship appears to be accidental rather than causal as the carotid chemoreceptors respond to changes in oxygen tension and not oxygen saturation.

Figure 7.3 Ventilatory stimulation by CO_2 and hypoxia

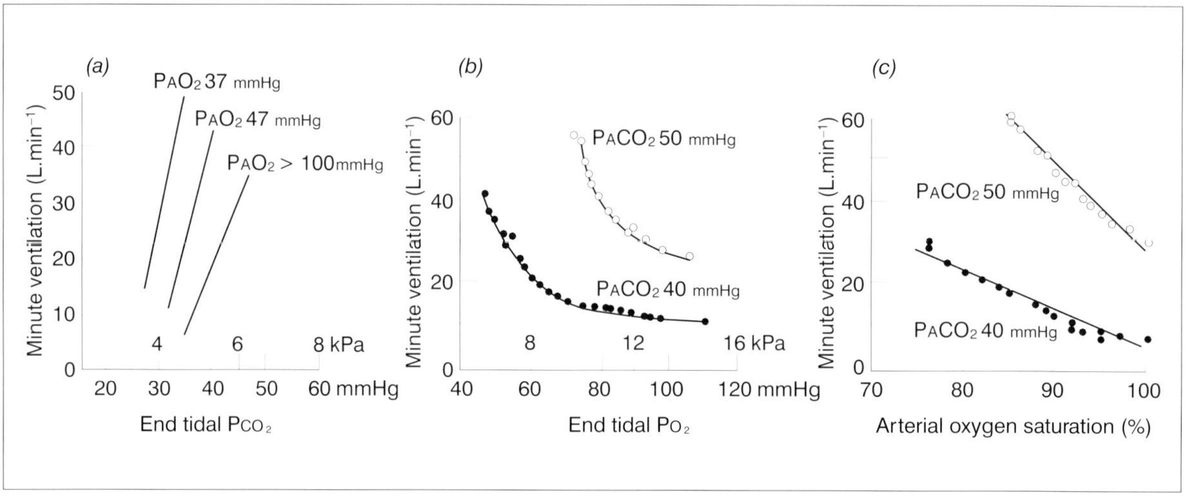

(a) P_{AO_2} 37 mmHg, P_{AO_2} 47 mmHg, P_{AO_2} > 100 mmHg — Minute ventilation (L.min^{-1}) vs End tidal P_{CO_2} (kPa / mmHg).

(b) P_{aCO_2} 50 mmHg, P_{aCO_2} 40 mmHg — Minute ventilation (L.min^{-1}) vs End tidal P_{O_2} (kPa / mmHg).

(c) P_{aCO_2} 50 mmHg, P_{aCO_2} 40 mmHg — Minute ventilation (L.min^{-1}) vs Arterial oxygen saturation (%).

(a) Reducing alveolar PO_2 (P_{AO_2}) shows how hypoxia greatly increases the ventilatory response to CO_2.

(b) Minute ventilation plotted against end-tidal PO_2 (~ arterial PO_2 in normal subjects) showing a curvilinear relationship for the rebreathing hypoxic ventilatory response and the potentiating effect of raising alveolar PCO_2.

(c) Same data as in (b) plotted against arterial oxygen saturation which gives a linear response.

CO_2 and hypoxia combined The interaction between low oxygen levels and high CO_2 is a potent one (Figure 7.3b and c) and serves to increase both responses. While this is physiologically desirable it complicates interpretation of ventilatory responses, particularly with respect to the slope of the hypoxic response where a few mmHg difference in CO_2 can have a substantial effect (Figure 7.3c). This is important when interpreting data from the literature.

Practical aspects of testing

A variety of methods of applying the stimulus and measuring the response have been developed (see Table 7.1). Applying an abnormal chemical stimulus is not as straightforward as it seems.

Changes in carbon dioxide tension in the blood are buffered by bicarbonate while the gas stores within the lungs (the gas resident within the alveoli at FRC) mean that the stimulus to breathe does not change immediately when an abnormal gas mixture is inhaled. Steady state CO_2 responses allow the comparison of ventilation at a normal and at a high level of CO_2, when a new equilibrium has been reached between body gas stores and added CO_2. This procedure can be repeated at the same levels of CO_2 but at a lower oxygen tension, the ratio of the two slopes being a measure of hypoxic sensitivity. Although this is a logical approach it is extremely time consuming for technician and patient alike. Most laboratories now use rebreathing techniques (Figure 7.4) where the subject breathes from a 5–6 liter anesthetic bag containing oxygen (typically 50% but often 90%) together with 7% CO_2. This method was devised by Read et al,[7] who calculated that after two to three large breaths the CSF and pulmonary venous CO_2 content would be similar and any subsequent rise in CO_2 would be linear, reflecting metabolic CO_2 production. Rebuck and Campbell[8] developed a rebreathing method to study progressive hypoxia which incorporates a soda lime CO_2 absorber in the circuit and, by monitoring end-tidal CO_2, could maintain this constant while oxygen fell. In individual laboratories CO_2 rebreathing is extremely reproducible while hypoxic tests show a greater coefficient of variation. The between day variation of both tests is greater than the immediate reproducibility.

In normal subjects data are usually reported in terms of the $\dot{V}_E/PetCO_2$ slope. Although theoretically interesting, data about the intercept with the abscissa

Figure 7.4 Rebreathing response to hypercapnia or hypoxia

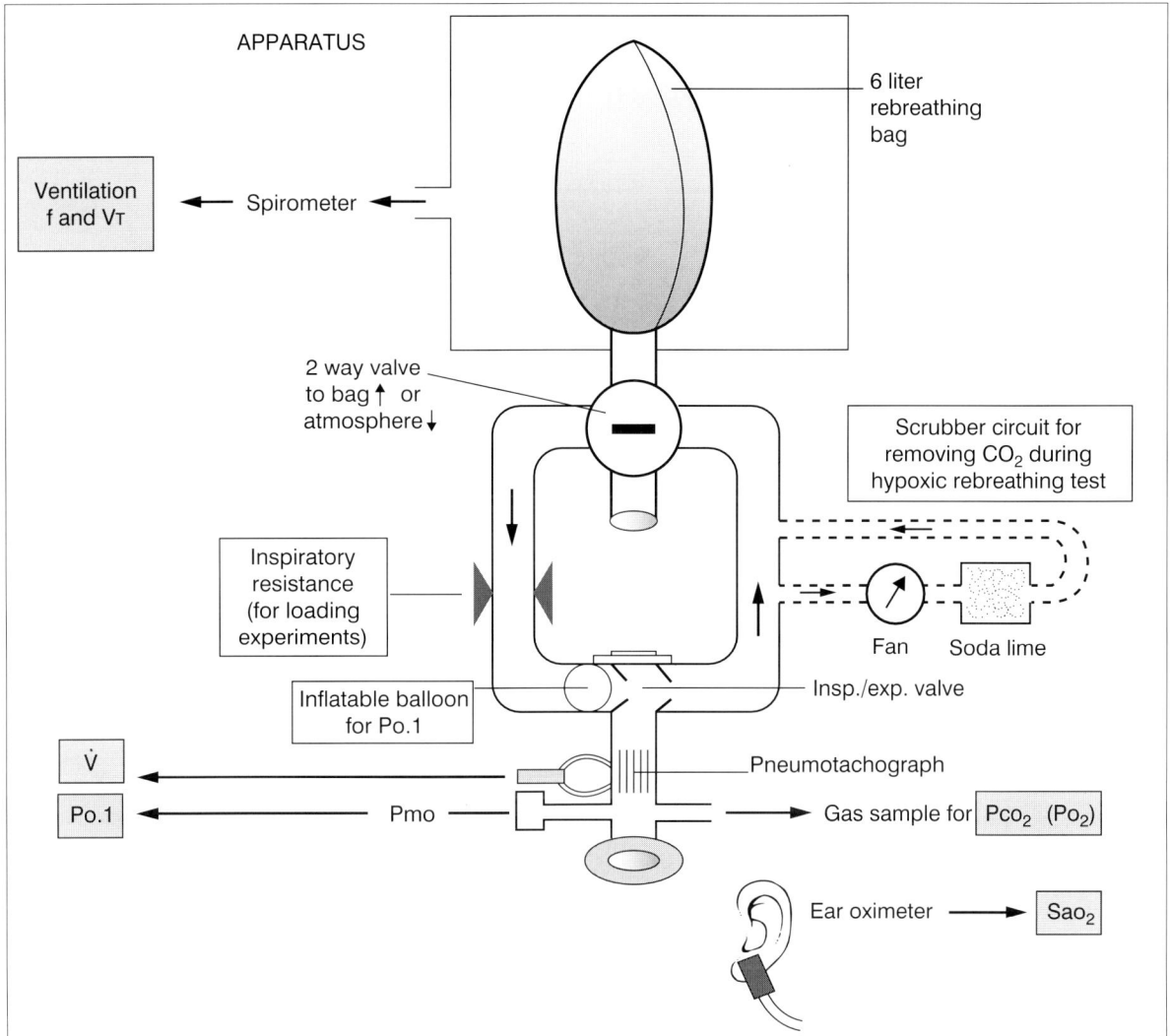

SUBJECT PREPARATION
1. Before testing the subject should avoid caffeinated drinks and empty bladder.
2. Subjects should be comfortable, relaxed, and not hyperventilating.
3. Time is needed to acclimatize to the equipment.
4. Earphones playing bland music in a quiet room help distract the subject.
5. Equipment should be screened from view.

ANALYSIS
   Plot ventilation and $P_{0.1}$ against bag PCO_2 and SaO_2 (or bag PO_2).
   Duplicate the tests – at least 10 minutes apart.
   Data analysis by computer software has removed much of the drudgery from these tests.

REBREATHING PROTOCOLS
Hypercapnic hyperoxic:
   When stable turn valve into rebreathing bag.
   Fill bag with 7% CO_2, 93% oxygen.
   Continue recording for up to 4 minutes.
   Record $P_{0.1}$ and Borg scale at rest then every minute.
Hypoxic isocapnic:
   As above, plus:
   Fill bag with 7% CO_2, 70% N_2 and balance O_2.
   Take 3 large breaths initially to encourage gas mixing.
   Maintain CO_2 by varying flow through scrubber circuit.
   Stop test if $SaO_2 < 75\%$ or subject distressed.

Table 7.1 Tests of ventilatory control

Test	Analysis	Effects of disease	Comment
Hyperoxic CO_2 rebreathing	$\dot{V}_E/PCO_2$ slope	Reduced in most diseases – increased in thyrotoxicosis and some acromegalics	Wide range of normal 1.0–4.0 L.min^{-1} mmHg^{-1} (0.13–0.53 L.min^{-1} kPa^{-1})
Steady state CO_2 response	$\dot{V}_E/PCO_2$	Reduced in most cases	Rarely used
Steady state CO_2 at two or more O_2 tensions	Ratio of slope $\dot{V}_E/PCO_2$ when hypoxic to when normoxic or hyperoxic	Limited data – reduced in COPD patients	Very difficult technically – problems with change in PCO_2 when hyperoxic
Progressive hypoxia with isocapnia (rebreathing)	Either curve fit of $\dot{V}_E/PO_2$ relationship or as slope $\dot{V}_E/SaO_2$	Variable reduction in airway disease	Choice of isocapnic PCO_2 for baseline is crucial; sensitive to drug effects; relative changes helpful – absolute value not
Mouth occlusion pressure	$P_{0.1}/PCO_2$ slope; $P_{0.1}$ = 0.5–1.5 cmH$_2$O at rest; can be added to chemical stimulation test	Usually increased; appears preserved in neuromuscular disease	Influenced by posture, lung volume, and maximum inspiratory pressure; useful when ventilation reduced by internal or external loading
Integrated EMG (usually diaphragm)	Arbitrary units; can be added to chemical stimulation test	Increased by added loads; natural and experimental	Relative changes helpful, absolute value not; specific to part of muscle sampled

are too variable to interpret. End-tidal CO_2 is assumed to reflect the gas tension in the alveoli and hence should be similar to the pulmonary capillary gas tensions. However, in rebreathing circuits there is almost no difference between the inspiratory and expiratory CO_2 tensions which may cause technical problems with modern infra-red CO_2 analyzers set to report end-tidal values.

Assessment of chemoresponsiveness

- Hypercapnia (PCO_2 ↑) and hypoxia (PO_2 ↓) interact to stimulate breathing.
- Response to CO_2 alone requires hyperoxic breathing (FiO_2 > 60%).
- Response to hypoxia alone requires constant PetCO$_2$ (isocapnia).
- Abnormal lung mechanics will lead to a reduced *ventilatory* response (Figure 7.5).

There has been some interest in transient gas changes, particularly with single breaths of nitrogen or oxygen, to try to either stimulate or abolish peripheral chemoreceptor action but the reproducibility of these tests is poor.

Mechanical loading

Types of load

Studying breathing when *external* loads are applied to increase mechanoreceptor stimulation can simulate some aspects of the more complex *internal* loading seen in disease.[9] In general the ventilatory response to chemical stimulation is reduced with loading but the drive to breathing, reflected by the $P_{0.1}$ or EMG responses, rises. Exact quantitative relationships remain unclear and are undoubtedly affected by patient mood. There are obvious differences between individuals in the response to loading but it is less clear how constant these are from day to day. Loads may be *resistive*, where the driving pressure for a given flow is increased, or *elastic*, where the pressure change per unit volume change increases, and can be applied during either inspiration or expiration. A third type of load is *threshold* loading in which a fixed pressure has to be developed before airflow begins but once flow starts it is unimpeded. This is similar to the type of resistor used in inspiratory muscle training and simulates PEEPi but produces different responses when used as a way of assessing ventilatory control.

Practical aspects

The most common studies involve inspiratory loads applied throughout inspiration as this is the more active part of the respiratory cycle reflecting the motor outflow from the respiratory center. Loading during expiration is harder to assess, but is influenced by the mechanical properties of the lungs and the degree to which the subject will permit his or her FRC to rise. Elastic loads are difficult to administer for more than one breath although some systems have been devised to do this. Laboratories usually build and calibrate their own resistances which vary from a few $cmH_2O.L^{-1}$ s to 25 or more $cmH_2O.L^{-1}$ s, with most being around 10 $cmH_2O.L^{-1}$ s. Care needs to be taken about the range of ventilation studied as most resistances have some curvilinearity. Information about resistive loading is likely to be qualitative as different intensities of load are applied in different laboratories, and the load applied will also vary depending upon the inspiratory flow rate.

Breathing patterns

Studies of respiratory loading during wakefulness and sleep give considerable insight into how the respiratory controller responds to changes in respiratory mechanics similar to those seen in disease states at rest, during exercise, and particularly in patients who are treated in the ICU (see later).

Healthy subjects breathing against isolated inspiratory resistances prolong the duty cycle (T_I/T_{TOT}) and reduce V_T/T_I. Conversely breathing against increases in inspiratory elastance alone produces a shortening of the duty cycle. In disease, there is a more complex mixture of inspiratory and expiratory resistive and elastic loading, and changes in duty cycle are seldom seen.

Breath-holding time (BHT)

This simple test only requires a nose clip and a stop watch. The subject, with the nose clip in place, breathes out to RV, inhales to TLC, and then holds his or her breath for as long as possible. Analysis of expired gas allows the stimulus (change in gas tension) to be related to breath-holding time. The test is repeated until the results are reproducible or the subject is exhausted. The test is repeatable between subjects and mean breath-holding time from TLC in young people is 78 seconds. However, this test does not assess simply respiratory control and the stimulus to breathe but is influenced by the motivation of the subject, inspiratory muscle strength, and the geometry of the chest wall. BHT is difficult to interpret in the presence of lung disease but is frequently less than 20 seconds in patients experiencing disproportionate breathlessness. Each laboratory should establish its own range of values if this test is to be used clinically. BHT is longer at large lung volumes, and it is prolonged by prior hyperoxia and hypocapnia.

VENTILATORY CONTROL IN DISEASE

Problems of interpretation

As noted above, the mechanical and gas exchange abnormalities characteristic of disease can interfere with the interpretation of any ventilatory control test, particularly in patients with chronic obstructive pulmonary disease (COPD). Typical problems include:

Impaired gas mixing

In COPD and chronic asthma lung gas stores are increased and mixing of fresh air and resident gas is not homogenous. Slowly ventilating areas of lung may not achieve the same gas concentrations as well ventilated ones and the normal near-equality (at rest) between end-tidal gas concentrations measured at the lips and arterial gas tension is distorted, at least when the FEV_1 is below 1 liter. This is a greater problem for non-invasive CO_2 measurements as SaO_2 can be non-invasively measured from a finger or ear probe using a pulse oximeter. Slower gas equilibration can theoretically effect the CO_2 response, particularly if there is increased cerebrospinal fluid (CSF) bicarbonate.

Mechanical inequalities

In many diseases gas exchange is abnormal because the time constants (resistance × compliance) of individual lung units are abnormal. In COPD time constants tend to be high so the pressure resulting from muscle contraction applied to the lungs may be delayed in reaching the mouth, making $P_{0.1}$ hard to interpret. In contrast, in interstitial lung disease time constants are short.

Changes in respiratory muscles

In chronic airways disease the chest wall is overinflated, shortening the diaphragm and reducing its mechanical efficiency. Conversely, in interstitial lung disease when the FRC is reduced, the diaphragm is lengthened and may improve its pressure generating capacity. Both changes alter the relationships between the degree of muscle activation and $P_{0.1}$. In neuromuscular disease $P_{0.1}$ values at rest are normal, but muscle weakness may limit the ability to generate higher pressures during stimulated breathing.

Mechanical loading

As noted already, minute ventilation may not reflect respiratory drive when the chest wall is stiff or the inspiratory muscles are weak due to primary muscle disease or their function is impaired by overinflation of the lungs. In these circumstances it is best to express measured responses as a percentage of the maximum attainable, e.g. ventilatory capacity or inspiratory esophageal pressure as % $P_{I}max$.

Specific diseases

Primary disorders of ventilatory control

Hypoventilation Ondine's curse or primary alveolar hypoventilation is a condition seen mainly in children where there is an absence of chemoreceptor responsiveness, compensated for during the day, which causes very shallow breathing and central apneas during sleep. CO_2 and hypoxic responses are absent even though lung mechanics are normal, but the ventilatory response to exercise is preserved.[10] Primary neoplasms or extensive vascular disease of the brain stem can simulate this problem. Inappropriate hypoventilation can be seen in patients recovering from severe head injuries with marked cortical damage where there is an undue dependence on peripheral chemoreceptor drive. In these circumstances inferences about ventilatory control are made from examining the breathing pattern of the individual and changes in the blood gas tensions, although establishing a definitive diagnosis is often difficult because of the presence of coexisting pulmonary and/or post-traumatic pathology.

Periodic breathing In periodic breathing, periods of apnea or hypopnea alternate with periods of hyperpnea. In its most frequently recognized form (Cheyne-Stokes respiration), tidal volume (and, to a lesser extent, frequency) increases progressively over 30–60 seconds to a maximum, followed by a similar progressive decrease – very much like a musical 'crescendo' and 'diminuendo'. Unlike primary alveolar hypoventilation, sensitivity to CO_2 is increased and the mean arterial PCO_2 is low. Periodic breathing is associated with disease above the medulla (pons to cerebral cortex), usually vascular in nature and often accompanied by heart disease. Cheyne-Stokes respiration also occurs in healthy subjects at altitude during sleep. It is analogous to the 'hunting' observed in servo-controlled systems. The supposition is that normally the mid-brain and cerebral cortex are able to minimize this oscillatory tendency.

Hyperventilation syndrome This is a controversial clinical entity which lacks clear diagnostic criteria. Many patients present with either excessive breathlessness on minimal exertion or unexplained exercise limitation. It is easiest to define these patients when spirometric measurements are normal but there is probably a spectrum of response, some individuals experiencing excessive symptoms with only a minor abnormality in lung mechanics. Such patients exhibit inappropriately high levels of ventilation at rest and unusually V_T as well as f is increased while the duty cycle is normal. The breathing pattern is often very irregular. End-tidal CO_2 is often at the lower limit of normal or reduced. Cardiopulmonary exercise testing shows that these patients are limited by ventilatory demand rather than cardiac causes. In the first two to three minutes of exercise their ventilation rises acutely and their CO_2 tensions fall, although as exercise continues end-tidal CO_2 tends to approach normal values again. There is usually marked and inappropriate hyperventilation and hypocapnia at the end of exercise. The natural history of this condition is poorly defined; therapy is usually directed at breathing control, with variable results.

Abnormalities of control due to abnormal respiratory mechanics

Chronic obstructive pulmonary disease[11] This is the most extensively studied condition and has led to the development of several of the new techniques described above. Fifty years ago the ventilatory response to steady state carbon dioxide testing was found to be reduced in COPD. Subsequent studies have generally confirmed this but with considerable variation between subjects in the extent of ventilatory depression. Patients with high levels of arterial CO_2 often have reduced hypoxic responses; however, expressing the results in terms of maximum ventilatory capacity, patients have an increased response compared to normal (Figure 7.5). $P_{0.1}$ values at rest (and during CO_2 rebreathing) are generally increased, although patients with both hypoxia and hypercapnia may increase $P_{0.1}$ less in response to rising CO_2 than patients with more normal blood gas tensions.[12]

Hypercapnia in COPD patients is related to the severity of the mechanical load on inspiration which is not directly described by the FEV_1. Most recent studies have not found chronic inspiratory muscle fatigue in COPD patients with stable hypercapnia. Nonetheless, reduction in inspiratory muscle strength is probably important, not least because it is related to the shallow, rapid breathing pattern adopted by these patients.[13]

The classic distinctions between 'pink and puffing' and 'blue and bloated' patients may reflect individual differences in internal mechanical load and in perception of breathlessness, which affects the interaction of central perceptual mechanisms and chemoreceptor responses. Patients with chronic hypoxemia may limit their breathlessness by adopting a rapid, shallow breathing pattern (Figure 7.6) that promotes CO_2 retention because with a small V_T the dead space/tidal volume ratio is higher.[12,14] Patients with more normal blood gas tensions accept a higher work of breathing because they are unable to make this compromise. To this extent both sides of the 'can't breathe, won't breathe' controversy are correct.

During acute exacerbations of COPD when there is a further increase in the work of breathing, and to a lesser extent when patients are clinically stable, increases in the inspired oxygen tension lead to a rise in $PaCO_2$. In general, the higher the inspired oxygen concentration the greater the CO_2 retention. This may be due to mismatching of ventilation and perfusion in the lungs but most people believe that therapeutic increases in oxygen tension reduce the input from the peripheral chemoreceptors, promoting a more shallow breathing pattern. Even a modest fall in ventilation in patients with lung disease and an elevated V_D/V_T ratio leads to further CO_2 retention.[15] The realization by Campbell that a middle course could be steered in which sufficient oxygen is administered to permit adequate oxygen delivery to the tissues, but not so much as to cause severe CO_2 retention, has been one of the most important practical outcomes from studies of the control of ventilation.

Bronchial asthma Asthma is also characterized by increased resistive and elastic loads to breathing but typically these loads vary throughout the day and from day to day depending upon degree of bronchoconstriction. Some asthmatics deteriorate acutely and there are good data now that these patients perceive the increasing chemical stimuli poorly.[16] Early studies showed that the ventilatory response to CO_2 was reduced in some asthmatics during the recovery phase from a severe exacerbation,[17] and in those where there is chronic loading both respiratory perception and the ventilatory responses to chemical stimuli are impaired.[18] It is important to identify such patients clinically as they are particularly at risk of sudden death from their asthma. However, most patients with asthma in remission have normal ventilatory control when the mechanical load is absent.

Interstitial lung disease This heterogeneous group of conditions is characterized by generalized fibrosis within the lungs. The principal problem is an increase in the elastic work of breathing. Arterial blood gas tensions are often normal at rest but there is marked oxygen desaturation during exercise; as disease progresses hypoxemia and sometimes hypercapnia at rest may eventually develop. Increase in the absolute

Figure 7.5 Hypercapnic rebreathing responses in 12 healthy subjects and 12 normocapnic COPD patients (mean FEV$_1$ 0.9 L)

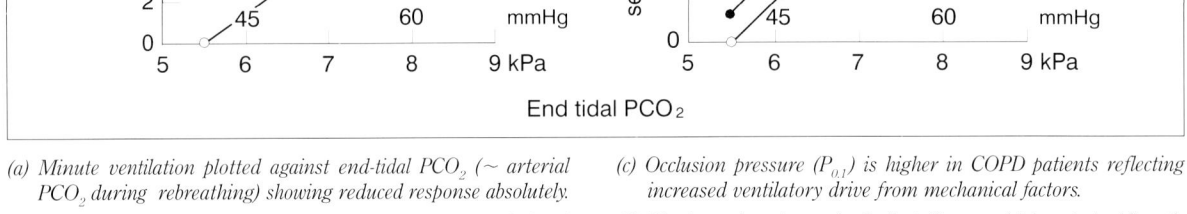

(a) Minute ventilation plotted against end-tidal PCO_2 (~ arterial PCO_2 during rebreathing) showing reduced response absolutely.

(b) As a percentage of maximum breathing capacity (calculated from FEV$_1$), COPD subjects appear to have a greater response than normal subjects.

(c) Occlusion pressure ($P_{0.1}$) is higher in COPD patients reflecting increased ventilatory drive from mechanical factors.

(d) The intensity of perceived effort (Borg scale) is not significantly different in COPD patients at a given CO_2 level even though the absolute ventilation produced is less. (From Calverley[11]).

values of ventilation in response to chemical stimuli is reduced while the $P_{0.1}$ responses at rest and during stimulated breathing are normal or high (see above). Breathing patterns are characteristically rapid and shallow.

Chest wall and neuromuscular disease Patients with chest wall deformities, especially kyphoscoliosis, have an increased elastic load to breathing and reduced strength of their inspiratory muscles. Patients with severe deformity are likely to develop CO_2 retention, initially at night and later by day.

Careful studies from the 1970s showed that the impaired ventilatory response to CO_2 was closely related to the reduction in compliance of the respiratory system and especially that of the chest wall,[19] while the breathing pattern is typically rapid and shallow. Treatment with nocturnal nasal ventilation can partially reverse these changes and improve exercise tolerance (see Chapter 13).

In neuromuscular disease such as the muscular dystrophies the lungs are relatively normal but the ability to develop pressure is limited because of muscle weakness. Despite the different etiology, the

Figure 7.6 Breathing pattern in patients with airflow obstruction

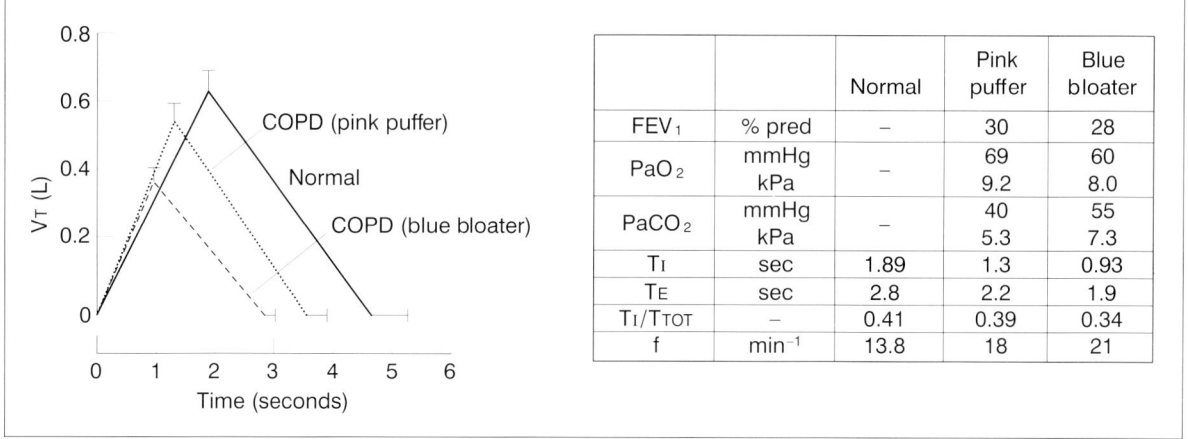

Note that patients with airflow obstruction have a more rapid and shallow breathing pattern, especially the so-called 'blue bloaters' who are hypercapnic and more hypoxemic. (From Gorini et al). Neural respiratory drive and neuromuscular coupling in patients with chronic pulmonary disease. Chest 1990; 98:1179–86, with permission.

changes in tests of ventilatory control are very similar to those seen in chest wall disease. The metabolic CO_2 production and oxygen consumption of these immobile and wasted patients is relatively small and so abnormal daytime blood gas tensions are infrequent, but an upper respiratory tract infection or an increase in upper airway resistance during sleep can rapidly compromise ventilation and gas exchange and lead to respiratory failure with hypoxemia and hypercapnia.

Sleep and breathing disorders The problems of ventilatory control during sleep have already been referred to and have been reviewed elsewhere.[20] In normal subjects there is a small rise in upper airway resistance during sleep, but in those with narrow upper airways for whatever reason, greater increases in resistance occur. Chronic snorers show 2 to 5 fold increases in upper airway resistance above the normal range. This produces a flutter in the surrounding tissues which is obvious as a snoring noise. The respiratory system responds with increased motor output and pleural pressure swings, although whether there is an equivalent increase in the drive to the upper airway during sleep is less certain. In some patients with particularly narrow upper airways occlusion occurs (obstructive sleep apnea); with no flow possible, oxygen tensions fall and CO_2 tensions rise during the apneic episode. This is paralleled by increasing efforts to overcome the absolute increase in upper airway resistance and, when a critical amount of respiratory effort is achieved, an arousal from sleep occurs. The extent to which these chemoreceptor-mediated responses explain the variability in apnea duration is not clear. Other factors, particularly the depth of sleep and the extent of prior sleep disruption, are relevant to the nocturnal arousal response. There is no relationship between the magnitude of the chemoreceptor responses measured during the day and any sleep related variable.

Changes in ventilatory control during sleep are relevant in other diseases. There are marked episodes of oxygen desaturation in COPD patients who are hypoxic during the day, particularly if they also retain carbon dioxide. Whether this reflects a global reduction in ventilatory responsiveness or is simply an exaggeration of a normal reduction in ventilatory drive during sleep in someone with daytime hypoxemia is still not fully resolved. In some people a combination of abnormal upper airways and obstructive lung disease is present. Some morbidly obese patients appear to preserve their upper airway patency but hypoventilate during the night. These subjects have blunted chemoreceptor responses when awake but chemoresponsiveness can be restored when the night-time hypoventilation is corrected by non-invasive ventilation.

CONCLUSION

At present an understanding of ventilatory control is largely of theoretical value and most laboratories do not need detailed assessment facilities. In future more severe asthmatics may need assessment of ventilatory control, as will patients with unexplained hypercapnia or nocturnal hypoventilation. Characterizing patients with objective evidence of hyperventilation is valuable in preventing the prescription of inappropriate treatment. In practice the arterial blood gases remain the best simple guide to abnormal ventilatory control.

References

1 Euler C von. Brain stem mechanisms for generation and control of breathing pattern. In: Cherniack NS & Widdicombe JG (eds) *Handbook of Physiology*, Vol. 2, Part II, Section 3, Control of Breathing. Bethesda: American Physiological Society 1986: 1–67.
2 Bisgard GE & Neubauer JA. Peripheral and central effects of hypoxia. In: Dempsey JA & Pack AI (eds) *Regulation of Breathing*, 2nd edn. New York: Marcel Dekker 1995: 617–68.
3 Cherniack NS. Respiratory sensation as a respiratory controller. In: Adams L & Guz A (eds) *Respiratory Sensation*. New York: Marcel Dekker 1996: 213–30.
4 Konno K & Mead J. Measurement of the separate volume changes of rib cage and abdomen during breathing. *J Appl Physiol* 1967; **22**: 407–22.
5 Maxwell DL, Cover D & Hughes JMB. Effect of respiratory apparatus on timing and depth of breathing in man. *Respir Physiol* 1985; **61**: 255–64.
6 Whitelaw WA & Derenne JP. Airway occlusion pressure. *J Appl Physiol* 1993; **74**: 1475–83.
7 Read DJC. A clinical method for assessing the ventilatory response to carbon dioxide. *Australas Ann Med* 1967; **16**: 20–32.
8 Rebuck AS & Campbell EJM. A clinical method for assessing the ventilatory response to hypoxia. *Am Rev Respir Dis* 1974; **109**: 345–50.
9 Cherniack NS & Milic-Emili J. Mechanical aspects of loaded breathing. In: Roussos C & Macklem PT (eds) *The Thorax*. New York: Marcel Dekker 1985: 751–86.
10 Shea SA, Andres LE, Shannon DC, Banzett RB. Ventilatory responses to exercise in humans lacking ventilatory chemosensitivity. *J Physiol (Lond)* 1993; **468**: 623–40.
11 Calverley PMA. Ventilatory control and dyspnea. In: Calverley PMA & Pride NB (eds) *Chronic Obstructive Pulmonary Disease*. London: Chapman and Hall 1995: 205–42.
12 Oliven A, Kelsen SG, Deal EC, Cherniack NS. Mechanisms of CO_2 retention during flow-resistive loading in patients with chronic obstructive pulmonary disease. *J Clin Invest* 1983; **71**: 1442–49.
13 Gorini M, Spinelli A, Ginanni R, Duranti R, Gigliotti F, Scano G. Neural respiratory drive and neuromuscular coupling in patients with chronic obstructive pulmonary disease. *Chest* 1990; **98**: 1179–86.
14 Loveridge B, West P, Anthonisen NR, Kryger MH. Breathing pattern in patients with chronic obstructive pulmonary disease. *Am Rev Respir Dis* 1984; **130**: 730–33.
15 Stradling JR. Hypercapnia during oxygen therapy in airways obstruction: a reappraisal. *Thorax* 1986; **41**: 897–902.
16 Kikuchi Y, Okabe S, Tamura G *et al*. Chemosensitivity and perception of dyspnea in patients with a history of near-fatal asthma. *N Engl J Med* 1994; **330**: 1329–43.
17 Rebuck AS & Read J. Patterns of ventilatory response to carbon dioxide during recovery from severe asthma. *Clin Sci* 1971; **41**: 13–21.
18 Altose MD, McCauley WC, Kelsen SG, Cherniack NS. Effects of hypercapnia and inspiratory flow resistive loading on respiratory activity in chronic airways obstruction. *J Clin Invest* 1987; **59**: 500–7.
19 Kafer E. Idiopathic scoliosis. Mechanical properties of the respiratory system and the ventilatory response to carbon dioxide. *J Clin Invest* 1975; **55**: 1153–63.
20 Stradling JR. *Handbook of Sleep Related Breathing Disorders*. Oxford: Oxford University Press 1993: 13–21.

8 Measurement of Breathlessness
P W Jones

- **INTRODUCTION**
- **DEFINITION OF BREATHLESSNESS**
- **MEASUREMENT OF BREATHLESSNESS**
  Indirect methods
  Medical Research Council Dyspnea Scale
  Oxygen Cost Diagram
  The Baseline Dyspnea Index and Transitional Dyspnea Index
  UCSD Shortness of Breath Questionnaire
  Comprehensive dyspnea questionnaires
  Clinical dyspnea scales – summary
  Direct methods
  Visual analogue scale (VAS)
  Borg scale
  VAS versus Borg CR-10 scale
  Reference variable for dyspnea measurements
  Application of direct measures
- **ANALYSIS OF DYSPNEA**
  Intensity versus distress
  Effect of experience on dyspnea scaling
  Dyspnea versus fatigue
- **SUMMARY**

INTRODUCTION

Breathlessness or dyspnea is the subjective experience of discomfort in breathing. Unlike pain, for which clearly defined neural pathways and centers have been identified within the brain, the pathways and systems by which breathlessness is perceived are much more complex. There are no specific breathlessness receptors, nerves, or areas in the brain that can be readily identified as 'breathlessness centers'. It is thought that the perception of breathlessness involves neural signals derived from the motor drive to breathe that arises in the brain stem respiratory centers coupled with feedback from receptors in the respiratory muscles and possibly the lung.[1] The sensation of breathlessness is perceived in the cerebral cortex and there is evidence that cognitive functions related to previous experience of dyspnea may influence the perception of breathlessness.

DEFINITION OF BREATHLESSNESS

The difficulty in identifying mechanisms responsible for breathlessness is matched by the difficulty in defining it. One commonly used definition is 'the sense of an uncomfortable need to breathe'. This has proved useful, but there is evidence that there are different types, or qualities, of breathlessness. For example, patients with cardiac and respiratory diseases have been shown to use a range of different descriptions for their breathlessness.[2] These descriptors can be clustered together and, to a degree, associated with different diseases. The three most common sensations associated with breathlessness are:

- the urge to breathe (sometimes called air hunger)
- a sense of respiratory effort
- sensations associated with chest tightness.

Patients with chronic obstructive pulmonary disease (COPD) usually report that they felt out of breath or that their breathing required effort. Patients with asthma also used those descriptions but also said that their chest felt tight. In contrast, patients with cardiac disease tend not to report wheeze or chest tightness. There has been discussion as to how much information these descriptions provide about the nature of the processes underlying breathlessness.[3] This is still unresolved, but this research into what patients mean by 'breathlessness' has shown that it is a complex and poorly understood symptom.

Descriptors of breathlessness

Sensation	Typical disease process
Urge to breathe	Several
Sense of effort	COPD
Chest tightness	Asthma

The term 'dyspnea' is often used to indicate the unpleasant sensations associated with the act of breathing. Some think this term should be limited to *breathlessness due to disease* and that the word 'breathlessness' should be restricted to the sensations experienced by normal subjects. This distinction implies that 'dypsnea' and 'breathlessness' have different mechanisms, but there is no evidence that this is the case. Furthermore it may be difficult to know when 'normal' breathlessness ends and dyspnea begins. For this reason the two terms will be used interchangeably.

Breathlessness has been measured in two basic ways. One method involves direct quantification of the sensation during physical activity; the second approach is more indirect and assesses the effect of breathlessness experienced during recent daily activities. Such scales frequently include the term 'dyspnea' in their name but they do not attempt to perform direct estimations of dyspnea, rather they measure its impact on mobility and physical function. They may best be thought of as being clinical rating scales. A number have been developed over the years and they vary in complexity.

MEASUREMENT OF BREATHLESSNESS

Indirect:	Direct:
MRC Dyspnea Scale	Visual analogue scale (VAS)
Oxygen Cost Diagram (OCD)	Borg CR-10 scale
Baseline/Transitional Dyspnea Index (BDI/TDI)	
UCSD Shortness of Breath Questionnaire	
Complex breathlessness questionnaires	

Indirect methods

Medical Research Council (MRC) Dyspnea Scale

This has appeared in a number of versions; one of the most widely used is illustrated in Table 8.1. This is a simple measure that can be completed by the patients themselves. It is standardized and very widely used. MRC dyspnea grades provide a useful way of defining impairment of activity due to breathlessness, both in individuals and in populations of patients. The major limitation is that the intervals between categories are quite wide, so the scale may be too insensitive to detect small but clinically worthwhile responses to treatment. Despite this theoretical limitation, improvements in MRC scores have been reported following lung volume reduction surgery and surgery for the removal of emphysematous bullae.

Table 8.1 MRC Dyspnea Scale for breathlessness during daily activities

Grade 0	No breathlessness
Grade 1	Breathless with strenuous exercise
Grade 2	Short of breath when hurrying on the level *or* walking up a slight hill
Grade 3	Walk slower than people of the same age on the level *or* stop for breath while walking at own pace on the level
Grade 4	Stop for breath after walking about 100 yards *or* after a few minutes on the level
Grade 5	Too breathless to leave the house *or* breathless when dressing or undressing

Oxygen Cost Diagram

The oxygen cost diagram (OCD) is a visual analogue scale with 13 activities listed along a 100 mm line,[4] as illustrated in Figure 8.1. The position of these activities along this vertical line corresponds approximately to their oxygen requirements. Patients are asked to indicate the level of activity at which they begin to experience dyspnea. The OCD score is measured in millimeters. The shorter the distance, the greater the breathlessness. This measure is simple to use and for this reason has been used quite widely.

The Baseline Dyspnea Index (BDI) and Transitional Dyspnea Index (TDI)

The Baseline and Transition Dyspnea Indexes are two related scales that use a different approach to most

Figure 8.1 Oxygen Cost Diagram for breathlessness during daily activities

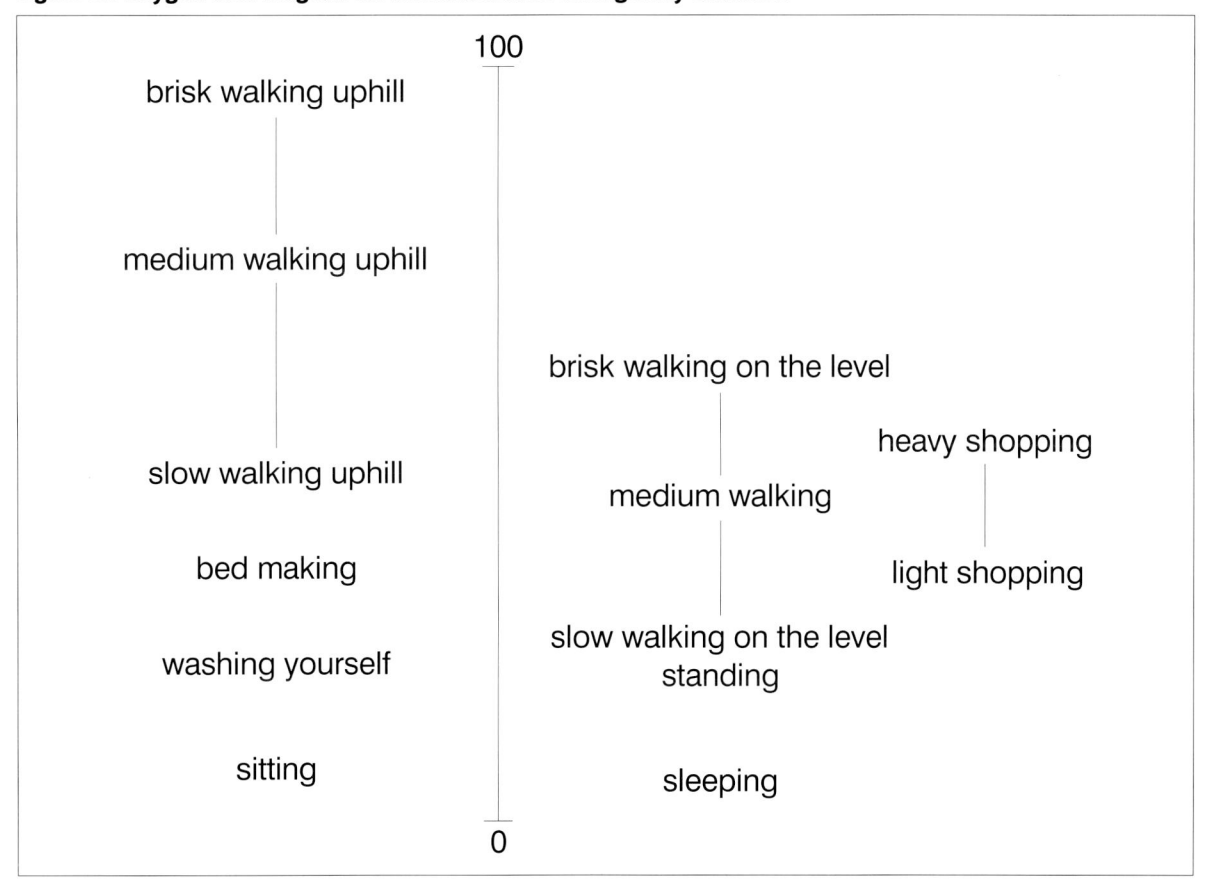

Subjects indicate on the 100 mm vertical line their level of breathlessness in daily life using the descriptions as a guide. Breathlessness is measured as the distance along the line. The shorter the distance, the greater the breathlessness.

other instruments of this type. They have three components. One assesses *functional impairment due to dyspnea* in a manner similar to other scales for indirect measurement of breathlessness. The other two components are largely unique to the BDI/TDI and assess the *magnitude of the task* and the *magnitude of effort* as factors that provoke breathlessness.[5] The BDI is designed to discriminate between different levels of breathlessness in different patients at a single point in time whereas the TDI measures changes from the baseline state. Unlike most of the instruments used to measure dyspnea, the BDI and TDI scores are obtained as part of an interview by a clinician with experience in taking medical histories from patients. This includes nurses and pulmonary function technicians.

When administering the BDI/TDI, the interviewer should ask open-ended questions about the patient's breathlessness and then select a grade for each component by matching the patient's responses with pre-set criteria. The grades for the functional impairment component are defined in Table 8.2; full details of the other components are given in Mahler et al.[5] The BDI total score is obtained by adding the scores, from zero (severe) to four (not impaired) for each of the three components. Thus the BDI score ranges from 0 to 12: the lower the score the greater the intensity of dyspnea. The TDI total score represents changes in dyspnea compared to the baseline condition according to seven possible grades from −3 (major deterioration) to +3 (major improvement) for each component. When using this scale, the interviewer should refer to the grades from the BDI and can remind the individual patient of his/her comments before selecting the component grades for the TDI.

The BDI and TDI have been recognized for clinical use by an Outcomes Committee of the American Association of Cardiovascular and Pulmonary Rehabilitation. In clinical trials, the TDI has been shown to detect changes in breathlessness following exercise training and pulmonary rehabilitation and following lung volume reduction surgery in patients with emphysema.

UCSD Shortness of Breath Questionnaire

This questionnaire was developed at the University of California, San Diego (UCSD). It is more complex than the MRC scale or OCD since it has 24 items concerned with breathlessness over the preceding week. It is a self-report, self-completed instrument whose items cover 21 standard activities.[6] There are also three global questions concerning overall limitation. The patient has to respond to each item using a six point scale. This instrument has been shown to be reliable and to be sensitive to improvements in dyspnea following pulmonary rehabilitation.

Comprehensive dyspnea questionnaires

Some questionnaires provide a very comprehensive inventory of the impact of breathlessness on daily function. These often have many items. They are closer in structure and size to questionnaires designed to measure 'quality of life' or health status, although they do not attempt to address the full range of dis-

Table 8.2 Baseline Dyspnea Index – functional impairment component

Grade 4: *No Impairment*
Able to carry out usual activities and occupation without shortness of breath.

Grade 3: *Slight Impairment*
Distinct impairment in at least one activity but no activities completely abandoned. Reduction, in activities at work or in usual activities, that seems slight or not clearly caused by shortness of breath.

Grade 2: *Moderate Impairment*
Patient has changed jobs and/or has abandoned at least one usual activity due to shortness of breath.

Grade 1: *Severe Impairment*
Patient unable to work or has given up most or all usual activities due to shortness of breath.

Grade 0: *Very Severe Impairment*
Unable to work and has given up most or all usual activities due to shortness of breath.

Note: Usual activities refer to requirements of daily living, maintenance or upkeep of residence, yard work, gardening, etc.
The clinician assessing the patient relates the patient's description of his/her limitations due to breathlessness to the grades contained in the questionnaire. Full details of this scale are given elsewhere.[5]

turbances to health covered by such instruments. Comprehensive dyspnea questionnaires include the Pulmonary Functional Status and Dyspnea Questionnaire[7] and the Pulmonary Function Status Scale.[8] They are both self-administered, but take rather longer to complete than the UCSD Shortness of Breath Questionnaire. They have both been shown to be valid and have adequate repeatability.

Clinical dyspnea scales – summary

These rating scales provide valid estimates of the impairment of patients lives due to dyspnea. Dyspnea scores obtained with some of these scales have been shown to correlate quite well with impaired quality of life. Clinical trial data show that they can detect changes in the impact of dyspnea or physical function following treatment. Several of these scales are quick and easy to use and they correlate with each other quite well. They also correlate quite well with exercise performance when measured using walking distance tests, but much more weakly with peak exercise performance on a cycle-ergometer.[9] Scales of this type provide a valuable method of making standardized measurements of the effect of breathlessness on physical activity, however they do not measure breathlessness directly. A different type of instrument is needed for that purpose.

Indirect measurements of breathlessness

Advantages	Disadvantages
Relate to habitual activities	Sensitivity may depend on the number of categories in the scale
Can detect change post-treatment	Relate to past experience of breathlessness
	May be unreliable if exercise limited by other disease, e.g. arthritis

Direct methods

In many clinical situations or studies, an assessment of the impact of breathlessness on a patient's daily physical activity may be the measurement of greatest interest. There are, however, circumstances where a direct measurement of breathlessness is needed. This applies particularly when investigating causes of breathlessness in an individual patient. Such measurements are also needed when studying mechanisms of dyspnea or evaluating treatments designed to reduce it. The indirect measurements of dyspnea described above all relate to the experience of breathlessness in the past. They depend upon the subject's sensation of breathlessness or experience of its effects in the context of some form of daily physical activity. In contrast, direct measures quantify breathlessness as felt by the subject at the time of measurement.

Visual analogue scale (VAS)

The visual analogue scale takes the form of a line that may be vertical or horizontal and has descriptors at either end of the scale to provide anchor or reference points between which all intermediate levels of the sensation are scaled.[10] VAS scales for dyspnea have been used with a number of differently worded reference points. The mild end is often labeled 'none' or 'not at all', and the severe end 'extreme breathlessness' or 'maximum imaginable' or 'as bad as can be' (Figure 8.2). The subjects are asked to indicate their level of breathlessness at that moment by selecting a point along the scale. A range of methods are used including pencil and paper, computer and electronic displays. The latter have employed two methods of graphical presentation, either a method analogous to the pencil and line approach or a thermometer type display. Both vertical and horizontal presentations have been used. In many exercise laboratories an electronic display is actuated by the subject using a rotating or sliding potentiometer placed at a convenient site on the ergometer. There has been little work to compare the different methods of presenting the VAS, although it has been shown that vertical and horizontal presentations give similar results. The repeatability of the VAS over time is moderately high in both normal subjects[11] and patients with lung disease.[12]

Borg scale

The Borg scale for dyspnea was developed from an earlier scale to measure perceived exertion – the *Ratio of Perceived Exertion* had a scaling range of 0–21. This unusual scaling range is due to the fact that it

Figure 8.2 Scales for measuring breathlessness during an exercise test

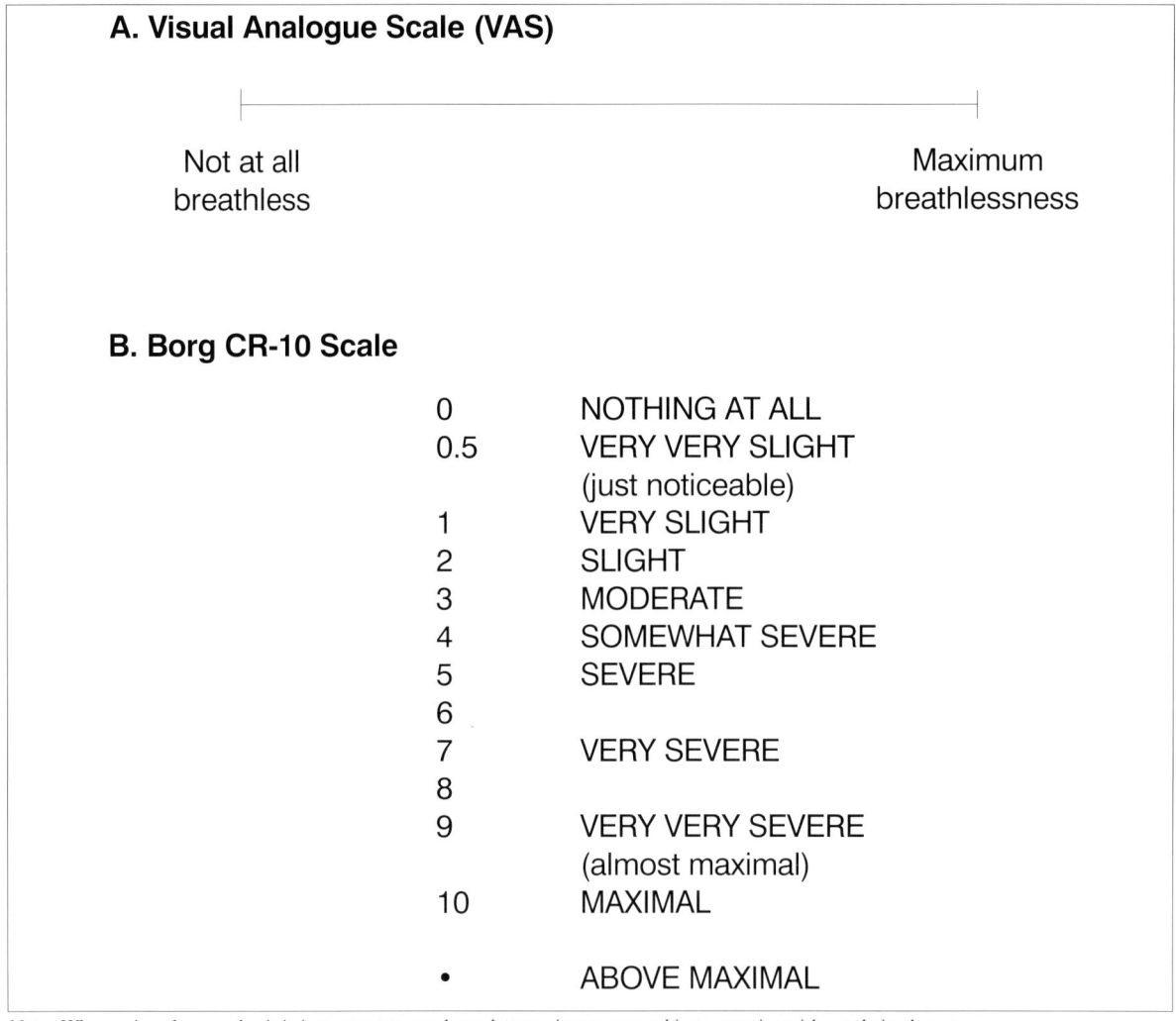

Note: When using these scales it is important to use large letters since many subjects exercise without their glasses.

was calibrated against the heart rate increase that occurs during exercise, 21 being the level of exertion experienced at the 'maximal' heart rate of 210 beats per minute. The Clinical Rating Scale for Dyspnea uses a range from 0 to 10 and is usually called the CR-10 scale.[13] It has a series of numbers from 0 to 10 with descriptors at certain points along its length (Figure 8.2). It will be noted that a value of 0.5 has been included to allow subjects to indicate a level of dyspnea that is just perceptible. The use of numbers and descriptors implies that this is a category scale, although it is permissible to indicate a level of dyspnea between two category levels and indicate that the current level of dyspnea is not an integer number, so scores such as 3.4 are permitted.

The Borg CR-10 scale (like the VAS) is closed. There is a finite upper limit, defined by the maximum value for the value 'maximum'. This leads to the problem of what the subject is to do if he/she experiences a level of dyspnea that surpasses the level of dyspnea that had, up to that moment, been judged to be 'maximal'. This led to the inclusion of a point in the CR-10 scale above maximum called 'supra-maximal'. Unfortunately this does not solve the problem. The use of a new upper limit must mean that all the sub-maximal levels of dyspnea are now judged with reference to a new anchor point and are therefore not comparable to previous dyspnea estimates in the same subject. This extreme case may occur relatively rarely, but it illustrates that none of the scaling methods used for the measurement of dyspnea is ideal.

VAS versus Borg CR-10 scale

The similarities between the VAS and CR-10 are much greater than their differences. Both have anchor points that indicate no breathlessness at one end and maximum breathlessness at the other. Both are closed and both may be used to produce a continuous scale (since the intervals between Borg CR-10 categories may be used). The use of descriptors may offer a particular advantage to the CR-10 scale since the use of terms such as 'slight', 'moderate', 'severe', etc. may permit standardization between subjects. This depends of course upon the assumption that all subjects use the descriptions in the same way and that they use the same semantic differentials (i.e. the perceptual distances between 'slight', 'moderate', and 'severe' are the same across all subjects). The assumption that different subjects use descriptors of intensity in the same way has never been tested formally in dyspnea, but it seems reasonable to assume that there may be more agreement between subjects over the intensity of dyspnea when it is defined in words rather than in VAS units (usually millimeters). A range of values for CR-10 scores obtained in normal subjects and patients with chronic airflow limitation has been published, which suggests that these descriptors may have some utility.[14]

One test of the validity of a measurement instrument is its repeatability. Both the VAS and the CR-10 scales have adequate reproducibility in patients with COPD when measured over days to a few weeks.[12,15] One of the problems in assessing the repeatability of dyspnea scores in patients is that breathlessness levels may be affected by changes in disease state. Medium and long-term stability of dyspnea scores can only be obtained in normal subjects. The CR-10 scale has been found to have slightly better medium and long-term repeatability than the VAS.[16]

Reference variable for dyspnea measurements

To be meaningful, direct measurements of breathlessness cannot be made in isolation, they must be related to something. They can be made at rest, to measure breathlessness in the resting unstimulated state, but are most often used during an exercise test. In this setting they may be used in two ways. The simplest technique is to record the level of dyspnea at peak exercise or peak oxygen consumption ($\dot{V}O_2$). Measurements may also be made at the end of a standard 6 or 12 minute walking test. Care must be taken in the interpretation of such measurements. A treatment may reduce the level of dyspnea during exercise and thus permit the patient to achieve a higher level of work for the same level of breathlessness. If the patient exercised to the same level of breathlessness it would appear that the dyspnea was unchanged whereas in fact the patient was able to achieve a higher maximum work rate. This highlights the need to standardize the level of breathlessness against another relevant physiological variable.

The source of the sensations responsible for the generation of dyspnea has not been fully identified. This makes the choice of reference variable a little difficult. There are theoretical grounds to suggest that dyspnea may be most closely related to the work of breathing, based upon a study that showed that nearly 70% of the variance in Borg CR-10 scores on incremental exercise could be accounted for by a parameter derived from a number of respiratory variables such as Ppl(min), V_T/VC ratio, inspiratory flow rate, and T_I/T_{TOT}. Such measurements are complex and not made routinely. Two more easily measured variables are commonly used as the denominator against which breathlessness measurements are standardized. One is minute ventilation ($\dot{V}_E$). The rationale for this is that the work of breathing is related to the level of ventilation, and this relationship should remain unchanged as long as airways resistance, dynamic lung compliance, and compliance of the chest wall remain unchanged. In many situations, this assumption may hold true for changes in $\dot{V}_E$ within individuals so $\dot{V}_E$ may provide an adequate surrogate for the work of breathing. An alternative approach, often favored by clinicians, is to argue that the relationship between breathlessness and external work capacity is more important in a patient's daily life than the relationship between ventilation and breathlessness. This has lead to the frequent adoption of ergometer work rate or $\dot{V}O_2$ as the denominator of breathlessness. Both of these approaches have advantages and the selection of the reference measure may depend on the purpose of any particular study. In practice, differences between

Figure 8.3 Perceived dyspnea versus ventilation in two normal subjects

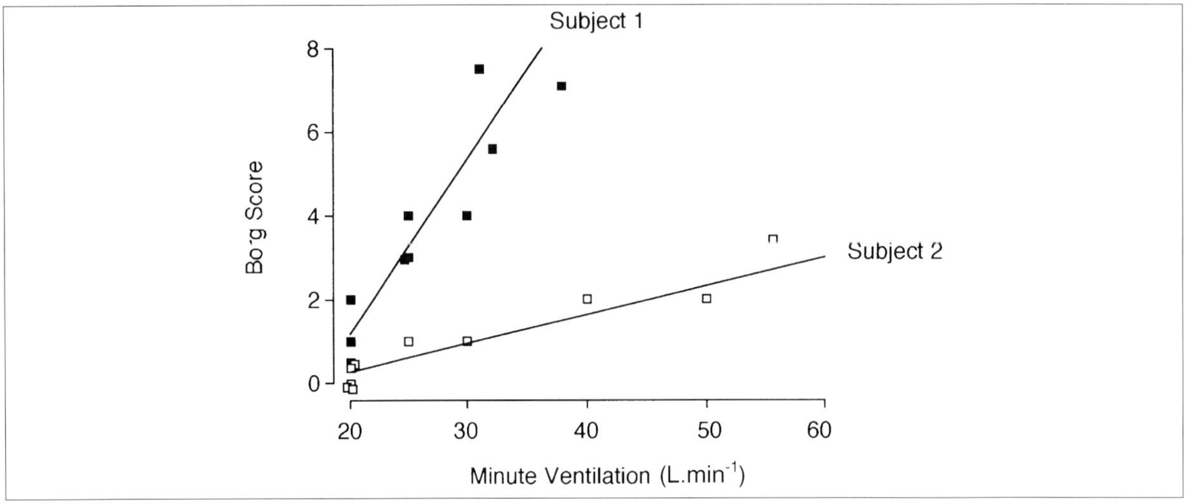

The relationship between dyspnea measured using the Borg CR-10 scale and minute ventilation during an incremental exercise test in two normal subjects. Wide discrepancies in rating of breathlessness are common even in normal, disease-free subjects.

the use of $\dot{V}_E$ or external work as denominators of breathlessness may be slight.

The use of a denominator such as $\dot{V}_E$ or $\dot{V}O_2$ is especially helpful since it provides a method by which a number of breathlessness measurements from a single exercise test may be analyzed, not just the peak level. This allows greater precision in the estimate of dyspnea, which is usually achieved by calculating the slope of the relationship between dyspnea and $\dot{V}_E$ or $\dot{V}O_2$, as illustrated in Figure 8.3. It will be noted that, in both of the subjects illustrated, the correlation for a linear regression between Borg score and $\dot{V}_E$ is high. This is usually the case; few subjects show a non-linear breathlessness-ventilation relationship, at least when studied during incremental exercise tests. Figure 8.3 also illustrates the wide variation between normal subjects in terms of their breathlessness-ventilation relationships. The reasons for this normal variation are not known but, importantly, this relationship is stable *within* subjects for quite long periods of time if nothing occurs that might change it.[17] The wide inter-individual variability may limit the degree to which breathlessness-ventilation relationships may be compared *across* subjects. Nevertheless, this technique has shown that the intensity of dyspnea during ergometer exercise is higher in patients with cardiopulmonary disease than in healthy subjects.

Direct measurements of breathlessness

Advantages	Disadvantages
Quantifies current perception	Response will depend on the instructions to the patient
Repeatable	May be dependent upon the anchor points at either end of scale
May be applied under standardized conditions	Not open-ended, so patients use of the scale may change with experience of maximum breathlessness
Can be related to a physiological variable such as $\dot{V}_E$ or $\dot{V}O_2$	May be unreliable if exercise limited by other disease, e.g. arthritis

Application of direct measures

Direct measurements of breathlessness have been used quite widely in clinical trials, especially in studies of pulmonary rehabilitation. For example, Borg CR-10 scores fell in patients completing exercise programs compared to control patients who received no rehabilitation. In another study, the slope of the relationship between breathlessness and work rate or $\dot{V}O_2$ fell following participation in an exercise program. The latter observation is of particular interest because it illustrates the different contributions of indirect and direct measurements of breathlessness to the understanding of dyspnea. Indirect measurements can show that physical rehabilitation may reduce impairment due to dyspnea in daily life but they do not identify the mechanism by which this happens. In contrast, direct measurement may provide some clues. The observation that the relationship between breathlessness and $\dot{V}O_2$ may be changed by exercise training directed to the legs suggests that the link between work rate and dyspnea may be altered by factors other than those related to the simple processing of respiratory motor activity and its associated sensory feedback. This has implications for future research into the mechanisms of breathlessness and methods of reducing dyspnea.

ANALYSIS OF DYSPNEA

Intensity versus distress

Breathlessness is usually measured in terms of its magnitude, but there is increasing evidence that this sensation may be more like pain, in which two components have been identified. These are intensity and an affective or emotional component that reflects the distress resulting from the pain. There is some evidence that a similar situation may exist in the perception of breathlessness. It has been shown that normal subjects may scale the intensity of their dyspnea differently from the amount of distress that it causes them.[18] This is illustrated in Figure 8.4. One subject rated distress due to breathlessness higher than the intensity of breathlessness. Another subject rated intensity above distress. The latter was more representative of the group as a whole in that scores for intensity were greater, on average, than corresponding scores for distress. While these observations may have importance for an understanding of the nature of breathlessness, they also have more immediate practical implications for the measurement of breathlessness since they show that the instructions to the subjects in terms of what aspect of breathlessness they should scale may have a significant effect on the breathlessness scores obtained.

Figure 8.4 Breathlessness versus distress in two normal subjects

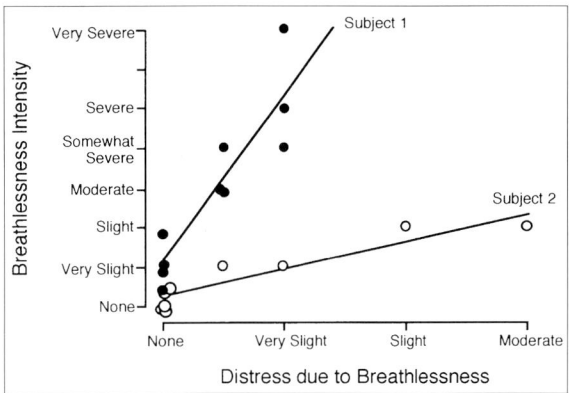

Relationship between the intensity of breathlessness and the distress associated with it in two normal subjects during an incremental exercise test. Most subjects follow the pattern illustrated by Subject 1 in that they indicate the intensity of breathlessness to be greater than its associated distress.

Effect of experience on dyspnea scaling

The process of scaling breathlessness must require memory and judgment since to scale a point on a VAS somewhere between 'no breathlessness' and 'extreme breathlessness' requires either that the subject has experienced extreme breathlessness or can imagine it. This requires judgment based upon experience. Two studies in normal subjects have shown evidence that prior experience of breathlessness may modify current estimates, both in the short term, over the time course of a single experiment, and over a period of several weeks or months.[19] The influence of experience and cognitive function upon estimates of breathlessness may explain why patients indicate a lower level of dyspnea for a given level of ventilation following pulmonary rehabilitation. It can be argued that they may have been deconditioned to breathlessness through the experience of regular periods of dyspnea during the exercise training. While this is an interesting hypothesis, the practical implication of these observations is that when breathlessness is measured during an exercise test,

Figure 8.5 Symptom intensity on cessation of exercise

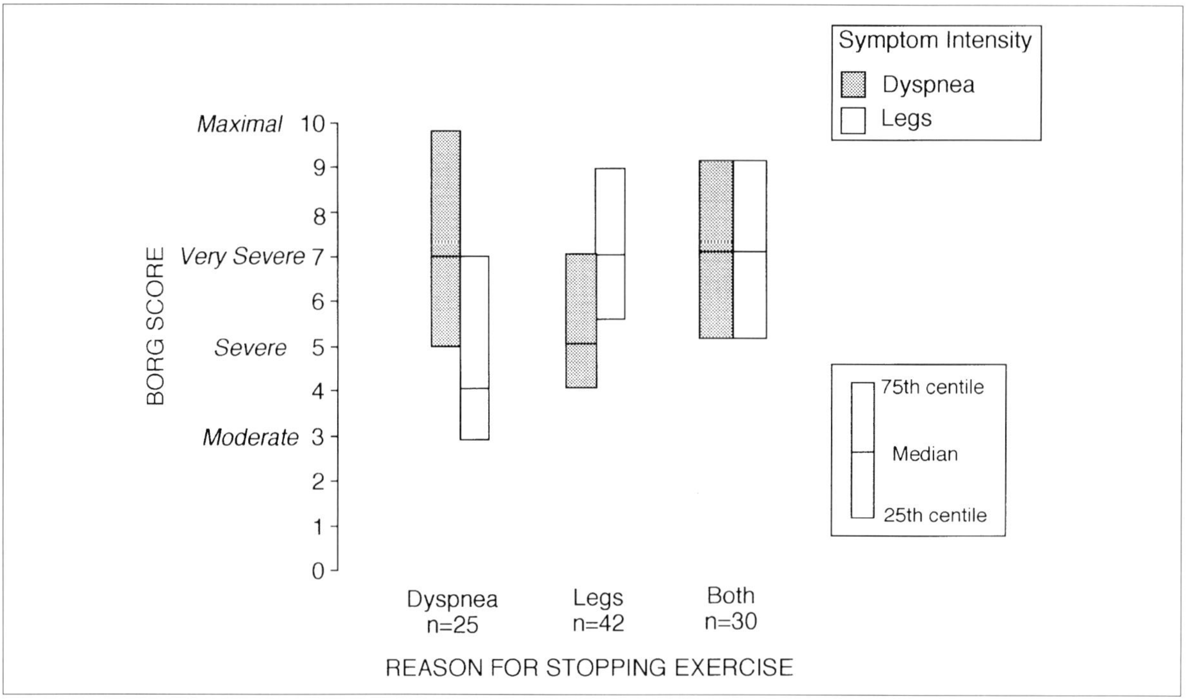

25 patients stopped exercising because of breathlessness. Their median score for dyspnea was 7, while the median score for their leg fatigue was 4. In contrast, the median score for breathlessness in the patients who stopped because of their legs was 5, while their median score for leg fatigue was 7. Those patients who stopped because of a combination of leg fatigue and dyspnea indicated a median score of 7 for both dyspnea and leg fatigue. (Data from Killian KJ, Leblanc P, Martin DH, Summers E, Jones NL, Campbell EJM. Exercise capacity and ventilatory, circulatory, and symptom limitation in patients with chronic airflow limitation. American Review of Respiratory Disease 1992; 146:935–40. © American Lung Association.)

not only the test but also the patient's recent experience of breathlessness prior to the test should be standardized. Thus it would not be correct to measure breathlessness on one occasion when the patient had been resting for an hour then test on another occasion shortly after he or she had walked up three flights of stairs. This is particularly important when breathlessness is measured before and after an experimental intervention.

Dyspnea versus fatigue

Direct measurements of leg fatigue may also be measured using the Borg CR-10 scale.[14] Using this approach, it has been observed that normal subjects and patients with COPD may stop exercising because of leg effort, dyspnea, or both (Figure 8.5). The proportion of subjects stopping for the different reasons were similar for both groups of subjects: leg effort 37–43%, dyspnea 22–26%, and both 31–42%. On average, subjects stopped exercising when their predominant symptom reached the level of 'very severe'. It is noteworthy that more patients with chronic lung disease stopped because of leg effort than dyspnea.

SUMMARY

Breathlessness may be measured both indirectly and directly. Both approaches have particular applications. Direct measurements have greatest application in the pulmonary function laboratory since they are best made under standardized conditions using a physiological variable such as work rate, $\dot{V}_E$, or $\dot{V}O_2$. The properties of direct measurements of dyspnea are summarized below:

- Direct measurements provide different information from indirect measures.
- Individuals scale breathlessness differently.
- Measurements are repeatable in the short and medium term.
- Most useful when related to a physiological variables such as $\dot{V}_E$ or $\dot{V}O_2$.
- Intensity of breathlessness and distress due to breathlessness are different.
- Breathlessness may be influenced by prior experience.
- Useful in the evaluation of exercise limitation due to lung disease.
- Can be used to measure changes due to treatment.

References

1 Eldridge FL & Chen Z. Respiratory sensation – a neurological perspective. In: Adams L & Guz A (eds) *Respiratory Sensation*. New York: Marcel Dekker 1996: 19–67.
2 Simon PM, Schwartzstein RM, Weiss JW, Fencl V, Teghtsoonian M, Weinberger SE. Distinguishable types of dyspnea in patients with shortness of breath. *Am Rev Respir Dis* 1990; **142**: 1009–14.
3 Mahler DA, Harver A, Lentine T, Scott JA, Beck K, Schwartzstein RM. Descriptors of breathlessness in cardiorespiratory diseases. *Am J Respir Crit Care Med* 1996; **154**: 1357–63.
4 McGavin CR, Artvinli M, Naoe H, McHardy GJR. Dyspnoea, disability and distance walked: comparison of estimates of exercise performance in respiratory disease. *BMJ* 1978; **2**: 241–3.
5 Mahler DA, Weinberg DH, Wells CK, Feinstein AR. The measurement of dyspnea: contents, interobserver agreement and physiological correlates of two new clinical scales. *Chest* 1984; **85**: 751–8.
6 Eakin EG, Prewitt LM, Ries AL, Kaplan RM. Validation of the UCSD shortness of breath questionnaire. *J Cardiopulm Rehab* 1994; **14**: 322.
7 Lareau S, Carrieri-Kohlman V, Janson-Bjerklie S, Roos PJ. Development and testing of the Pulmonary Functional Status and Dyspnea Questionnaire (PFSDQ). *Heart and Lung* 1994; **23**: 242–50.
8 Weaver TE & Narsavage GL. Physiological and psychological variables related to functional status in COPD. *Nursing Research* 1992; **41**: 286–91.
9 Guyatt GH, Thompson PJ, Berman LB, Sullivan MJ, Townsend M, Jones NL, Pugsley SO. How should we measure function in patients with chronic lung disease? *J Chron Dis* 1985; **38**: 517–24.
10 Adams L, Chronos N, Lane R, Guz A. The measurement of breathlessness induced in normal subjects: validity of two scaling techniques. *Clin Sci* 1985; **69**: 7–16.
11 Wilson RC & Jones PW. A comparison of the visual analogue scale and modified Borg scale for the measurement of dyspnoea during exercise. *Clin Sci* 1989; **76**: 277–82.
12 Mador MJ & Kufel TJ. Reproducibility of visual analogue scale measurement of dyspnea in patients with chronic obstructive pulmonary disease. *Am Rev Respir Dis* 1992; **146**: 82–7.
13 Schwartzstein RM, Manning HL, Weiss JW, Weinberger SE. Dyspnea: a sensory experience. *Lung* 1990; **168**: 185–99.
14 Killian KJ, Leblanc P, Martin DH, Summers E, Jones NL, Campbell EJM. Exercise capacity and ventilatory, circulatory, and symptom limitation in patients with chronic airflow limitation. *Am Rev Respir Dis* 1992; **146**: 935–40.
15 Muza SR, Silverman MT, Gilmore GC, Hellerstein HK. Comparison of scales used to quantitate the sense of effort to breathe in patients with chronic obstructive pulmonary disease. *Am Rev Respir Dis* 1990; **141**: 909–13.
16 Wilson RC & Jones PW. Long-term reproducibility of Borg scale estimates of breathlessness during exercise. *Clin Sci* 1991; **80**: 309–12.
17 Leblanc P, Bowie DM, Summers NL, Jones NL, Killian KJ. Breathlessness and exercise in patients with cardiorespiratory disease. *Am Rev Respir Dis* 1986; **133**: 21–5.
18 Wilson RC & Jones PW. Differentiation between the intensity of breathlessness and the distress it evokes in normal subjects during exercise. *Clin Sci* 1991; **80**: 65–70.
19 Wilson RC, Oldfield WLG, Jones PW. Effect of residence at altitude on the perception of breathlessness on return to sea level in normal subjects. *Clin Sci* 1993; **84**: 159–67.

9 Exercise Testing
M D L Morgan

- **RATIONALE FOR EXERCISE TESTING**
  The exercise response in health and lung disease
  Limits to exercise in lung disease
  Assessment of disability

- **THE SPECTRUM OF EXERCISE TESTING**
  Field exercise tests
  The conduct of six minute and shuttle walk tests
  Laboratory exercise testing
  Equipment
  Data presentation
  Quality control
  Safety and conduct
  Protocols
  Normal values
  Identification of $\dot{V}O_2$max or $\dot{V}O_2$peak
  Anaerobic threshold
  Ventilatory limit
  Submaximal testing

- **CLINICAL SITUATIONS**
  Cardiac versus lung disease
  Preoperative evaluation
  Asthma

- **THE INTERPRETATION AND REPORTING OF EXERCISE TESTS**
  Patterns of abnormal response to exercise in different conditions
  Normal response to peak exercise

  Interpretative questions
  Cooperation and motivation
  Reason for stopping
  Physiological response

- **CONCLUSIONS**

RATIONALE FOR EXERCISE TESTING

In the context of lung disease the testing of exercise capacity has five major functions:

1. the differential diagnosis of exertional dyspnea
2. the objective measurement of disability
3. preoperative assessment
4. the assessment of treatment
5. the identification of exercise induced asthma.

In recent years sophisticated equipment for assessing the cardiorespiratory responses to exercise has become available. Although this is a welcome development, there is a belief that exercise testing is complex, technically demanding and difficult to interpret. This chapter aims to show that exercise testing for lung disease can be simply understood and need not always depend upon expensive technology or require a specific protocol.

The value of exercise testing lies in the observation that physicians are poor at predicting exercise capacity from clinical examination and static lung function tests. In patients with lung disease there is likely to be a general relationship between the deterioration in lung function and exercise performance. Numerous studies have tried to identify predictive relationships without success and patients with similar lung function may have widely different degrees of exercise capacity.[1,2] Some of this discrepancy may be accounted for by the observation that exercise may be limited as much by fatigue or circulatory factors, as by breathlessness, in patients with severe lung disease.

The exercise response in health and lung disease

The demands of exercise are driven by the appetite of muscle cells for oxygen which is delivered to them by the cardiovascular system in order to regenerate adenosine triphosphate (ATP). This cellular oxygen requirement may rise by a factor of 40, demands which are satisfied by increased ventilation, increased cardiac output, and redistribution of blood to the appropriate musculature. Ventilation and cardiac output increase linearly with progressive exercise though their components (breathing frequency, tidal volume, and heart rate and stroke volume) may contribute differently. In addition, the wasted fraction of ventilation (V_D/V_T) may halve as alveolar ventilation becomes more efficient. Oxygen uptake ($\dot{V}O_2$) rises steadily with work rate but begins to slow down at higher workloads as anaerobic respiration, marked by a progressive increase in lactate production, occurs. Eventually, in well motivated healthy subjects, $\dot{V}O_2$ reaches a plateau although workload, ventilation, and cardiac output continue to increase for a time. Meanwhile, since CO_2 production continues, the respiratory exchange ratio (RER = $\dot{V}CO_2/\dot{V}O_2$) will rise. This plateau of oxygen consumption is the maximal aerobic capacity ($\dot{V}O_2$ max), which is usually determined by the capacity of the circulation to deliver oxygen to respiring muscle (Figure 9.1). Blood gas tensions remain fairly stable throughout exercise but hyperventilation induced by lactic acidosis and pulmonary $\dot{V}_A/\dot{Q}$ adjustments may result in a slight fall in $PaCO_2$ and rise in PaO_2. In health, diffusion limitation of gas exchange from the lung to blood, as the cause of exercise-induced arterial hypoxemia, occurs only in elite athletes at peak exercise or when exercising at a low FiO_2.

The limits of constant submaximal or endurance exercise are not determined solely by the aerobic capacity ($\dot{V}O_2$ max). The ability to sustain exercise at a certain fraction of maximal aerobic capacity is influenced by nutrition, substrate, training, and thermoregulation as well as motivation and confidence.

> **During incremental exercise in healthy subjects:**
>
> - Minute ventilation ($\dot{V}E$) and cardiac output ($\dot{Q}$) increase linearly with work rate.
> - Oxygen consumption ($\dot{V}O_2$) reaches a plateau ($\dot{V}O_2$ max) in motivated subjects.
> - PaO_2 and $PaCO_2$ remain relatively stable.
> - Maximal exercise is limited by the circulatory delivery of oxygen, not the lungs.

Limits to exercise in lung disease

The development of disease increases the likelihood that exercise may be limited by pathology in the lung or chest wall. However, it is important to remember that exercise capacity is commonly limit-

Figure 9.1 $\dot{V}O_2$max versus $\dot{V}O_2$peak

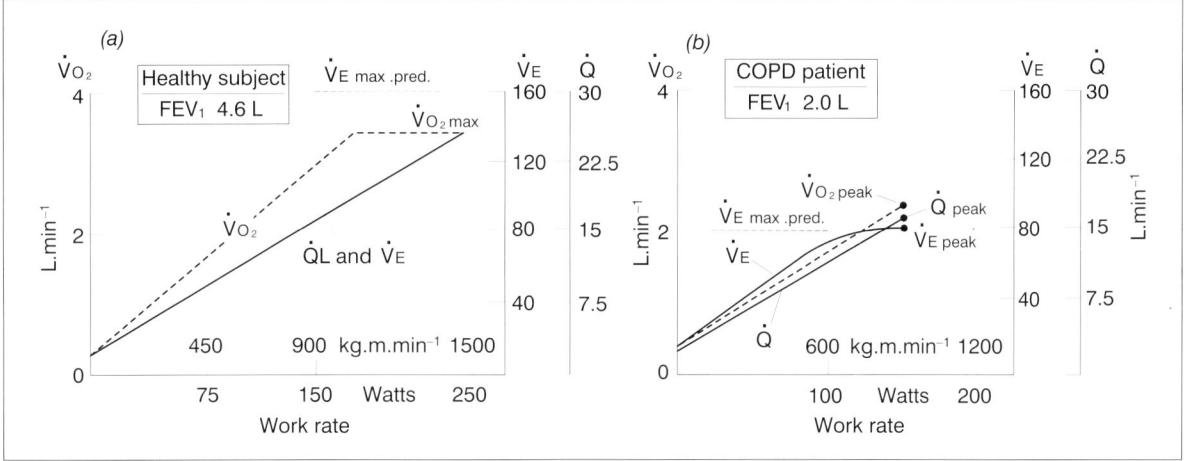

Ventilation ($\dot{V}_E$), cardiac output ($\dot{Q}$), and oxygen consumption ($\dot{V}O_2$) all increase with increasing work rate. Towards the end of incremental exercise, $\dot{V}O_2$ in motivated healthy subjects reaches a plateau ($\dot{V}O_2$max) while $\dot{V}_E$ and $\dot{Q}$ still continue to increase.

In patients with lung disease, particularly COPD, the $\dot{V}O_2$ fails to demonstrate a plateau ($\dot{V}O_2$peak) since exercise may be prematurely terminated by a ventilatory limit (low FEV_1).

ed primarily by limb muscle fatigue or chest pain, even in patients with respiratory disease. This can be identified by inquiring about the cause of exercise cessation. Respiratory interference with exercise function can occur from ventilatory inadequacy or, less commonly, from gas exchange failure. Patients with significant lung disease will not be able to reach a true aerobic capacity as demonstrated by a plateau of $\dot{V}O_2$ (Figure 9.1). When exercise is curtailed prematurely by ventilatory limitation or deconditioning, the highest $\dot{V}O_2$ is termed $\dot{V}O_2$peak to distinguish it from a true maximal performance. In many patients with severe disease it is also difficult to demonstrate a lactate or anaerobic threshold (AT) (i.e. the onset of blood lactate accumulation) (see later section on Clinical Situations).

Assessment of disability

Exercise testing is often used, for legal or prognostic reasons, to make an objective assessment of a patient's work capacity. Appropriate information concerning maximal capacity or submaximal efficiency can be obtained from laboratory testing. There is, however, some lack of agreement about the terminology and the methods of identifying disability. The WHO defines *impairment* as the physiological damage resulting from illness (e.g. airway obstruction). *Disability* is the effect of impairment on physical functioning (e.g. inability to climb stairs through breathlessness). *Handicap* is the social impact of the disability (e.g. inability to work).

There is still debate as to whether exercise testing assesses impairment or disability or both. Impairment of exercise capacity is equivalent to reduction of aerobic capacity [$\dot{V}O_2$max]. Maximal performance, on the other hand, is affected by factors other than ventilatory limitation (e.g. fatigue) and respiratory disability could also be related to the efficiency of ventilation

Maximal exercise in lung disease

- Maximal capacity may be reduced by a ventilatory limit from airway obstruction, interstitial lung disease or chest wall restriction.
- Fatigue, skeletal muscle deconditioning, or circulatory factors may still limit performance in a large proportion of patients with lung disease.
- Anaerobic threshold may be reduced or may not be reached.
- Progressive fall in SaO_2 may occur in interstitial or pulmonary vascular disease.

during submaximal exercise at a reference $\dot{V}O_2$, e.g. 1.0 L.min^{-1}. Disability is reduction of social functioning and should be measured by a standardized performance test with some relevance to real life, e.g. shuttle walk test, 6 minute walk test, or endurance capacity.

Human physical activity is not confined to the artificial circumstances in which it is often tested. The symptom limited maximal exercise test defines the upper limit of physical performance and describes what the subject is capable of achieving. It can, for example, identify an individual who will never be an elite athlete. However, maximal capacity is irrelevant to the everyday life of most people. A more relevant assessment of disability may be the percentage of $\dot{V}O_2$max which could be sustained for a prolonged period or the efficiency with which a constant workload task can be achieved. It follows that the mode of testing should try to recreate the circumstances of the disability as closely as possible.

Endurance tests	Maximal capacity tests
6 minute walk test (MWT)	20 meter shuttle run
Endurance walk	10 meter shuttle walk test (SWT)
Step test	Paced incremental step test

THE SPECTRUM OF EXERCISE TESTING

Field exercise tests

Field exercise tests are often simple performance measures of endurance or maximal capacity which can be carried out at remote sites without reliance on a fixed laboratory. They can be simple in concept but not necessarily unsophisticated since it is now possible to make virtually every laboratory measurement in the field with appropriate portable equipment (e.g. $\dot{V}O_2$, $\dot{V}E$, HR, SaO_2, etc). The spectrum of field testing covers the range from unstructured free endurance walking to complex, paced incremental tests which relate closely to laboratory tests of maximal capacity.

The unpaced endurance tests such as the 6MWT are realistic and 'mimic real life' since no pressure is applied to the subject to complete the test. However, this implies that reproducibility can only be achieved after a number of practice walks. By contrast the shuttle walk and run tests are highly reproducible and correlate well with maximal aerobic capacity.[3,4] In general the unpaced tests, in spite of realism, tend to underestimate subject's performance and are affected by mood and encouragement. Nevertheless, both the maximal capacity SWT walk test and the endurance 6MWT have proved sensitive enough to detect changes as a result of treatment. Therefore they are valuable performance measures which have a role in the assessment of interventions such as rehabilitation, drug therapy, or lung volume reduction surgery. In certain circumstances, for example in athletes, it may be desirable to take the laboratory to the patient and use portable equipment to make metabolic measurements. However, in the majority of cases where metabolic measurements are required the laboratory is the more appropriate place.

The conduct of six minute and shuttle walk tests

Both of these tests require very basic equipment; they are suitable for studying disabled patients with restricted exercise capacity. In the 6MWT the subject is asked to cover a long corridor walk with instructions to cover as much ground as possible in six minutes. No formal encouragement may be given since this has been shown to influence the results. The results are expressed in terms of the distance traveled in the time (i.e. meters). The 6MWT distance increases with practice and at least three attempts should be performed to ensure stability. SaO_2 with pulse oximetry is easily measured at the beginning and end of the test. The 6MWT can also be used to assess domiciliary oxygen requirements (see Chapter 13) with the patient breathing from a portable cylinder containing air or 100% oxygen (and preferably not knowing which is which).

By contrast the shuttle walk test is an incremental test of maximal capacity which is achieved by walking the subject around two cones 10 meters apart and increasing the paced walking speed every minute. The pace is provided by an audio tape which 'beeps' at progressively shorter time intervals. The result is expressed in meters or number of shuttles. The SWT is reproducible after one practice test and the heart rate response to the SWT can easily be obtained by the addition of a pulse monitor (e.g. Sportstester or oximeter). The choice of field test depends upon the question that is being asked. The SWT is akin to the standard incremental laboratory test of maximal performance while the 6MWT may reflect more everyday activity which may be influenced by mood. Both are sensitive to interventions but the SWT is more reproducible.

Laboratory exercise testing

Equipment

Although the study of exercise is necessarily more complex than static lung function measurements it can still be achieved simply with a minimum of expensive equipment. Many laboratories now have access to automated systems however, and there is a risk that the results will be accepted without full understanding of the underlying principles. The basic exercise laboratory (Figure 9.2) contains:

- Platforms for exercise (treadmill or cycle).
- Method for measuring ventilation ($\dot{V}_E$).
- Expired gas analysis ($\dot{V}O_2$ and $\dot{V}CO_2$).
- Facilities for estimating arterial blood gases, SaO_2 and blood lactate.
- EKG and BP monitors.
- Dyspnea and fatigue score charts.
- Processing, analysis, presentation, and reporting facilities.
- Resuscitation equipment including a defibrillator and drug box.

There is no universally satisfactory platform for exercise. Most laboratories contain either a cycle ergometer or a treadmill, though both are desirable. In other circumstances the exercise platform may be customized to a different activity such as upper body exercise or rowing to reflect the purpose of the test. For the average laboratory there is no clear choice between a treadmill or cycle ergometer (Table 9.1).

It is desirable to have both platforms: the treadmill is better for obtaining the best performance in healthy people (a larger muscle mass is utilized) but this advantage disappears in patients with severe lung disease where the support of the cycle may become important.[5] A major advantage of the cycle ergometer is the measurement of work rate (in watts [SI] or kg.m.min^{-1} [× 0.163 for conversion to watts]). There are predictions for maximal exercise capacity for men and women as a function of age and height;[6] work rate (watts or kg.m.min^{-1}) can predict $\dot{V}O_2$ and cardiac output to a degree which is useful in clinical situations.

When purchasing a treadmill the belt length is an important consideration, especially if it is intended to test normal subjects or athletes while running, when the treadmill should be the biggest that can be afforded. Similarly, an electronically braked cycle ergometer is useful since it removes the dependence on keeping cadence (pedaling frequency) for sustaining workload. For comparison, patients should be retested on the same platform.

Ventilation ($\dot{V}_E$) is usually measured on either the expiratory or inspiratory side of a one-way valve. Initially, Douglas bags were used to collect expired gas in one minute aliquots and then passed through a dry gas meter. Nowadays, a flow meter such as a pneumotachograph, turbine, or hot wire anemometer is used to record individual breaths. The mechanism for collecting the expired gas should have minimal interference with breathing and may need to be mechanically supported by a headpiece or gantry. In most cases mouthpiece and nose clips will be acceptable but a face mask can be used provided it does not leak. Flow transducers which sense bi-directional flow or volume can be positioned near the mouthpiece, eliminating the need for a non-rebreathing valve and reducing apparatus dead space, but pneumotachograph screens are best placed well away from the mouthpiece because of their dependence on laminar

Table 9.1 Treadmill versus cycle ergometer

	Advantages	Disadvantages
Treadmill	Familiar exercise	Instability
	Higher $\dot{V}O_2$max	No direct measure of work
	Calibration	Cost
Cycle	Stable platform	Lower $\dot{V}O_2$max
	Work measured	Pedalling control
	Safety	Unfamiliar exercise

Figure 9.2 Basic design of a laboratory exercise system

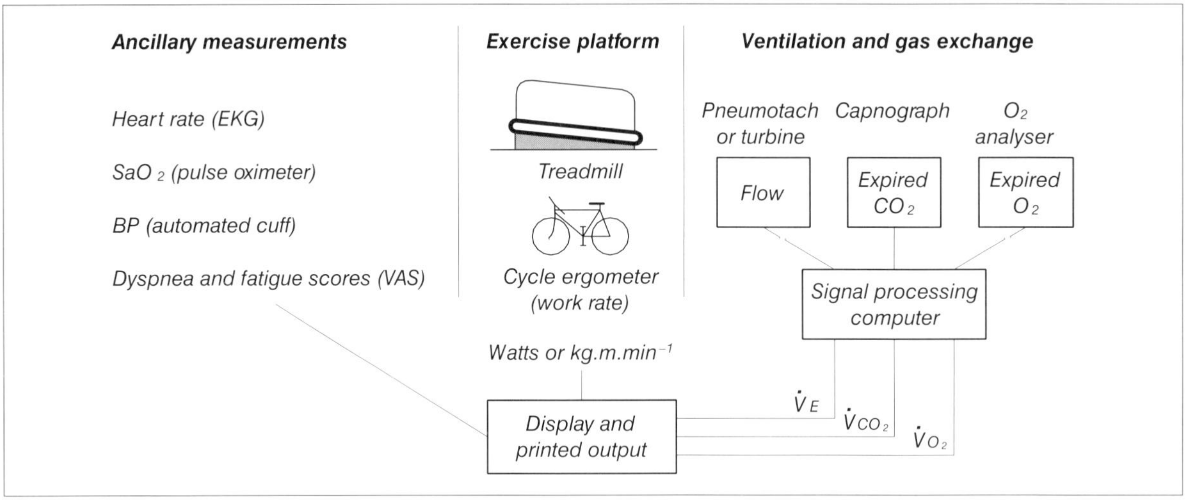

Ancillary measurements
- Heart rate (EKG)
- SaO$_2$ (pulse oximeter)
- BP (automated cuff)
- Dyspnea and fatigue scores (VAS)

Exercise platform
- Treadmill
- Cycle ergometer (work rate)
- Watts or kg.m.min^{-1}

Ventilation and gas exchange
- Pneumotach or turbine → Flow
- Capnograph → Expired CO$_2$
- O$_2$ analyser → Expired O$_2$
- Signal processing computer → $\dot{V}_E$, $\dot{V}_{CO_2}$, $\dot{V}_{O_2}$
- Display and printed output

---

flow regimes and constant temperature (although they are often heated). Sputum impaction affects their performance, so they are often positioned on the inspiratory limb of the circuit and measure inspired ventilation, which differs from expired ventilation except when RER = 1 due to the nitrogen balance.

Expired gas analysis ($\dot{V}_{O_2}$, $\dot{V}_{CO_2}$) is now generally carried out on-line by rapid response analyzers, such as a respiratory mass spectrometer or separate zirconium cell oxygen and infra-red carbon dioxide analyzers. All of these are capable of producing a 'breath-by-breath' $\dot{V}_{O_2}$ and $\dot{V}_{CO_2}$. This is achieved by breaking down each expiration into discrete time intervals (Δt) and computing total breath $\dot{V}_{O_2}$ and $\dot{V}_{CO_2}$ from the sum:

$$\Delta t \times F_E CO_2 \ \{or \ ([F_I - F_E]O_2)\} \times \dot{V}_{exp}$$

where $\dot{V}_{exp}$ is the instantaneous expiratory flow. A correction must be made for the delay between the time at which the gas is sampled at the mouth and the time at which the concentration is measured within the gas analyzer (~ 0.25 s). Slower analyzers can be used with a mixing box downstream but the response time is slow, and breath-by-breath analysis is replacing it. In practice, the breath-by-breath data must be averaged to minimize fluctuations and it is common to present results as 30 or 60 second averages. (For further details and references, consult the ERS Task Force document [Bibliography F].)

Additional measurements should include a record of heart rate, EKG, and blood pressure. The dedicated EKG monitors are usually stabilized to remove motion artifact but separate EKG monitoring can be added for a combined cardiac and respiratory stress test. Blood pressure measurement is easier with an automatic system. Pulse oximetry provides basic information during exercise but care should be taken over the siting of the probe since quality of the signal may deteriorate as exercise progresses. The earlobe may be the most reliable site. Ideally, arterial blood gases should be obtained during the exercise test but the insertion of an arterial cannula may be considered to be excessively invasive. A compromise is to obtain repeated earlobe capillary samples which can also be used for lactate estimation if required. This is obviously easier to perform on the cycle ergometer than the bouncing treadmill though skill and experience are required for both! Some centers have also used

---

Measurements during laboratory exercise tests

- Heart rate (EKG), BP.
- Power output (watts on cycle ergometer).
- Oxygen saturation (SaO$_2$); arterial blood gas analysis (PaO$_2$, P(A–a)O$_2$, PaCO$_2$).
- Minute ventilation ($\dot{V}_E$) and tidal volume and frequency.
- Metabolic gas exchange ($\dot{V}_{O_2}$, $\dot{V}_{CO_2}$, RER).
- Dyspnea and fatigue ratings.

Data presentation

Presentation of exercise data

- Summary sheet containing peak values of $\dot{V}O_2$ (total and ml.kg^{-1}), $\dot{V}_E$, WR, HR, RER, blood gases or pulse oximetry (SpO$_2$), peak lactate, oxygen pulse and anaerobic threshold. Technical comments, including reasons for stopping and possible artifacts.

- Selected plots of continuous output (Figure 9.3)
  $\dot{V}_E$ (ordinate) versus $\dot{V}O_2$ (abscissa) $\dot{V}CO_2$ (ordinate) versus $\dot{V}O_2$ (abscissa)
  RER (ordinate) versus $\dot{V}O_2$ (abscissa)   HR versus $\dot{V}O_2$ (oxygen pulse)
  V_T (ordinate) versus $\dot{V}_E$ PetO$_2$ or PetCO$_2$ versus $\dot{V}O_2$

- Line by line (30 s) numerical output of WR, $\dot{V}O_2$, HR, $\dot{V}_E$, RER accompanied by statements of BP, sensation, and test events.

- *Consult ERS Task Force document (see Bibliography F) for further details of physiology of exercise, equipment requirements and specifications, and data presentation (e.g. Figure 7).*

Figure 9.3 Graphical displays of incremental exercise protocols

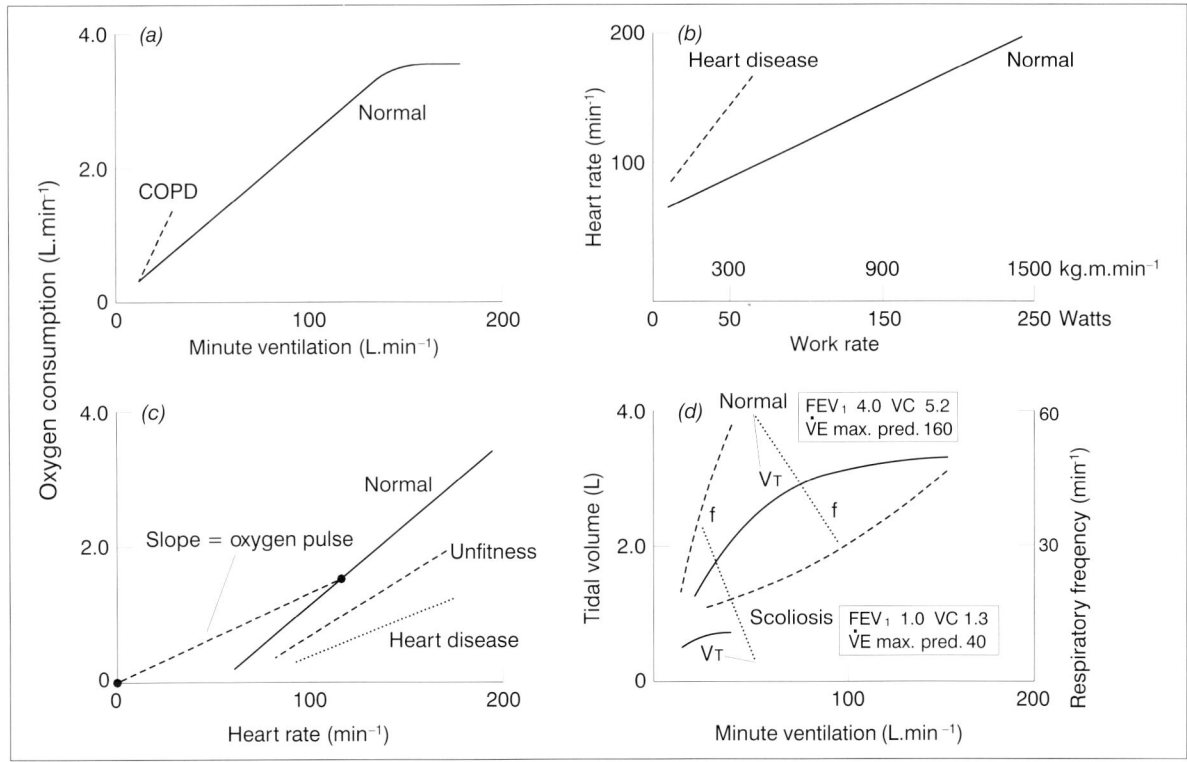

(a) The slope ($\dot{V}O_2/\dot{V}_E$) is the ventilatory equivalent for O_2. In many lung diseases, such as COPD, $\dot{V}O_2$ and $\dot{V}_E$ may be prematurely capped and the high ventilatory equivalent reflects increased oxygen cost of breathing or increased dead space.

(b) Heart rate rises linearly with exercise. In heart disease, there may be a resting tachycardia and a rapid rise in heart rate on exercise associated with an impaired stroke volume response, resulting in a low maximal work rate.

(c) Slope from origin equals oxygen pulse ($\dot{V}O_2/HR$) which may be reduced in physical deconditioning (unfitness) and also in heart disease.

(d) $\dot{V}_E$ increase is associated with a steady rise in tidal volume until V_T reaches about 66% of predicted vital capacity. In chest wall restriction, such as scoliosis, V_T plateau occurs much earlier; further increases in $\dot{V}_E$ occur via a rapid increase in respiratory rate.

transcutaneous blood gas measurements which can follow the trend but need to be calibrated from arterial blood samples for accuracy.

It is important to identify the factors which limit exercise performance throughout the test. This can be achieved by the regular presentation of Borg scales for dyspnea and perceived exertion throughout the test. The Borg scales are particularly suitable for exercise work since they present a categorical description to the subject but can also be scored numerically. Alternatively the 10 cm visual analogue scale (VAS) may be a useful method with the advantage that it could describe any sensation (e.g. How sore are your feet?). The reason for stopping the test (e.g. chest pain, leg fatigue, etc.) should also be recorded.[7] See Chapter 8 for further discussion of breathlessness scoring.

Most modern systems are now automated, and manual analysis is retained only for teachers and enthusiasts. Nevertheless, automated systems which align the signals from the various sources make assumptions which may produce a different result from the manual analysis. The continuous output of an exercise test commonly includes work rate (WR), $\dot{V}O_2$, $\dot{V}CO_2$, V_E, HR, f, V_T, RER, and SaO_2. In addition there are regular statements of BP, blood gases, and sensation. Derivative data such as oxygen pulse, ventilatory equivalent, and anaerobic threshold are also available.

Quality control

Calibration and quality control are important (see Bibliography F). Calibration of the gas analyzers is straightforward and the treadmill speed can be checked with a mark and timer to count the revolutions. Automated exercise systems are very complex and therefore overall quality control can be quite difficult. Ideally, the integrated system results should be compared to a Douglas bag or Tissot spirometer collection of expired gas for separate analysis. This simultaneous collection can be performed during steady state exercise at three levels of $\dot{V}O_2$. In practice this form of quality control is difficult to achieve and an alternative is for laboratory technicians to perform regular multistage tests on themselves, when the acceptable variability is about 6%.

Safety and conduct

Information about the precise risks of respiratory exercise testing is hard to obtain. Patients with lung disease generally discontinue exercise through dyspnea or fatigue before the cardiovascular system is challenged; the risk is likely to be much lower than the mortality rate of 1:10 000 which is quoted for cardiac stress testing. Routine pulmonary function should be measured beforehand. The relative and absolute contraindications for exercise testing (Table 9.2) should be included on the exercise test request form, together with a declaration as to whether physician or technician supervision is necessary. Technician supervision is satisfactory in most cases where there is no relative contraindication, but the laboratory should be fully equipped with resuscitation equipment, and medical support should be readily available. There should normally be two technicians present who are trained in cardiopulmonary resuscitation. Written procedures, understood by all staff, should be kept in the laboratory and regularly reviewed. The necessity for formal written consent is usually a local decision.

The provision of clear written instructions for the subject is very important since most complaints arise from misunderstanding of the test procedure. The information should contain details of the test together with instructions to continue regular medication,

Quality control and safety

- Calibrate gas analyzers and treadmill speed.
- Perform regular biological calibration (self testing).
- Resuscitation must be available.
- Operators must be trained in cardiopulmonary resuscitation (CPR).

Table 9.2 Contra-indications to exercise testing

Absolute:	Febrile illness
	IHD
	Unstable angina
	Aortic stenosis
	Uncontrolled hypertension
	Uncontrolled asthma
	Respiratory failure ($SaO_2 < 85\%$)
Relative:	Epilepsy
	Stable cardiac disease
	Locomotor disorder
	Hypertension
	Mental impairment

wear loose clothes and appropriate footwear, and not to eat immediately prior to the test. Ideally changing and showering facilities should be provided. The endpoint of the test should be explained and appropriate encouragement should be provided. A symptom limited test should be discontinued at the agreed signal with, if possible, a few seconds warning.

Indications to stop the test prematurely include:

- Chest pain
- Faintness or pallor
- Significant EKG abnormalities
- Fall in systolic BP > 20 mmHg from resting value
- Rise in systolic BP to > 250 mmHg (> 120 mmHg diastolic)
- Severe desaturation (SaO_2 < 80% – but check probe!)
- Achievement of maximum predicted HR (discretionary).

Protocols

Laboratory exercise testing has a variety of symptom limited maximal incremental protocols. The details of the protocol are not so important as the need for a steady increase in workload over an optimum period of 6–12 minutes while measurements are made. Most protocols are compromises and increments are usually made at one or three minute intervals, or as a steady, continuous increase (ramp). A true steady state is not generally obtained during each increment. The size of the increment (generally 5–15 watts for a patient with lung disease) should be determined individually for the patient to obtain the optimum length of test. When a true maximal response is required, the final increments can be reduced or suspended while the plateau of $\dot{V}O_2$ is obtained. The protocol should begin with measurements at rest, followed by a three minute warm–up period of unloaded exercise prior to the main protocol, and finish with a similar unloaded cool-down session with recovery measurements. Occasionally, multistage tests with longer duration increments may be useful for quality control or rehabilitation programs. When using the treadmill, the principle of steady, graded exercise should also apply. For that reason the Bruce protocol (Table 9.3) is too steep for patients with lung disease though the abrupt changes are good at provoking angina in others. The more gentle Balke protocol is to be preferred and can be easily modified to suit. The average laboratory will have protocols which strike a balance between familiarity and the individual subject's requirement.

Table 9.3 Exercise protocols

Treadmill	Bruce	3 minute increments ↑ speed and gradient
	Balke	1 minute increments Constant speed ↑ gradient (1–2%)
Cycle	Increment	5–15 watts/min for patients 25–50 watts/min for healthy/athletes
	Ramp	Test time 6–10 minutes

Athletic subjects Athletes with possible respiratory problems may be difficult subjects to study. First, the symptoms may only appear in specific circumstances and, second, they may be unduly sensitive to even a minor loss of performance. Where possible the athlete should be tested on the platform appropriate to the activity, e.g. athletes on the treadmill, cyclists on the cycle, etc. Compared to patients with lung disease or even normal subjects, the athlete may be capable of testing the limits of normal equipment and errors may occur at extremes. Athletes are also more likely to achieve a true $\dot{V}O_2$ max and this can be facilitated by holding the last increment until $\dot{V}O_2$ reaches a plateau. The value of testing serious athletes when problems arise lies in:

- identifying underlying pathology (e.g. asthma, cardiac arrhythmias)
- confirming fitness
- identifying a maximal capacity which is in keeping with the athlete's ambitions.

Normal values

Reference values for exercise performance have to be selected with even more care than those for static lung function tests since they have not been so well standardized. Normal values exist for the common measurements (e.g. $\dot{V}O_2$, $\dot{V}E$, HR, AT) but the selection of the reference populations may differ from your local characteristics.[7-9] In general, $\dot{V}O_2$ max decreases with age but is better preserved in the physically active. When corrected for weight, $\dot{V}O_2$ max is approximately 15% lower in females.

Factors affecting $\dot{V}O_2$max:

Age	Physical fitness
Gender	Population characteristics
Mode of testing	

The reference values are less reliable at the extremes of height and age, and there is debate concerning the effect of obesity which appears to increase the predicted $\dot{V}O_2$ max by 6 ml.kg^{-1} on the cycle. The highest $\dot{V}O_2$ max will normally be achieved on the treadmill, with 10% reduction for cycling or 30% reduction for upper body exercise. Remember, in patients with limitation of exercise not due to $\dot{V}O_2$ max, the platform which produces the best $\dot{V}O_2$ peak may not be predictable but the same apparatus should always be used for retesting. The reference values for children are not yet well developed, and reference values for submaximal performance are also lacking.

Identification of $\dot{V}O_2$max or $\dot{V}O_2$peak

The derivation of maximal oxygen ($\dot{V}O_2$ max) uptake depends upon the demonstration of a plateau of oxygen uptake with continued work to exhaustion. Since this is uncomfortable, it is usually only genuinely achieved in well motivated or athletic subjects. The $\dot{V}O_2$ peak is usually very close to $\dot{V}O_2$ max but a true plateau is seldom seen. It is therefore important to identify whether a test has been completed to maximum effort by the subject before making a judgment about performance.

After a familiarization test, the reproducibility of $\dot{V}O_2$ peak measurement is about 6% in both normal subjects and patients with COPD. The $\dot{V}O_2$ peak is usually expressed as total oxygen uptake (L or ml.min^{-1}) normalized to body weight (ml.min^{-1} kg^{-1}), but lean muscle mass and surface area have also been suggested as alternative denominators.

Indicators of maximum effort

- Plateau of $\dot{V}O_2$ max
- Patient exhaustion
- HR or $\dot{V}E$ close to predicted maximum
- Blood lactate > 4 mM
- Respiratory exchange ratio > 1.2.

Anaerobic (lactate) threshold

The concept and the measurement of the anaerobic threshold (AT) have generated much debate in recent years. The simple premise is that, above a certain work rate threshold, anaerobic metabolism, marked by lactate production, supplements and eventually overtakes aerobic metabolism. The position of this threshold in terms of $\dot{V}O_2$ may be determined by disease or the state of physical fitness and may be an aid to diagnosis and training prescription. The physiological meaning and the relevance of the AT may be debatable but the presence of lactic acidemia is an extremely useful guide to the individual degree of performance. Since lactate can only be assayed retrospectively by invasive arterial or capillary sampling, some non-invasive indicator of the lactate threshold is desirable. If direct evidence of lactic acidemia is required, however, a single earlobe capillary sample, taken 2 minutes post exercise, will suffice.

Non-invasive measures of anaerobic threshold are based upon the observation that CO_2 production increases as lactate is buffered by bicarbonate. This can be recognized by a number of methods of inspection of the $\dot{V}O_2$, $\dot{V}CO_2$ and $\dot{V}E$ patterns. Of the several methods, a change in slope on a plot of $\dot{V}CO_2$ vs $\dot{V}O_2$ (Figure 9.4a) is the most popular because it can be calculated manually and is now incorporated in most computerized systems.[10] There are discrepancies between different methods of detecting the slope change reproducibly in the same patients; these are the result of both experimental and observer error. When the AT is obtained from the automated analysis it is important to check that it appears to be sensible compared to the $\dot{V}O_2/\dot{V}CO_2$ plot. There is also an alternative, but time consuming, method which involves multiple 6 minute, steady state exercise tests at different levels to identify the continuous rise in $\dot{V}O_2$ that occurs once the level is above the anaerobic threshold (Figure 9.4b).

The AT is expressed as a percentage of $\dot{V}O_2$ max and may vary from 40–60%, depending on the degree of physical conditioning. An anaerobic threshold of < 40% may indicate cardiac disease but the distinction from deconditioning (lack of fitness) may be so difficult that interpretation algorithms which are entirely dependent on AT should be viewed with caution. In lung disease, where patients are limited by ventilation, the detection of AT may be difficult. Only 25–50% of patients with moderate to severe COPD demonstrate an anaerobic threshold, and it is usually absent in severe disease. For these reasons, the AT should be used with circumspection when making clinical decisions in patients with lung disease.

Anaerobic threshold

- Detects the $\dot{V}O_2$ threshold for increased lactate production.
- Is usually identified as the 'break' in the linear $\dot{V}O_2/\dot{V}CO_2$ plot.
- AT normally occurs at 40–60% of predicted $\dot{V}O_2$ max.
- May rise with training and fall with age.
- AT < 40% predicted $\dot{V}O_2$ max is seen in cardiac disease.
- AT may not be recorded in severe lung disease.

Ventilatory limit

In healthy subjects, ventilation increases with oxygen uptake and is not limiting. The increase in ventilation is achieved at first mainly by a rise in tidal volume, due to both a reduction in the end-expiratory lung volume and an increase in end-inspired volume, until V_T reaches a plateau at approximately two thirds of the VC. Further increase in $\dot{V}_E$ is achieved by an increase in respiratory rate. The maximum ventilatory capacity is the highest ventilation that can be achieved under the operating physiological conditions. A ventilatory limitation means that the subject cannot increase alveolar or total ventilation any further in response to demand. When ventilation is compromised by lung disease, the patients predicted maximum ventilation is reached at a

Figure 9.4 Derivation of anaerobic threshold (healthy subject)

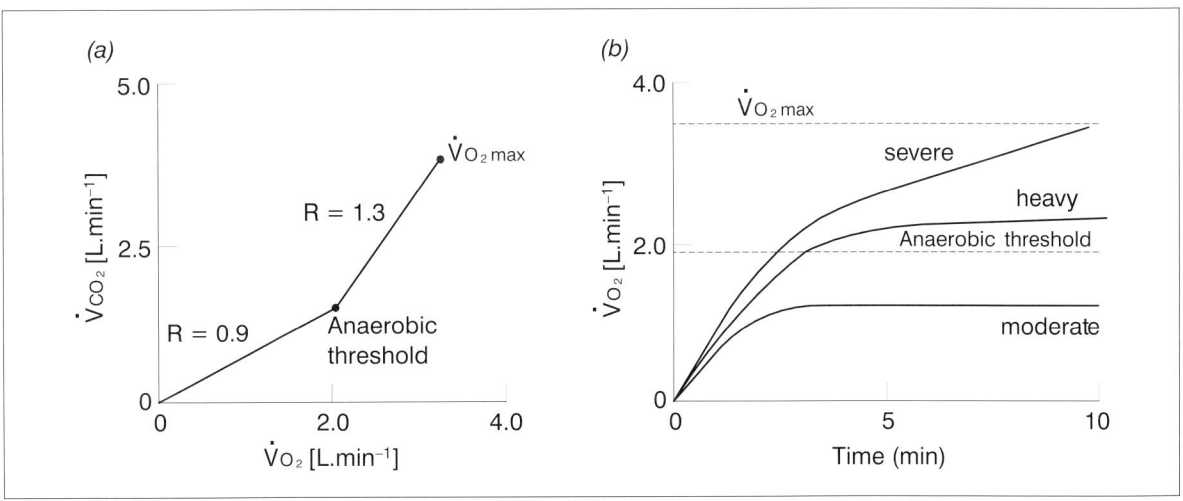

(a) In incremental exercise the AT is usually obtained from the inflexion on the $\dot{V}O_2/\dot{V}CO_2$ plot.

(b) AT can also be derived from a series of constant load exercise tests at moderate, heavy and severe work intensities; a plateau of $\dot{V}O_2$ occurs below the AT, but a continuous rise in $\dot{V}O_2$ is seen above the anaerobic threshold. At severe work intensity, $\dot{V}O_2$ max is reached even though higher work rates could have been achieved on shorter incremental test protocols.

time when the heart rate is considerably less than its maximum, i.e. heart rate reserves greatly exceed ventilatory reserves. The maximum ventilatory capacity on exercise can be predicted from measurements of maximum voluntary ventilation (MVV) or FEV_1 at rest.

> **Identification of ventilatory limit to exercise**
>
> ■ $\dot{V}_E$max > 80% $\dot{V}_E$max.$_{pred}$
>
> ■ Ventilatory reserve ($\dot{V}_E$max.$_{pred}$ − $\dot{V}_E$max) < 11 L.min^{-1}
>
> ■ V_T > 50–70% of VC
>
> ■ Breathing frequency > 50 min^{-1}.

The calculation of predicted $\dot{V}_E$max is obviously critical to the identification of a ventilatory limit but it is controversial. $\dot{V}_E$max can be calculated from a measurement of isocapnic MVV over 4 minutes or extrapolated from a 12–15 s non-isocapnic 'sprint' measurement, or calculated indirectly from the FEV_1. There have been several recommendations for calculating $\dot{V}_E$max; $FEV_1 \times 40$ seems to be suitable for normal subjects, but it underestimates exercise ventilation in subjects with airflow obstruction and a severely reduced FEV_1. In COPD, there are theoretical reasons why maximal exercise ventilation should differ from predictions made at rest because of the occurrence of dynamic hyperinflation during exercise (see Chapter 1). In patients with interstitial lung disease, maximum flow-volume loops at rest have been compared with tidal flow-volume loops on maximal exercise, taking into account changes of end-expiratory lung volume.[11] These may provide better prediction of $\dot{V}_E$max but are not yet routine.

Submaximal testing

Submaximal exercise testing is not as popular as maximal testing but may have some important roles in both the laboratory and the field. In the laboratory there may be several uses for single or multistage submaximal testing, including:

- laboratory quality control
- precise determinations of AT
- investigation of gas exchange kinetics
- investigation of endurance exercise
- more sensitive assessment of treatment
- provocation of exercise induced asthma.

The repeated assessment of submaximal exercise is a more sensitive indicator of improvement after treatment in patients with lung disease since the factors which produce a ventilatory limit to *maximal* exercise are unlikely to be improved. Repeated testing at a proportion of $\dot{V}O_2$ peak (e.g. 50% $\dot{V}O_2$peak) can demonstrate dramatic improvements. In fact, patients with chronic lung disease are able to sustain a relatively higher *percentage* of their $\dot{V}O_2$ peak than normal subjects.[12] Submaximal performance after training in more healthy subjects may be assessed at the same relative proportion of either the original or the current $\dot{V}O_2$max.

CLINICAL SITUATIONS

Ventilatory limitation is characteristic of many respiratory diseases but the individual mechanisms may be varied and multiple. For example, in COPD the increased airway resistance, coupled to the hyperventilation of exercise, may lead to hyperinflation which increases the elastic work of breathing and shortens inspiratory muscle fiber length and the efficiency of contraction. By contrast, in interstitial lung disease, the ventilatory limit may be reached because of loss of lung volume; in addition, hypoxemia may occur from a restricted pulmonary microcirculation (a low D_{LCO}) leading to increased capillary transit time. It is difficult to predict the limits to exercise in individual patients with lung disease without testing them, and several mechanisms may coexist.

Cardiac versus lung disease

The distinction between cardiac and pulmonary limitation is a common clinical dilemma made more difficult by the frequent coexistence of the two conditions. One obvious pointer to cardiac disease is the termination of the test by chest pain, arrhythmia or EKG abnormality. The heart rate responses provide important evidence for cardiac disease with high resting rate, excessive rise with work, and early achievement of HR max (prediction: 220 min^{-1} minus age in years). The oxygen pulse (oxygen uptake per heart beat [$\dot{V}O_2$/HR]) is an indirect reflection of stroke volume and is reduced in cardiac failure (Table 9.4).

Table 9.4 Distinction between cardiac and lung disease

	Cardiac limitation	Pulmonary limitation
At peak exercise		
$\dot{V}O_2$	Reduced	Reduced
Oxygen pulse	Reduced	Slightly reduced
Anaerobic threshold	Reduced	Normal or not reached
Heart rate reserve	Low	High
SaO_2	No fall	May fall

It may be difficult to distinguish cardiac disease from poor performance due to unfitness, though both may be present. The value of exercise testing in cardiac disease lies in the differential diagnosis as well as the assessment of function in patients with cardiac failure or transplantation.

Exercise testing for preoperative evaluation

Preoperative assessment before thoracic surgery is discussed in Chapter 15. Exercise testing may have value in the emphysematous patient with borderline function who is being considered for lung volume reduction surgery. 200 m on the 6MWT or 180 m on the SWT have been suggested as the lowest acceptable values for surgery. For pulmonary resection (lobectomy or pneumonectomy) patients with $FEV_1 <$ 50% predicted should undergo maximal exercise testing.[14] Where the $\dot{V}O_2$ peak is greater than 75% predicted the risk is low; a $\dot{V}O_2$ peak below 60% predicted carries excessive risk[13].

Asthma

Activity-induced bronchospasm immediately after strenuous exercise occurs in the majority of patients with asthma and may be the only symptom in some. It may also remain a problem when asthma is otherwise adequately treated. Exercise testing has a role in identifying the condition and assessing treatment.

Exercise testing can confirm the presence of asthma in patients who complain of wheeze and breathlessness occurring with or after exertion. Formal demonstration of a fall in PEF or $FEV_1 > 15\%$ baseline after exercise is significant. The recommended protocol is a warm-up period followed by at least 4 minutes of treadmill exercise at an intensity of at least 40–60% $\dot{V}_Emax$ or 80% HR max.[15] There is initial bronchodilatation during exercise so FEV_1 should be measured at five minute intervals for at least 30 minutes post exercise. Although short-burst running is a potent stimulus for bronchoconstriction in asthmatic subjects, the conditions of the laboratory may still not recreate the exact cold, damp sporting environment. The shuttle running test and peak flow meter is a useful alternative for field use. Tests can be repeated to study the effects of treatment. (See the ERS Task Force document [Bibliography F] for more details on the assessment of exercise-induced bronchoconstriction.)

Abnormalities of gas exchange during exercise can be demonstrated for up to one month after an acute severe asthmatic attack, but most exercise intolerance in patients when in remission is due to lack of physical fitness rather than asthma per se.[14]

THE INTERPRETATION AND REPORTING OF EXERCISE TESTS

The interpretation of complex cardiorespiratory exercise tests is often more difficult than the measurement itself. If the exercise test was done to assess performance, the result of the appropriate field test is quoted, assuming the correct habituation or practice tests have been performed.

There is no standardization of interpretation of the symptom limited maximal laboratory test. There are two broad approaches. First, the algorithm or flow-chart approach, primarily recommended by Wasserman, takes the interpreter through paths determined by the $\dot{V}O_2$ max and AT. This method has the advantage that it can be automated but the disadvantage that clinical decisions may rely heavily on the single measurement of anaerobic threshold. The alternative is the recognition of different patterns of abnormality associated with distinctive pathologies (see Table 9.5).

Patterns of abnormal response to maximal exercise in different conditions

Table 9.5	$\dot{V}O_2$peak	AT as % pred $\dot{V}O_2$max	$\dot{V}_E$ reserve	$\dot{V}_E/\dot{V}O_2$	ΔSaO_2	O_2 pulse $\dot{V}O_2$/HR	HR reserve
Cardiac disease (chest pain may limit)	Low	Low	High	High	No fall	Low	Low/nil
Pulmonary vascular disease	Low	Low	High	High	Fall	Low	Low/nil
Airway obstruction	Low	Normal/absent	Low/nil	High	May fall	Normal/low	High
Interstitial lung disease	Low	Normal/low	Low	High	Fall	Normal/low	High/normal
Chest wall restriction	Low	Normal/absent	Low	High	Fall	Normal	High
Unfitness	Low	Normal/low	Normal/high	High	No fall	Low	Normal
Poor effort	Low	Normal/absent	High	Normal	No fall	Normal	High

HR reserve: (HR max predicted – HR max exercise); $\dot{V}_E$ reserve: ($\dot{V}_E$ max predicted – $\dot{V}_E$ max exercise)

Normal response to peak exercise

$\dot{V}O_2$
$\dot{V}O_2$ max > 84% predicted
AT > 40% $\dot{V}O_2$ max pred

Ventilation
$\dot{V}_E$max/$\dot{V}_E$max pred > 0.75
Ventilatory reserve [$\dot{V}_E$max pred – $\dot{V}_E$max]
   > 11 L. min^{-1}
Breathing frequency < 50 min^{-1}

Cardiac
Oxygen pulse > 80% predicted
Heart rate reserve
   [HR max pred – HR max ex] < 15 min^{-1}
BP < 220/90 mmHg

In view of the complexity of the response to exercise, it is difficult to identify a single value which implies normality if achieved. The pattern outlined in the shaded box would suggest a normal response:

It is important to realize that these values are context specific. For example, you would expect a club athlete to have a $\dot{V}O_2$max well in excess of 100 % predicted.

Interpretative questions

Cooperation and motivation

The identification of maximal effort has already been described. How does one distinguish subjects who stop prematurely through lack of conditioning or motivation, or malingering? In the first two categories, the cardiorespiratory responses are usually normal up until the break point. In addition to premature failure, patients who are very anxious or malingering fail to reach AT and demonstrate hyperventilation, breath-holding and variable RER.

Reason for stopping

It is important to ask this question since the answer (chest or leg pain) may not relate to cardiopulmonary fitness. If there is no clear answer when the performance is subnormal, the pattern of physiological response may suggest the reason.

Physiological response

The graphical and tabulated data must be inspected (Table 9.5). If the responses are completely within normal limits until submaximal discontinuation the reason is likely to be poor effort. Other patterns of response are characteristic of different diseases. These patterns relate to values achieved at peak exercise and a more considered analysis will involve examination of steady state submaximal performance. This is obtained either from visual inspection of the graphs or by comparison at fixed points. A $\dot{V}O_2$ of 1.0 L.min^{-1} and the $\dot{V}E$ of 30 L.min^{-1} have been proposed as suitable levels to measure.

CONCLUSIONS

Exercise testing in lung disease offers the opportunity to examine the response of the cardiorespiratory system under circumstances which recreate the patient's symptoms. This form of examination can assess disability and progress as well as determining cause.

In summary:

- The assessment of disability in lung disease should be objective to be accurate.
- Progressive work rate tests are more reproducible but do not reflect 'real life' activity.
- Submaximal tests are more sensitive to changes following treatment.
- Unpaced tests may underestimate true capacity.
- Field tests (generally walking) provide a cheap and practical assessment of disability in rehabilitation programs.

Bibliography

A Wasserman K, Hansen JE, Sue DY, Whipp BJ, Casaburi R. *Principles of Exercise Testing and Interpretation*, 2nd edn. Philadelphia: Lea and Febiger 1994.

B Whipp BJ, Wasserman K (eds) *Exercise: Pulmonary Physiology and Pathophysiology. Lung Biology in Health and Disease*, Vol. 52. New York: Marcel Dekker 1991.

C Weisman IM, Zeballos RJ (eds) *Clinical Exercise Testing*. Clinics in Chest Medicine, Vol. 15 (2). Philadelphia: W B Saunders 1994.

D Jones NL. *Clinical Exercise Testing*, 3rd edn. Philadelphia: W B Saunders 1988.

E Belman MJ. Exercise in patients with chronic obstructive pulmonary disease. *Thorax* 1993; **48**: 936–46.

F Roca J, Whipp BJ *et al*. Clinical exercise testing with reference to lung diseases: indications, standardization and interpretation strategies. ERS Task Force Report. *Eur Respir J* 1997; **10**: 2662–89.

References

1 Cotes JE, Zedja J & King B. Lung function impairment as a guide to exercise limitation in work-related lung disorders. *Am Rev Respir Dis* 1988; **137**: 1089–93.

2 Ortega F, Montemayor T, Sanchez A, Cabello F, Castillo J. Role of cardiopulmonary exercise testing and the criteria used to determine disability in patients with severe chronic obstructive pulmonary disease. *Am J Respir Crit Care Med* 1994; **150**: 747–51.

3 Singh SJ, Morgan MDL, Hardman AE, Rowe C, Bardsley PA. Comparison of oxygen uptake during conventional treadmill test and shuttle walk test in patients with chronic airflow limitation. *Eur Resp J* 1994; **7**: 2016–20.

4 Leger LA, Lambert JA. Maximal multi-stage 20m shuttle run test to predict VO$_2$ max. *Eur J Appl Physiol* 1982; **49**: 1–12.

5 Mathur RS, Revill SM, Vara DD, Walton RM, Morgan MDL. Comparison of peak oxygen consumption during cycle and treadmill exercise in severe chronic obstructive pulmonary disease. *Thorax* 1995; **50**: 829–33.

6 Jones NL, Makrides L, Hitchcock C *et al*. Normal standards for an incremental progressive cycle ergometer test. *Am Rev Respir Dis* 1985; **131**: 700–8.

7 Killian KJ, Leblanc P, Martin DH, Summers E, Jones NL, Campbell EJM. Exercise capacity and ventilatory, circulatory, and symptom limitation in patients with chronic airflow limitation. *Am Rev Respir Dis* 1992; **146**: 935–40.

8 Jones NL, Summers E, Killian KJ. Influence of age on exercise capacity during incremental cycle ergometry in men and women. *Am Rev Respir Dis* 1989; **140**: 1373–80.

9 Hansen JE, Sue DY, Wasserman K. Predicted values for clinical exercise testing. *Am Rev Respir Dis* 1984; **129**: S49–55.

10 Sue DY, Wasserman K, Moricca RB *et al*. Metabolic acidosis during exercise in patients with chronic obstructive pulmonary disease. Use of v-slope method for anaerobic threshold determination. *Chest* 1988; **94**: 931–8.

11 Marciniuk DD, Sridhar G, Clemens RE, Zintel TA, Gallagher CG. Lung volumes and expiratory flow limitation during exercise in interstitial lung disease. *J Appl Physiol* 1994; **77**: 963–73.
12 Punzal PA, Ries AL, Kaplan RM, Prewitt LM. Maximum intensity exercise training in patients with chronic obstructive pulmonary disease. *Chest* 1991; **100**: 618–23.
13 Bolliger CT, Jordan P, Soler M *et al.* Exercise capacity as a predictor of postoperative complications in lung resection candidates. *Am J Respir Crit Care Med* 1995; **151**:1472–80
14 Garfinkel SK, Kesten S, Chapman KR *et al.* Physiological and non-physiological determinants of aerobic fitness in mild to moderate asthma. *Am Rev Respir Dis* 1992; **145**: 741–5.
15 Sterk PJ, Fabbri LM, Quanjer PhH *et al.* Airway responsiveness. In: Standardised lung function testing. *Eur Resp J* 1993; **6**: (Suppl 16), 64–6.

Section III
APPLICATIONS OUTSIDE THE ROUTINE LABORATORY

10 Sleep-Disordered Breathing
J R Stradling

- **INTRODUCTION**
- **THE OBSTRUCTIVE SLEEP APNEA SYNDROME**
  What is obstructive sleep apnea?
  Pharyngeal narrowing and collapse
  The spectrum of upper airway narrowing
  Predisposing factors
  Why treat obstructive sleep apnea?
  How is sleep apnea defined?
- **THE PERFORMANCE OF RESPIRATORY SLEEP STUDIES**
  What are the essential features?
  What techniques are available to measure inspiratory effort?
  Snoring
  Flow limitation on inspiration
  Abdominal versus rib cage movements
  Intrathoracic effects on blood pressure
  What techniques are available to measure sleep fragmentation?
  Assessment of body movement
  Arousal-induced blood pressure changes
- **CLINICAL APPLICATIONS**
  Approach to respiratory sleep studies
  How is the sleep study used to guide clinical management?
  Treatment of obstructive sleep apnea
  Trial of continuous positive airway pressure
- **CONCLUSIONS**

INTRODUCTION

Sleep medicine is a new area in respiratory clinical practice, particularly in the United Kingdom. Although a few neurologists and psychiatrists have long been interested in sleep, there was only limited value to studying it in terms of making a diagnosis and designing treatment. The recognition of a common, disabling, and treatable respiratory condition, obstructive sleep apnea (OSA), has changed all this.[1]

The demand for sleep studies has risen astronomically and this rise is due to the requirement for respiratory sleep studies looking for OSA and its variants. Respiration during sleep has become an exciting new area in respiratory physiology, able to utilize many older techniques but in a new field. The diagnostic and therapeutic workload is largely undertaken by respiratory departments because this is a disorder of the upper airway and breathing; it can interact with lung disease to produce respiratory failure,[2] and its treatment involves an understanding of respiratory physiology. In many respiratory units the investigation and management of these patients devolves upon lung function technicians or specially trained nurses. It is the author's view that where this happens there still needs to be significant consultant input into sleep study reporting and decisions over treatment. This is because there are many clinical decisions to be made that cannot be based simply on numbers generated from a sleep study.

Although clear guidelines can be drawn up for the provision and use of lung function tests (and equipment specifications) this is unfortunately not yet the case for the investigation of sleep related breathing disorders because our understanding of them is at present incomplete.

THE OBSTRUCTIVE SLEEP APNEA SYNDROME

What is obstructive sleep apnoea?

Pharyngeal narrowing and collapse

Obstructive sleep apnea and its variants are due to failure of the pharyngeal airway to maintain adequate patency during sleep. This means that the pharyngeal airway narrows with sleep onset, initially producing harsh inspiratory breathing with some evidence of inspiratory flow limitation (Figure 10.1), then with further narrowing snoring is generated, and finally there is complete collapse which produces a full apnea. This narrowing is mainly retroglossal but occasionally can be at the palatal level. The body's main defense against this upper airway narrowing is to arouse and reactivate the upper airway muscles to allow adequate airflow once more. The stimulus for this arousal appears to be mainly the increased inspiratory effort that the respiratory center generates in response to the increased respiratory loading and deterioration in blood gases.[3] Thus complete apnea is not necessary to produce an arousal, only the generation of increased inspiratory effort which can occur during snoring alone, and occasionally even without snoring, particularly in women.[4]

The pharyngeal lumen is surrounded by many muscles with geometrically complex shapes and actions: functioning in concert, most of them defend

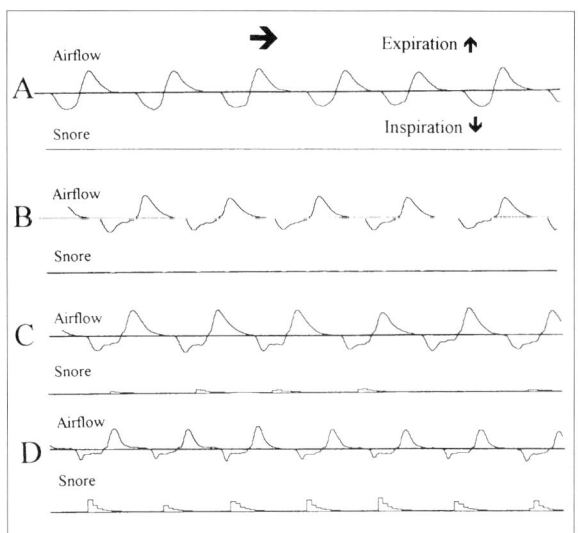

Figure 10.1 Development of inspiratory flow limitation during sleep

A. Non-flow limited inspiration (downwards), left to right, horizontal line is zero flow. The inspiratory flow profile is rounded and there is no snoring (lower line).

B. Flow limitation just developing with 'scalloping' of the latter half of the inspiratory flow curve; snoring has not yet developed.

C. Inspiratory flow limitation is more severe and snoring is now appearing.

D. Severe flow limitation with only a brief inspiratory spike of flow with a plateau thereafter, in association with louder snoring (synchronous with flow limitation).

Recorded with nasal pressure probe and throat microphone, RM50 recorder, Parametric Recorders, London, UK.

pharyngeal patency by dilating (e.g. genioglossus, stylopharyngeus) or stiffening the walls (e.g. the pharyngeal constrictors). Although a primary failure of these muscles was originally thought to be a common cause of OSA, it is now realized that these muscles are actually working harder than normal to defend the compromised airway both awake and asleep.

The spectrum of upper airway narrowing

Slight pharyngeal narrowing is seen in normal people at sleep onset, although there is a spectrum of responsiveness;[5] further narrowing produces inspiratory flow limitation, then snoring, and finally full sleep apnea. They are all on a continuum of pharyngeal incompetence during sleep (Figure 10.2). The two easily and clearly identifiable points on this con-

Figure 10.2 Progression of upper airway narrowing

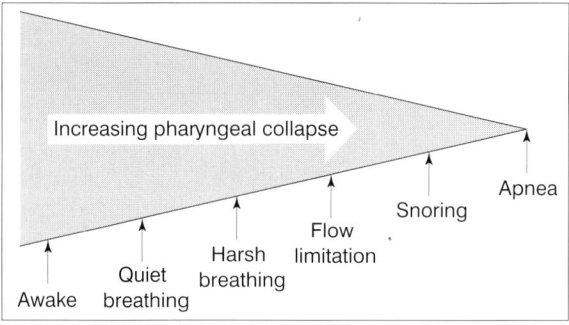

As pharynx narrows from awake state to sleep, breathing becomes noisier and, in sequence, flow limitation, snoring, and finally apnea occur.

Figure 10.3 Progression to symptomatic sleep apnea as age and weight increase

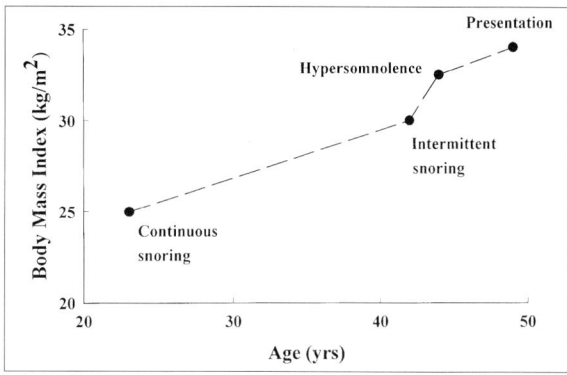

Retrospective survey of 118 patients. Typical story is of presentation to a sleep clinic at 50 years old having gained 40% in weight since age 22 years, with a 28 year history of snoring, intermittent in the last 9 years, and with symptoms of hypersomnolence for 6 years. (Redrawn from Lugaresi et al.)[8]

tinuum are the onset of snoring and complete airway closure. The existence of these two specific points on the spectrum tends to obscure a realization that the underlying pathology is continuously distributed and that individuals can move up and down this spectrum depending on such factors as body weight, alcohol consumption, sleep deprivation, sleeping posture, hormone status (especially thyroid), and age. Age and body weight are probably the dominant factors that produce evolution across this spectrum (Figure 10.3).

Predisposing factors

Increasing body weight provokes OSA, probably through increased fat deposition in the neck.[6] This is likely to act through external pressure on the pharynx, producing both a reduction in starting size of the pharynx (so that it is already narrowed even during wakefulness) and also an extra load which the pharyngeal dilators can no longer fend off when their tone is reduced at sleep onset. Subtle changes in the shape of the lower face (essentially a retropositioned lower jaw) can also narrow the upper airway and may be the factor that produces the inherited tendency to OSA.[7] Other important factors are significantly enlarged tonsils, hypothyroidism, and acromegaly.

Many studies have demonstrated differences in the shape of both bony and soft tissues of the head and neck between normal subjects and those with OSA. For example, lateral head radiographs (cephalometry) demonstrate a relative downward and backward positioning of the mandible. However the overlap between normal subjects and patients with OSA is considerable. These measurements are therefore useful for research studies on the pathogenesis of OSA, but rarely help in its clinical investigation. For example, such measurements have not been shown to diagnose OSA with any accuracy, or to usefully predict the outcome of surgical treatments.

Predisposing factors for obstructive sleep apnea

- Obese middle-aged male
- Retropositioning of lower jaw
- Large tonsils
- Crowded pharynx
- High alcohol/sedative consumption

Why treat obstructive sleep apnea?

Just as it is impossible for normal awake people to hold their breath for a dangerous length of time, it is also usually the case that during sleep patients do not stop breathing for dangerous lengths of time. Each episode of apnea in its own right is very rarely a dangerous event, what is important is that too many of them provoke arousals and produce symptoms worthy of treatment. This is true in the vast majority of patients unless the resulting hypoxemia is very considerable (SaO_2 < 60%) and associated with ischemic heart disease, when significant arrhythmias can be generated. Thus treatment for obstructive sleep apnea and its variants is instituted largely for its symptoms of gross sleep fragmentation, i.e. daytime sleepiness, poor concentration, low quality of life, and driving accidents through falling asleep at the wheel.[9] Although much has been written recently on the cardiovascular consequences of obstructive sleep apnea (heart attacks, strokes, etc.), there is still no good evidence that such possible sequelae should be considered when deciding whether to treat someone for OSA,[10] with the exception of nocturnal angina.

The obstructive sleep apnea *syndrome* should be thought of as the combination of recurrent obstructive events leading to arousal at night, *combined* with significant daytime symptoms due to this sleep fragmentation. Epidemiological surveys trying to assess the prevalence of OSA have often failed to grasp this fundamental point. In the most widely quoted prevalence study, the occurrence of recurrent apneas at night was astonishingly high. However, the occurrence of daytime sleepiness in this subgroup of the population was not significantly higher than in the rest of the population.[11] Of course, daytime sleepiness can be due to many other causes, most commonly shift work, depression, alcohol and coffee abuse, and, less commonly, narcolepsy.

The problem of poor association between sleep study findings and symptomatic disease in OSA has made assessment of the true prevalence, and thus the health burden, of this condition very difficult. Recent studies have estimated that perhaps 0.5–2% of middle-aged men have significant symptomatic disease worthy of treatment.[12] This is an enormous number of patients and probably explains why, despite a considerable expansion of sleep study facilities in many countries, there are usually long waiting lists for their services.

Consequences of obstructive sleep apnea

- Sleep fragmentation
- Daytime sleepiness
- Poor concentration and vigilance
- Driving accidents

How is sleep apnea defined?

Our understanding of the relationship between daytime symptoms and the features on the sleep study that cause them is so poor that it is unrealistic to expect current investigative techniques to provide clear answers in all cases. There are fixed definitions of OSA based on, for example, the numbers of apneas of a certain length (usually 10 seconds) occurring per hour of sleep. Consequently arousals due to heavy snoring are missed. How many apneas should there be to justify a trial of CPAP, especially when the number occurring can vary enormously from night to night, particularly in the moderate sufferers?

If we abandon an approach based on indirect and unreliable numerical measures, what are the alternatives? In the author's view obstructive sleep apnea (OSA) and its variants (heavy snoring with arousals, upper airway resistance syndrome) should be defined as *symptomatic sleep disturbance due to pharyngeal incompetence during sleep*, or 'hypnogogic stenosis' as Lugaresi called it. This definition requires the association of relevant symptoms gathered during history taking, combined with reasonable evidence on a sleep study that sleep is being disrupted through upper airway narrowing. We find the Epworth Sleepiness score quite useful as a simple measure of a patient's daytime sleepiness. This score asks about tendency to fall asleep in eight situations of varying stimulation (e.g. watching television, talking to someone). Each situation is graded 'never', 'slight', 'moderate', or 'high', ascribed the numbers 0 to 3 respectively, and totaled. A score of less than 9 is regarded as within the normal range; most OSA patients score in the teens. As there is a poor association between nocturnal events and daytime symptoms, it is not possible to set reliable thresholds to sleep indices that will indicate whether an individual's symptoms are, or are not, due to upper airway induced arousals. Hence no 'numbers' are attached to this working definition. How to handle this uncertainty will be discussed later.

THE PERFORMANCE OF RESPIRATORY SLEEP STUDIES

What are the essential features?

Early approaches to assessing sleep disordered breathing stressed the identification of obstructive versus central apneas. The former were due to upper airway collapse and the latter to failure of inspiratory drive. Much apparent central apnea, present in individuals with primarily obstructive events, is secondary. For example, each arousal caused by an obstruction can lead to brief hyperventilation with hypocapnia which provokes a central apnea when sleep is quickly re-established, the so-called mixed apnea. Sometimes upper airway collapse provokes a reflex cessation of inspiratory effort which is by definition central but 'obstructive' in origin. Thus the counting of central versus obstructive apneas is rarely clinically useful.[13] Most primary central apneas occur in patients with primary disorders of ventilatory control (damage to the brain stem for example) and neuromuscular disorders, and they usually present very different clinical features. The important exception is the central apnea/periodic respiration of heart failure (Cheyne-Stokes breathing). These individuals can have secondarily obstructed airways at the end of each primary central apnea (passive collapse due to withdrawal of inspiratory drive) and this may cause diagnostic confusion; once again, the history should help sort out the real diagnosis, although a repeat sleep study on nasal continuous positive airway pressure (NCPAP) is sometimes required to remove any obstructive component and see what is left.

Earlier on it was mentioned that the stimulus to arousal was probably the increase in inspiratory effort generated in response to the added upper airway resistance.[3] This cannot be the only arousal stimulus since in central apnea, where no inspiratory effort is made, hypoxemia is probably the arousal stimulus. In most situations, therefore, it would be useful to have a measure of inspiratory effort, and indeed some laboratories routinely use some form of esophageal pressure monitoring as a consequence. Many of the monitoring systems in use measure respiratory effort, but only very indirectly. Traditionally, respiratory 'effort' is assessed from rib cage and abdominal movement transducers to identify any apneas and whether they are *central* (no signal) or *obstructive* (inspiratory paradox signal). An alternative would be to measure upper airway resistance itself, although this is still once removed from the arousing stimulus of increased inspiratory effort. One way or another, a sleep study system needs to measure, or infer, inspiratory effort and a later section deals with the many ways in which this could be done.

The other important information to derive from a respiratory sleep study is sleep quality. This was originally done through classic sleep staging of electroencephalogram (EEG) tracings. However, now that sleep fragmentation is realized to be the most important cause of poor sleep leading to daytime symptoms, several other approaches are being explored that may turn out to be as good as, if not better than, EEG based techniques.

Important variables in a sleep study

- A measure of sleep fragmentation
- A measure of (increased) inspiratory effort
- A measure of hypoxemia

What techniques are available to measure inspiratory effort?

Snoring

Increases in inspiratory effort, or the upper airway narrowing that provoked it, can be measured by several different approaches. Snoring itself is an indicator of a narrowing of the upper airway but does not necessarily imply increased effort and hence not all snoring leads to sleep disturbance. This has occurred after surgery to reconstruct the soft palate (uvulopalatopharyngoplasty [UPPP]) for snoring or sleep apnea. Conversely, maybe more so in women, significant upper airway narrowing and inspiratory flow limitation with increased inspiratory effort can occur without snoring – only harsher breath sounds.[4] Despite these limitations, snoring still remains a highly valuable signal to monitor, particularly since it is so easy to perform, although there are problems with quantitative measurements and calibration.

Flow limitation on inspiration

Inspiratory flow limitation[14] can be detected fairly consistently by looking at the profile of the inspiratory flow curve (Figure 10.1). Just as in standard flow volume loops, a flattening of the inspiratory flow profile indicates flow limitation in the upper airway. This can be measured by a tight-fitting face mask and pneumotachograph, or almost as well by a pressure probe inserted into the nasal entrance. The square root of this pressure signal looks very similar to a pneumotachograph tracing (see Figure 10.1), and yields the same information about inspiratory flow limitation. Using a thermistor to measure airflow produces too damped a signal and does not allow an estimation of airflow limitation.

Abdominal versus rib cage movements

Asynchronous movement of the abdomen and rib cage often implies increased effort due to upper airway inspiratory loading.[15] This is because the power of the diaphragm and of the intercostal muscles are rarely equal and, under load, one or the other will lead during inspiration (so-called 'phase shift'). During complete apneas of course the movement of these two compartments is equal and opposite (in terms of volume) – so-called 'respiratory paradox'. Unfortunately, the quality of these surface measurements can be severely impaired in the very obese.

Transducers are available that measure inward drawing of the suprasternal notch or supraclavicular fossa. When there is increased effort these surfaces are sucked harder into the chest and follow inspiratory effort. These measurements can only be regarded as qualitative and also work less well in the obese. A bed, from which electrostatic charges can be recorded, may serve as a movement monitor, one derivative being the fast component of rib cage and abdominal movements present during obstructed breathing; this might prove to be a useful signal to monitor.

Intrathoracic effects on blood pressure

An alternative approach is to utilize a physiological correlate of swings in intrathoracic pressure – the beat-to-beat blood pressure (pulsus paradoxus). Because the heart is in the chest, the arterial blood pressure reflects intrathoracic pressure swings.[16] There are, of course, physiological mechanisms to dampen such swings but they do not seem to operate over the time scale of a single breath. These swings in beat-to-beat blood pressure can be measured non-invasively with an ingenious device called the Finapres™, which produces a tracing similar to that available from an intra-arterial line. It does this by compressing the digital arteries with an external inflatable cuff on a millisecond to millisecond basis to keep the volume of blood in the arteries constant by employing photoplethysmography (based on infra-red light absorption). To do this, the pressure in the cuff

Figure 10.4 Blood pressure variation in presence and absence of pharyngeal collapse

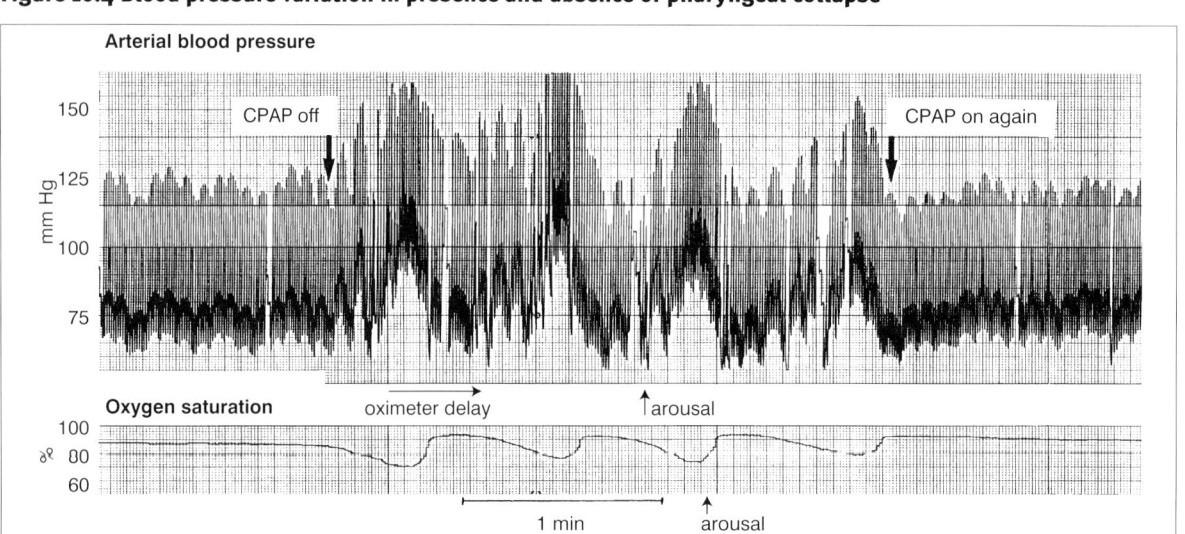

Beat-to-beat arterial blood pressure using the Finapres device (Ohmeda) from a patient on nasal CPAP at the beginning of the tracing (left hand edge). After one minute the CPAP pressure is reduced to below that necessary to splint open the pharynx, and the apneas with oxygen desaturation return. Note the large sustained rises in BP that result from arousals, and the smaller regular oscillations that result from swings in pleural pressure. The bottom tracing shows the oxygen saturation from a pulse oximeter on the finger, and the signal is therefore delayed relative to the Finapres by about 15 s.

Techniques for assessing increased inspiratory effort or airflow limitation

Physiological variable	Technique
Snoring	Microphone: in room or on skin (over pharynx)
Airflow*	Oronasal pressure transducer
Intrathoracic pressure swings	Esophageal balloon or via pulsus paradoxus (Finapres or pulse transit time)
Chest and abdominal paradox	Surface transducers (inductance bands, or piezo strain gauges)
Chest surface indrawing	Supraclavicular deformation transducer
Hypoxic dipping*	Oximetry

* These also reflect central apneas/hypoventilation

has to match the millisecond to millisecond changes in pressure in the artery, thus recreating the intra-arterial pressure. Figure 10.4 shows a tracing made using the Finapres in a patient with sleep apnea while on NCPAP. It can be shown that the arterial blood pressure swings measured using this device are in phase with the intrathoracic pressure swings.[17] The size of this device means that measurements must be made in the laboratory; no really portable equivalent has been devised. Beat-to-beat changes in blood pressure can be inferred from another technique, measurement of pulse transit time (PTT) – the time from aortic valve opening to the arrival of the pulse wave at a peripheral site (Figure 10.5). The speed of this shock wave depends on the stiffness or tension in the arterial wall, which in turn depends (in the short term) on the arterial pressure: as the pressure goes up, the arterial wall tenses, the pulse shock wave travels faster and the pulse transit time decreases. In practice this time interval is measured from the R-wave of the EKG (as a surrogate of aortic valve opening) to the arrival of the pulse wave at the finger detected photometrically with an oximeter finger probe: thus it can be derived from EKG electrodes and an oximeter probe that is already being used to measure SaO_2.

Other measurements, such as oronasal airflow or arterial oxygen saturation, indicate that less air is going in and out of the lungs, but do not indicate whether this is attended by increased effort. Using oronasal airflow, in combination with measures of respiratory effort, an attempt can be made to differentiate obstructive events from central events, such as occurs in Cheyne-Stokes breathing due to heart failure. Such a differentiation is usually possible from the history.

Figure 10.5 Pulse transit time recordings

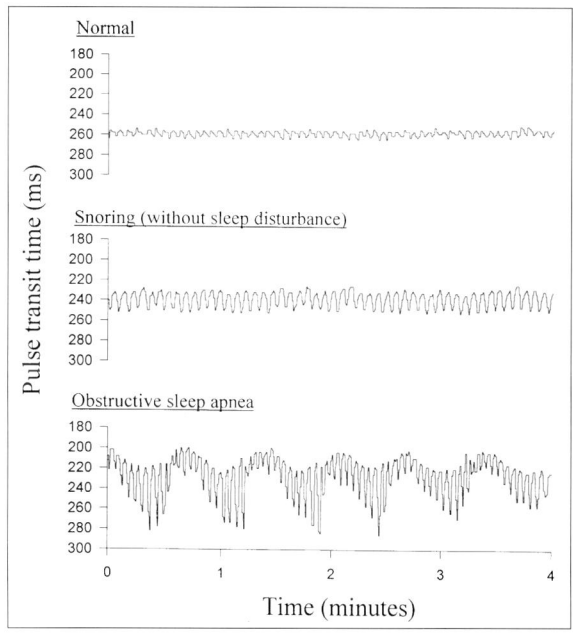

Tracings of beat-to-beat pulse transit time (from R wave of ECG and pulse oximetry) during sleep – inversely related to systolic blood pressure – in a normal subject, a snorer, and a patient with obstructive sleep apnea. Note the normal subject has only small 'blood pressure' swings, the snorer has bigger oscillations (due to bigger pleural pressure changes) and the patient with OSA has the biggest rises and falls in 'blood pressure' (as shown by falls and rises in pulse transit time, note the inverted scale) which are caused by each arousal.

What techniques are available to measure sleep fragmentation?

Several non-EEG techniques have been evaluated to assess sleep disturbance or fragmentation. The problem arises – what is the gold standard? Although EEG tracings can be hand scored for micro-arousals,[18] it is far from clear what events are significant in terms of producing daytime symptoms. For example, is it the length, 'height', or frequency of arousals that is important, or their distribution within the sleep stages, or the length of the undisturbed interval between them? It is likely to be a complex combination of all of these features and may vary between individuals. New markers of sleep fragmentation should be tested for their ability to predict daytime symptoms, rather than mimic EEG micro-arousal scoring. In most studies there has been little to choose between EEG and respiratory based markers of 'events' and their ability to predict sleepiness – both being fairly poor.[19]

Assessment of body movement

Alternatives to EEG have been based mainly on body movement, for example the wrist worn activity monitor or actigraph. The electrostatic mattress and video processing techniques have also been used. Movements correlate quite well with EEG micro-arousals (in excess of two seconds) but there is no evidence that they are better at predicting daytime sleepiness. Two techniques already mentioned in the context of inspiratory loading (airflow limitation and rib cage/abdominal phase angle changes) can also be used to monitor arousals from this situation. For example, the sudden disappearance of either flow limitation or rib cage/abdominal paradox implies that arousal is likely to have restored pharyngeal patency.[20]

Arousal-induced blood pressure changes

An alternative approach is to look at autonomic markers of arousal such as changes in heart rate and blood pressure. The process of arousal starts in the brain stem (where incoming sensory signals arrive) and radiates through to the cortex. Not all arousing stimuli lead to cortical arousal – for example we eventually 'learn' to sleep in noisy environments. However, these arousing stimuli do still seem to activate the cardiovascular center, leading to pulse rate and blood pressure rises. We and others have shown that auditory stimuli can provoke blood pressure rises of 10 mmHg or more with no cortical involvement at all.[21] Whether recurrent 'arousals' that do not propagate to the cortex can produce daytime symptoms is not clear, but they may. If they do, then counting them might provide a better index of whether respiratory events are disturbing sleep and producing daytime symptoms than superficial cortical EEG tracings.

Figure 10.4 shows the rises in blood pressure caused by the arousals that terminate each apnea. Note the slow rises over 10–20 seconds or so referred to earlier. Although these rises in blood pressure at the end of apnea were thought to be due to hypoxemia, the arousal process is far and away the more important cause. The blood pressure rises can be used as markers of sleep fragmentation; Figure 10.6 shows the relationship between the degree of cortical EEG arousal induced by an auditory stimulus and the consequent rise in blood pressure.[21] Once again these blood pressure rises can be followed with the technique based on pulse transit time described earlier. Figure 10.5 shows typical PTT tracings from a normal subject, a snorer without arousals, and a patient with OSA.[22]

It is serendipitous that beat-to-beat blood pressure tracings contain information about both inspiratory effort and arousals, two of the key features of a respiratory sleep study. Work with both the Finapres and PTT measurements has demonstrated that they can differentiate normal subjects from snorers (with and without arousals) and those with OSA.[22,23] In addition, there are clear changes with treatment.

Figure 10.6 Blood pressure response to induced arousals

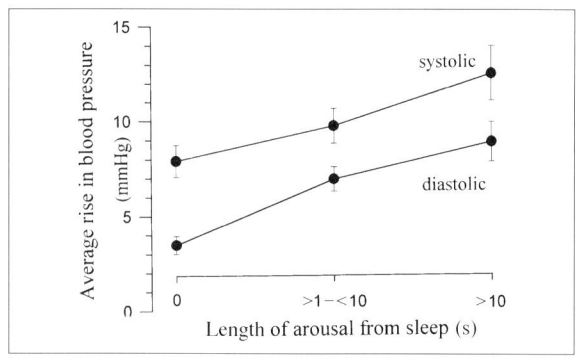

Relationship between high frequency EEG activity (defining arousals) as length in seconds of arousal in response to deliberate sounds, and the consequent rise in systolic and diastolic blood pressure (mean and SEM) (5 normal subjects) over the 10 s following the arousal stimulus, measured non-invasively by the Finapres device (Ohmeda). (From Davies RJO et al. J Appl Physiol 1993; 74:1123, with permission)[21]

Measurement techniques for assessing or implying sleep fragmentation

Physiological variable	Technique
Cerebral activation	EEG
Body movement	E.g. actigraphy/video
Apneas/hypopneas	Oronasal airflow
Hypoxic dips	Oximetry
Abrupt reversal of inspiratory airflow limitation	Oronasal airflow
Heart rate rises	EKG/oximetry
Blood pressure rises	Finapres/pulse transit time

CLINICAL APPLICATIONS

Approach to respiratory sleep studies

Conventional polysomnography usually involves measuring many signals: EEG, eye movements, electro-oculogram (EOG); chin muscle electromyogram (EMG) – to sleep stage into 20 or 30 epochs; oronasal airflow – to measure apneas and hypopneas; oxygen saturation; rib cage and abdominal movements – to measure apneas and hypopneas; leg EMG – to detect recurrent leg movements; and sometimes snoring. This plethora of signals certainly goes some way to help one understand whether a patient has a sleep related breathing disorder leading to abnormal sleep fragmentation. However, it is expensive and laborious and does not directly address the primary abnormalities of upper airway narrowing, increased inspiratory effort, and recurrent brief sleep fragmentation. This form of polysomnography missed heavy snoring with micro-arousals (but without apneas, hypopneas, or hypoxemia) for years.

When contemplating purchasing contemporary sleep study equipment (of which there are many different types) one must ask the question, can I detect sleep disruption and upper airway narrowing with increased inspiratory effort – directly or indirectly? Oximetry alone was advocated for a while and there is no doubt that overnight tracings can be diagnostic, particularly in more severe cases. The addition of snoring and body movements will add enormously, particularly if the pulse is monitored as well: movement and pulse rate being markers of sleep disturbance, snoring and hypoxia being markers of upper airway problems and hypoventilation as a consequence. Another way to get similar information is from a video recording that can be processed to derive body movements (Figure 10.7). There are many systems on the market that record rib cage/abdominal movements and oronasal airflow (to document apneas and hypopneas), some with snoring, heart rate, and movement. These kinds of signals can be processed to derive numerical outputs with minimal effort.

Figure 10.7 Sleep study tracing in OSA using video recordings and pulse oximetry

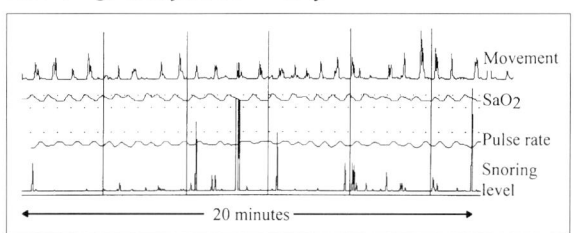

The top line is body movement, derived from digital processing of the video signal (VISI lab, Stowood Scientific Instruments, Oxford), and shows the movement associated with each arousal. The second line is oximetry, here oscillating between 90 and 95% SaO_2, the third is pulse rate (again showing recurrent 'arousals'), oscillating between about 50 and 65 bpm, and the fourth is sound level (or snoring). A normal tracing would be four flat lines.

Ultimately the value of all these systems depends on the skill of the interpreter: the operator is more important that the equipment. Operators become familiar with their equipment and learn to 'pattern recognize' its output; they are confused by other equipment's signals until they become familiar with them. I do not think there is a 'right' or 'best' system at present, nor is there likely to be for some time, owing to our uncertainty over the best measures of sleep disturbance.

How is the sleep study used to guide clinical management?

When faced with a patient complaining of excessive daytime sleepiness and heavy snoring, the aim of a sleep study is to establish whether the patient's symptoms are likely to be due to a problem of upper airway narrowing and sleep fragmentation. The sleep study might reveal periodic movements of the legs, or nothing at all, in which case a careful history is necessary to find out why the patient is sleepy. In patients with snoring and sleep apnea the relationship between findings on a sleep study and daytime symptoms is so poor that one has to have a qualitative approach to sleep studies: there is no magic cut-off measurement that allows one to say that this patient has a problem and this one does not.

Treatment of obstructive sleep apnea

Trial of continuous positive airway pressure

In practice the clinical problem is whether the patient's symptoms are bad enough to warrant treatment. If symptoms are bad, a trial of nasal CPAP may be appropriate: usually the patient is the best person to be asked about this. In our practice the patient is given a trial of CPAP if the sleep study shows something that could explain the patient's symptoms (which could just be heavy snoring with evidence of sleep disturbance), and the symptoms are bad enough to make the patient want to try CPAP, even when the difficulties of it have been fully explained. It is stressed that this is a trial and that the patient is under no obligation to keep the system if he feels the benefits do not outweigh the disadvantages. Of course, a very good CPAP support service is required so that the trial is not a failure simply because there were unresolved technical or emotional problems. The usual reasons for failure of the patient to be able to tolerate CPAP are its inappropriate use in the first place (i.e. inadequate symptoms), mask discomfort, claustrophobia, nasal obstruction or profuse rhinorrhea, psychological problems (usually embarrassment at having to wear the mask), and insufficient input from the prescribing team. Once a patient is established on CPAP there is no need to repeat sleep studies unless symptoms return for no obvious reason, or there has been potential improvement for other reasons (e.g. weight loss, hypothyroidism treated) and it seems likely that the patient now requires a much lower and hence more comfortable pressure.

As with diagnostic sleep studies, there is wide variation in the approach taken by different laboratories when starting patients on NCPAP. Some labs carefully adjust the pressure at the CPAP mask during sleep to just abolish the apneas and snoring, with constant minor adjustments throughout the night. Others send patients home on a fixed pressure (e.g. 10 cmH$_2$O) and it is altered at a later stage on the basis of symptom resolution and reports from the bed partner. Recently NCPAP machines that automatically adjust their pressures have been made. Essentially they monitor various signals, such as snoring, inspiratory air flow limitation, and flow reductions, and raise the pressure until these are improved to some predetermined level. The pressure is then slowly reduced until problems return and then raised again. Thus the system hunts around the correct pressure all night. The 'best' pressure can thus be read off the following morning from the all night data and the patient sent home on a fixed pressure machine set at this level. The pressures found by these auto-CPAP machines are remarkably similar to those found by experienced technicians. The pressures prescribed vary between 5 and 15 cmH$_2$O and seem to depend mainly on degree of obesity (neck circumference) and the original severity of the sleep apnea.

Sometimes we are not at all sure if a patient's symptoms are really due to the snoring and sleep disturbance we may have seen on a sleep study. In this situation a trial of CPAP is almost being used as a diagnostic tool, to establish if the problem is indeed CPAP responsive and therefore likely to be due to problems of upper airway collapse.

This symptom-based approach to the instigation of CPAP is only appropriate because CPAP is being prescribed for the daytime problems of sleepiness. If it is shown in future that OSA produces significant cardiovascular mortality, then this policy may need to be reassessed. However, there would have to be very powerful reasons to persuade a non-sleepy 40 year old man to wear a CPAP mask every night when the only benefits are in the dim and distant future: how many people would use CPAP every night for 30 years (assuming nothing else better replaces it) to prevent one stroke or heart attack amongst their number?

Until recently NCPAP was the only really effective treatment for OSA apart from tracheostomy. Palatal surgery has never been very successful except in carefully selected cases who usually have large tonsils.

Clinical approach

- History of hypersomnolence, snoring, and other OSA symptoms.
- Assess obesity (neck circumference), pharyngeal size, jaw size, and nasal patency.
- Sleep study reveals evidence of upper airway narrowing.
- Sleep study reveals evidence of sleep fragmentation.
- Trial of nasal CPAP.

Recent work has suggested that intraoral devices worn at night (mandibular advancement devices) that hold the lower jaw forward and closed can open up the pharyngeal lumen and be very effective in some cases. They clearly reduce snoring and improve mild to moderated OSA but their place in severe OSA has not yet been established.

CONCLUSIONS

- The approach to sleep related breathing disorders has evolved enormously over the last ten years. We have moved on from an ill-informed, rigid, and inflexible sleep study-based approach, to a more flexible one that admits the poor relationship between sleep study findings and symptoms, and places greater emphasis on the latter.[24]
- The tools necessary to implement the above approach are simpler than the conventional ones, particularly if they concentrate on measuring the key physiological problems – upper airway narrowing, increased inspiratory effort, and sleep fragmentation. It is not yet possible to work with the same level of precision that is appropriate in a lung function laboratory where the procedure for most of the routine tests is well established.
- Running a sleep service requires expertise, familiarity with the equipment in use, and a flexible approach to treatment, backed up by a high quality CPAP service that supports patients undergoing this therapy.

References

1. Gastaut H, Tassinari CA & Duron B. Etude polygraphique des manifestations épisodiques (hypniques et respiratoires), diurnes et nocturnes, du syndrome de Pickwick. *Rev Neurol* 1965; **112**: 568–79.
2. Weitzenblum E, Krieger J, Apprill M *et al*. Daytime pulmonary hypertension in patients with obstructive sleep apnea syndrome. *Am Rev Respir Dis* 1988; **138**: 345–9.
3. Gleeson K, Zwillich CW & White DP. The influence of increasing ventilatory effort on arousal from sleep. *Am Rev Respir Dis* 1990; **142**: 295–300.
4. Guilleminault C, Stoohs R, Clerk A, Cetel M, Maistros P. A cause of excessive daytime sleepiness. The upper airway resistance syndrome. *Chest* 1993; **104**: 781–7.
5. Wiegand L, Zwillich CW & White D. Collapsibility of the human upper airway during normal sleep. *J Appl Physiol* 1989; **66**: 1800–8.
6. Davies RJO, Ali NJ & Stradling JR. Neck circumference and other clinical features in the diagnosis of the obstructive sleep apnoea syndrome. *Thorax* 1992; **47**: 101–5.
7. Mathur R & Douglas NJ. Family studies in patients with the sleep apnea–hypopnea syndrome. *Ann Intern Med* 1995; **122**: 174–8.
8. Lugaresi E, Cirignotta F, Gerardi R, Montagna P. Snoring and sleep apnea: natural history of heavy snorers disease. In: Guilleminault C & Partinen M(eds) *Obstructive Sleep Apnea Syndrome: Clinical Research and Treatment*. New York: Raven Press 1990: 25–36.
9. Findley LJ, Weiss JW & Jabour ER. Drivers with untreated sleep apnea. A cause of death and serious injury. *Arch Intern Med* 1991; **151**: 1451–2.
10. Working group on OSA and hypertension. Carlson J, Davies R *et al*. Obstructive sleep apnea and blood pressure elevation. What is the relationship? *Blood Press* 1993; **2**: 166–82.
11. Young T, Palta M, Dempsey J, Skatrud J, Weber S, Badr S. Occurrence of sleep disordered breathing among middle-aged adults. *N Engl J Med* 1993; **328**: 1230–5.
12. Stradling JR. Obstructive sleep apnoea: definitions, epidemiology and natural history. *Thorax* 1995; **50**: 683–9.
13. Stradling JR, Davies RJO & Pitson DJ. New approaches to monitoring sleep related breathing disorders. *Sleep* 1996; **19**: S77–S84.
14. Condos R, Norman RG, Krishnasamy I, Peduzzi N, Goldring RM, Rapaport DM. Flow limitation as a non-invasive assessment of residual upper-airway resistance during continuous positive airway pressure therapy of obstructive sleep apnea. *Am J Respir Crit Care Med* 1994; **150**: 475–80.
15. Montserrat JM, Ballester E, Olivi H *et al*. Time-course of stepwise CPAP titration. Behavior of respiratory and neurological variables. *Am J Respir Crit Care Med* 1995; **152**: 1854–9.
16. Lea S, Ali NJ, Goldman M, Loh L, Fleetham J, Stradling JR. Systolic blood pressure swings reflect inspiratory effort during simulated obstructive sleep apnoea. In: Horne J (ed) *Sleep 90*. Bochum: Pontenagel Press 1990: 178–81.
17. Brock J, Pitson D & Stradling JR. Use of pulse transit time as a measure of changes in inspiratory effort. *J Amb Mon* 1993; **6**: 295–302.

18 Bonnet M, Carley D, Carskadon M *et al*. EEG arousals: scoring rules and examples. A preliminary report from the Sleep Disorders Atlas Task Force of the American Sleep Disorders Association. *Sleep* 1992; **15**: 173–84.
19 Cheshire K, Engleman H, Deary I, Shapiro C, Douglas NJ. Factors impairing daytime performance in patients with the sleep apnoea/hypopnoea syndrome. *Arch Intern Med* 1992; **152**: 538–41.
20 Atkins NCM, Stone PA, Davies J, Smith E, Woodcock A. The development and resolution of paradox in relation to respiratory events during sleep. *Am Rev Respir Dis* 1992; **145**: A173.
21 Davies RJO, Belt PJ, Robert SJ, Ali NJ, Stradling JR. Arterial blood pressure responses to graded transient arousal from sleep in normal humans. *J Appl Physiol* 1993; **74**: 1123–30.
22 Pitson DJ & Stradling JR. Evaluation of pulse transit time as a screening respiratory sleep study. *Am J Respir Crit Care Med* 1995; **151**: A250.
23 Davies RJO, Vardi-Visy K, Clarke M, Stradling JR. Identification of sleep disruption and sleep disordered breathing from the systolic blood pressure profile. *Thorax* 1993; **48**: 1242–7.
24 Stradling JR. *Handbook of Sleep-related Breathing Disorders*. Oxford: Oxford University Press 1993.

11 Pediatric Pulmonary Function

M Silverman and J Stocks

- **INTRODUCTION**
  Developmental physiology
  Clinical physiology

- **ASSESSMENT OF RESPIRATORY FUNCTION IN INFANTS**
  Why measure respiratory function in infants?
  Differences in the assessment of infants compared with adults/older children
  Equipment requirements
  Measurement conditions
  Airway function
  Esophageal manometry
  Plethysmography
  Forced oscillation technique
  Occlusion techniques
  Indices of forced expiratory flow
  Tidal breathing
  Body surface measurements
  Lung volumes
  Lung and chest wall elasticity
  Non-invasive determination of blood gases
  Distribution of ventilation
  Cardiorespiratory polygraphic monitoring
  Control of breathing

- **ASSESSMENT OF RESPIRATORY FUNCTION IN UNSEDATED PRE-SCHOOL CHILDREN**
  Background
  Laboratory conditions
  Techniques available
  Airway function
  Other lung function techniques

- **MEASUREMENT IN SCHOOL CHILDREN**
  Clinical situations in school children
  Asthma
  Cystic fibrosis
  Chest wall disorders
  Obstructive sleep apnea

- **GUIDANCE TO INTERPRETATION OF RESULTS**

- **CONCLUSIONS**

INTRODUCTION

Respiratory disease is the major cause of morbidity in infants and young children in the UK, with up to 40% of infants wheezing during the first year of life. Disturbances of the mechanical function of the respiratory system are central to many disorders in newborns and infants[1] and may be the direct result of lung disease, for instance in infantile asthma, pulmonary hypoplasia, or neonatal hyaline membrane disease, or result indirectly from cardiovascular or neuromuscular disorders.

Developmental physiology

An understanding of developmental anatomy and physiology is essential for clinical measurement and interpretation of pulmonary function tests in infants and young children.[2,3(pp S15-S17)] The respiratory system undergoes dramatic functional changes during the first few hours after birth with rapid aeration of the lungs, clearance of lung fluid, and establishment of a resting lung volume. These changes are accompanied by a rapid rise in compliance and fall in resistance with relatively stable values being achieved within 12 hours of birth. Although respiratory problems are common during the neonatal period, especially if the infant is delivered prematurely,[1] under normal circumstances there is rapid and complete adaptation to extra-uterine life.

In healthy individuals, most parameters of respiratory function remain remarkably constant when related to either surface area or body size, reflecting the fact that respiration is closely attuned to the metabolic requirements of the body (Table 11.1).

The underlying factors determining these parameters may however vary considerably according to age.[3(pp S15-S17),4(pp 1-18)] Interpretation of lung function measurements in infancy (Table 11.2) may be confounded by an unstable end-expiratory level, compliant chest wall, the dominance of the upper airways, shunting of gas flow in the oropharynx, difficulty in achieving flow limitation in healthy infants, and variability of respiratory, lung, or airway resistance (possibly related to the upper airways) which increases the difficulty of assessing the significance of changes in resistance as a result of treatment or challenge.

Airway responsiveness to histamine and methacholine can be measured from early infancy. However, its role in wheezing lower respiratory illnesses in young infants may be over-shadowed by other factors such as congenital differences in airway geometry and lung mechanics or by pathological changes such as airway edema and mucous hypersecretion.[3] Although some remodeling of the lung may occur during the first year of life following prenatal and perinatal challenges, there appears to be considerable tracking of lung function from the end of the first year of life to late childhood (i.e. those with diminished function in infancy retain it thereafter). Alveolization is complete

Table 11.1 'Typical' values of lung function in healthy individuals

	Preterm	Newborn	1 year	7 year	Adult
Body weight (kg)	1	3	10	25	70
Crown–heel length (cm)	35	50	75	120	175
Respiratory rate (min^{-1})	60	45	30	20	15
Tidal volume (ml)	7	21	70	180	500
Anatomic dead space (ml)	3	6	20	50	150
Maximal flow at FRC (ml.s^{-1})	80	150	300	—	—
Functional residual capacity (FRC) (ml)	25	85	250	750	2100
Lung compliance (ml.cmH$_2$O^{-1})	1.5	5	15	50	200
Airway resistance (cmH$_2$O.L^{-1} s)	80	40	15	4	2
Specific compliance (cmH$_2$O^{-1})	0.06	0.06	0.06	0.07	0.08
Specific conductance (s^{-1} cmH$_2$O^{-1})	0.50	0.29	0.27	0.27	0.23

Note: Multiply compliance, and specific compliance by 10 to obtain values in SI units ml.kPa^{-1} and kPa^{-1} respectively, divide resistance by 10 to obtain values as kPa.L^{-1} s; multiply specific conductance by 10 to obtain values in s^{-1} kPa^{-1}.

Pediatric Pulmonary Function   165

Table 11.2 Major differences in respiratory physiology in the infant compared with adult

Chest wall	Preferential nose breathers	Dynamic elevation of end-expiratory lung volume (EELV)	Respiratory reflexes
• **Configuration**: horizontally placed ribs; more flexible • **Fewer type 1 oxidative fibers** in diaphragm ⇒ predisposes to fatigue • **High compliance:** low outward recoil of chest wall at FRC results in limited distending pressure Ppl −1.5 cmH_2O (0.15 kPa) in infants cf −7 cmH_2O in adults Effects include: − **Reduced EELV** during passive expiration and tendency to atelectasis − **Airway closure** during tidal breathing with ↑ tendency to peripheral airway obstruction, and hence − **Impaired gas exchange** (ventilation–perfusion imbalance) − **Increased work of breathing** due to chest wall retraction (asynchronous/paradoxical rib cage-abdominal movement)	• Most assessments of airway, lung, and respiratory resistance will include **nasal resistance**. Since this comprises about 50% total resistance, the sensitivity of these tests in detecting lower airway disease or response to therapeutic interventions is diminished. • Any upper airway **infection** will distort results. Hence infant RFTs should be deferred at least 3 weeks following a cold. • **Pharmacological challenges** by aerosol (bronchodilators or constrictors) may be preferentially deposited in the nose and may have major effects on nasal resistance, and reduced action in lower respiratory tract.	• To counteract tendency of lung to collapse to very low volumes, young infants adopt a strategy of modulating expiratory flow. A short expiratory time (rapid respiratory rate) plus prolonged expiratory time constant (achieved by laryngeal braking or post-inspiratory diaphragmatic activity) result in **dynamic elevation of EELV** above that passively determined by the outward recoil of chest wall and inward recoil of lung. • Transition to a more **relaxed** pattern of expiration occurs between 6 and 12 months of age. • **Unstable EELV**, particularly during rapid eye movement sleep, may invalidate some measurements of lung and airway function. Infant RFTs should ideally be confined to periods of quiet sleep.	• The strength of many respiratory reflexes, particularly those in the upper airways and those responsible for stretch receptor activity is greater in young infants than adults, e.g. infants have an **active Hering–Breuer reflex (HBR)** during tidal breathing, such that airway occlusion at end inspiration evokes a brief expiratory pause. Measurements of passive respiratory mechanics in infants are dependent on the presence of the HBR to induce an expiratory pause with muscle relaxation.

Note: Virtually all lung function measurements are made in infants while asleep (with or without sedation), and during nose breathing. EELV = End expired lung volume

by the end of the third postnatal year.[2] Thereafter lung volume increases by enlargement of lung spaces. Airways do not grow in proportion to air spaces (i.e. growth is 'dysynaptic') and there are sex differences even in young children. Girls have relatively wider airways than boys in early childhood with greater volume corrected maximum flows; the situation reverses after puberty.

Lung growth continues until the completion of skeletal growth in girls and for two to three years beyond in boys. Patterns of change during adolescence are complex, and the need to take into account the stage of pubertal development in addition to body size and sex remains controversial.[5]

Clinical physiology

Lung function tests are used in **clinical practice** to answer management questions concerning diagnosis, severity, trend, and response to therapy or to provide clues to prognosis. A specific diagnosis is rarely achieved this way, because physiological dysfunction is rarely specific. The exception is asthma, the physiological definition of which is 'airway obstruction varying spontaneously or in response to treatment'. Tests of bronchoconstrictor and bronchodilator responsiveness, and day-to-day peak flow (PEF) variability over weeks, may all contribute to the diagnosis.

The range of clinical problems commonly encountered in a specialist center dealing with childhood respiratory illness is wide (Table 11.3). Chronic obstructive pulmonary disease (COPD), suppurative conditions (except cystic fibrosis and ciliary dysfunction), interstitial lung disease, and lung cancer which are common in adults are rare in children. Investigations are rarely performed for diagnostic purposes, especially in infants, but rather to monitor severity or to assess the response to treatment (both physical, such as mechanical ventilation, and pharmacological).

Lung function tests must take their place among the other investigative techniques. If, for instance, tracheal obstruction is suspected, it may be more appropriate to perform bronchoscopy and CT or MRI to visualize the problem, than to measure its effects. Conversely, in a teenage child with asthma in whom laryngeal dysfunction is suspected, simply performing inspiratory (as well as expiratory) flow-volume curves may provide the answer, without the need for any imaging or more complex lung function measurements.

Epidemiological studies employing pulmonary function measurements during infancy provide important clues to the pathogenesis of pulmonary disease. The adverse effect of maternal smoking during pregnancy on fetal lung development and the relationship between pulmonary function at birth and subsequent recurrent wheezing in infancy are recent examples.[4] Awareness of the fetal and infantile origins of chronic airflow obstruction in adults has renewed interest in early pulmonary development.

Measurements of airway function and airway responsiveness in infancy are also contributing to a better understanding of the **pathophysiology** of wheezing disorders of infancy and chronic lung disease of prematurity. In the clinical realm, measurements of lung mechanics have had little influence on diagnosis since with few exceptions only simple, non-specific techniques are widely available. Thus, whereas in adults, asthma management is usually based on clinical symptoms, and the change in airway obstruction assessed by forced expiratory maneuvers, there is as yet no simple equivalent to PEF or FEV_1 in early childhood. Nevertheless, there are several highly technical methods which can be applied in the laboratory, and a few simpler techniques for domiciliary use (see below).

Since, for many respiratory diseases the lung cannot be described as a single compartment, integrative measures of lung function may prove more useful than mechanical parameters. For example, transcutaneous measurements of oxygenation appear to be a useful surrogate for airway function in detecting response to bronchial challenge in pre-school children (see later).

Measurements of respiratory function have found wide application as measures of outcome in **therapeutic trials** in children of all ages. As prospects for early intervention based on antenatal diagnosis or on gene therapy for specific defects become more widespread, the contribution of measurements of lung mechanics to outcome measurement will increase.

Pulmonary function testing has not yet achieved widespread clinical application in infants and pre-school children.[4(pp 521–550, 551–562)] This is related to:

- difficulties in testing and expertise required
- the lack of standardized methodologies
- inadequate reference data
- limited information concerning sensitivity and specificity.

Table 11.3 Common clinical situations in childhood

Clinical problem	Infancy	Pre-school child	School child
Acute respiratory failure (intensive care)	• hyaline membrane disease (IRDS)* • massive aspiration • acute viral or bacterial pneumonitis (e.g. bronchiolitis) §*	• drowning • foreign body aspiration • overwhelming infection (ARDS)	• ARDS* • acute severe asthma or anaphylaxis* • acute lung infection
Chronic respiratory failure	• CLD§* • neuromuscular disease (weakness) §*	• neuromuscular disease (weakness) §*	• neuromuscular disease (weakness)§* • skeletal disorder (kyphoscoliosis) § • cystic fibrosis §* • host defense disease §*
Chronic recurrent wheeze	• viral episodic wheeze (wheezy bronchitis)* • atopic asthma* • CLD§* • congenital heart and airways disease • recurrent aspiration	• asthma†* • foreign body aspiration	• asthma†*
Stridor (a) acute	• laryngotracheitis • epiglottitis	• acute laryngotracheitis • foreign body or other aspiration • 'spasmodic' croup similar to infancy	• angioedema (anaphylaxis) • smoke inhalation
(b) chronic	• congenital anomaly • neuromuscular disease§ (floppy upper airway)		• 'functional' (laryngeal dysfunction)† • neuromuscular disease §* • postoperative or post-infective scarring §
Cough (a) acute	• acute infection • foreign body aspiration	• acute infection • aspirated foreign body or substance	• infective or allergic cause
(b) chronic	• cystic fibrosis • wheezy bronchitis • perinatal infection • congenital anomaly of airways • recurrent aspiration	• whooping cough • wheezy bronchitis • congenital anomaly† (usually neuromuscular basis)	• complicating other diseases (asthma, cystic fibrosis)† • bronchiectasis† • habitual† • anatomical anomaly†
Sleep apnea and obstructive episodes	• prematurity and CLD†* • neuromuscular and CNS causes of floppiness† • fits • congenital anomalies (e.g. Pierre-Robin syndrome)	• upper airway obstruction†* (e.g. ↑ tonsils) • neuromuscular disease†	• fits or faints • 'hyperventilation' syndrome • upper airway obstruction (anatomical or neuromuscular)
Tachypnea (chronic)	• hypoplastic lungs §† • interstitial lung disease • metabolic acidosis	—	—

Note: Key:

CLD chronic lung disease (of prematurity)
IRDS infantile respiratory distress syndrome
ARDS adult respiratory distress syndrome

† lung function tests may be needed in diagnosis
§ tests are useful to monitor progress
* the response to treatment can be assessed by lung function tests

ASSESSMENT OF RESPIRATORY FUNCTION IN INFANTS

Until recently, the lack of suitable equipment and the complexity of measuring small uncooperative subjects limited infant respiratory function tests to specialized research establishments. Less invasive tests which are easier to perform have now been developed.[4] Between the ages of 2 and 5 years, assessments are more difficult, since such children are too young to cooperate but too old to be sedated. Thereafter, the procedures developed for adults and described elsewhere in this book can usually be applied.

Why measure respiratory function in infants?

Reasons for assessing respiratory function in infants are summarized in Table 11.4. The clinical applications of infant respiratory function tests in individual patients remain controversial. In particular, it should be remembered that the tests are rarely diagnostic, reference data are limited, serial tests are more valuable than single assessments, and results must be interpreted in the light of all other clinical information.

Since lung function tests in infants are far more complex and time consuming than in children or adults and may involve sedation, it is essential that the reason for the test is clearly defined and that there is a good chance of a successful outcome. Consequently, it is important to consider the age and clinical state of the infant, what information is required, and which tests are most relevant. Factors that must be taken into account when interpreting results are summarized in Table 11.5 (facing page).

Differences in the assessment of infants compared with adults/older children

Measurements in infants and young children under two years are usually made in the supine position while breathing nasally through a face mask. Since infants are unable to cooperate, most measurements must be made during sleep which, in infants beyond four weeks postnatal age, frequently requires sedation (e.g. with chloral hydrate or the related but more palatable agent, triclofos sodium). The inability of babies to perform special respiratory maneuvers means that many of the measurements are limited to the tidal breathing range, although innovative techniques allow measurements at raised lung volumes.[4(pp 379–409)] A lung function test in a baby can take up to three hours, thereby limiting the number of subjects that can be tested. The lack of appropriate commercially available equipment and standardized software for data collection and analysis also currently limits the extent to which data from different laboratories can be collated.

Table 11.4 Reasons for assessing respiratory function in infants

Research applications	Clinical applications
• *Influence of early life events* (e.g. passive tobacco smoke exposure, ventilator or oxygen therapy, air pollution, premature delivery) on lung development and on relative risk of developing respiratory disease	• *Early recognition of disease,* e.g. cystic fibrosis screening, effects of neuromuscular weakness
	• *Identification of iatrogenic damage* – intermittent positive pressure ventilation, O_2 therapy
• *Determinants of lung function* - body size, age, maturity, gender, ethnic group, family history of atopy	• *Determination of type and severity* of pulmonary defect
• *Evaluation of therapeutic interventions* - drug therapy (surfactant, steroids, bronchodilators), mode of ventilatory support, surgery, etc.	• *Efficacy of treatment,* e.g. bronchodilator therapy, steroids, surgical procedures on upper airway

Table 11.5 Interpretation of results: technical and biological factors

- Body size (accurate weight and length required)
- Lung size
- Sleep state (+ sedation)
- Upper airways including nose (nasal airway resistance ⩾ 50% Raw in infants)
- Posture
- Sex
- Ethnic group
- Gestational age
- Postnatal age
- Potential influence of equipment

For further details see Gaultier et al.[4(pp 29-44)]

Equipment requirements

Although increasing numbers of automated lung function carts are now available for use, these tend to be less sophisticated and more inflexible than those available for adult use, and many specialist laboratories still rely on home-made equipment. Full details of equipment requirements for infant respiratory function testing have been reported recently.[4(pp 45-116)] The characteristics of all equipment must accommodate the rapid respiratory rate of infants (up to 100 per minute for pre-term babies), combined with the need to miniaturize equipment so that dead space is reduced without unduly increasing resistance. This places special demands on the frequency characteristics. The need to dismantle such apparatus for adequate sterilization between each measurement adds further to the constraints.

Measurement conditions

When measuring young infants, standardization of measurement conditions is crucial for the infant's safety, accuracy of the test, and reproducibility of the data. Standardization of measurement conditions must address both laboratory conditions and the infant's state, with respect to factors such as posture, sedation, and sleep state. Recommendations have been published recently.[4(pp 29-44)]

The connection with the recording instruments is usually made via an oronasal (face) mask in infants. This should fit snugly and not leak at the line of contact with the face. A leak-free seal may be facilitated using Vaseline (petroleum jelly) or therapeutic silicone putty. The connection should always be tested for leaks prior to commencing measurements. Tidal volume can be measured by using a spirometer or inductance plethysmograph (see later) but is more commonly obtained by integration of a flow signal from a pneumotachograph.

Airway function

Assessment of airway function is useful in some infants with upper or lower airway obstruction, as a means of locating the site (upper, large, or small airways) and severity. In wheezy infants, measurements before and after therapeutic agents (e.g. bronchodilator aerosols) can help to guide management. In general, however, these tests are used in clinical research, to elucidate mechanisms of disease or to determine the general role of treatments. A number of techniques exist (Table 11.6), as described below.

Esophageal manometry

Dynamic lung resistance (R_L) (tissues plus airway) and compliance (C_L) can be measured in infants using esophageal manometry (see chapter 2). Pleural pressure can be measured in the lower third of the esophagus as in adults, using an esophageal balloon, fluid filled catheter or one of the recently introduced flexible catheter tipped microtransducers.[4(pp 241-282)] As in adults, the catheter or balloon is passed into the stomach and gradually withdrawn until negative pressure swings are seen on inspiration. Reliability of esophageal pressure (Pes) measurement should always be checked by comparing pressure changes with those recorded at the airway opening (ΔPao) during respiratory efforts against a briefly occluded airway. The two should agree within 5% (i.e. ΔPes:ΔPao ratio of 0.95–1.05). Calculations of R_L have conventionally been performed between points of mid isovolume using the method of Mead and Whittenberger. However, with the introduction of computerized data acquisition and analysis, there is increasing emphasis on the use of more reliable multiple linear regression techniques.[4(pp 258-281, 445-484)] With care, reliable measurements can be obtained even in small, sick pre-term infants. Nevertheless this technique remains technically demanding, and the need to pass an esophageal catheter (which is poorly tolerated by older infants and young children) has limited the application of this technique to early infancy.

Table 11.6 Comparison of techniques for assessing airway function

Technique	ICU	NBI	Sed	Advantages	Limitations
Esophageal manometry (R_L/C_L)	✓	✓	(✓)	• Continuous rapid data collection with simultaneous C_L measures • Minimum interference with baby once catheter in situ • Analysis using multiple linear regression allows complex modeling if required	• Technically demanding • Esophageal catheters poorly tolerated by older infants • Results must be validated by occlusion test since ΔPes may not always represent ΔPpl • Includes nasal resistance
Plethysmography (Raw)	✗	✓	✓	• Simultaneous measure of lung volume and resistance • Resistance measured throughout entire breath • P-V curves can distinguish upper and lower airway disease	• Expensive, complex equipment • Technically demanding • Not applicable to intubated infants • Accuracy dependent or achieving BTPS conditions • Includes nasal resistance
Forced oscillation (Rrs)	✗	✓	✓	• Non-invasive, applicable to wide age range	• Results invalidated by shunting into upper airways if input impedance used • Includes nasal resistance • Wide range normal values
Single-breath technique (Rrs/Crs)	✓	✓	✓	• Simple, cheap equipment • Simultaneous measures of Crs	• Numerous assumptions which are unlikely to be valid in intubated infants and those with airway disease (see Table 11.7) • Expiratory resistance only • Includes nasal resistance
Rapid thoraco-abdominal compression technique ($MEF_{FRC} + FEV_t$)	✗	✓	✓	• Largely independent of upper airway • Does not rely on single compartment model – therefore not invalidated in wheezy infants • Relatively simple data collection and analysis, and inexpensive equipment	• Wide range normal values • Flow limitation may not always occur in healthy infants • Dependent on stable FRC

Key: ICU Intensive Care Unit, i.e. intubated, ventilated infants
      NBI unsedated newborn infants (< 6 weeks)
      Sed sedated spontaneously breathing infants (> 6 weeks)

Plethysmography

Airway resistance can be measured throughout the breathing cycle using a whole body plethysmograph.[4(pp 190–240)] The technique is very similar to that described for adults with the exception that, as infants cannot be instructed to pant in order to minimize changes in temperature and humidity of the respired gas, they breathe for a short time through a face mask connected via a pneumotachograph to a heated rebreathing bag containing gas under BTPS conditions (Figure 11.1). The infant whole body plethysmograph is a valuable tool for obtaining simultaneous measurements of lung volume and airway resistance and may be particularly useful for discriminating between upper airway disease (in which there is a characteristic rise in inspiratory airway resistance (Raw) during inspiration), and lower airway disease, where the major increase in Raw is during late expiration (Figure 11.2). It is technically demanding however and its use is restricted to relatively few specialized laboratories.

Forced oscillation technique

Measurement of total respiratory resistance (Rrs) by the forced oscillation technique[4(pp 355–378)] is potentially applicable to a wide age range. Again, the technique used in infants has been adapted from that developed for adults (see chapter 2), wherein the impedance of the total respiratory system is determined by applying single or multiple frequency pressure oscillations to the respiratory system – usually using a loudspeaker, via a mask or headbox – and measuring the resultant flow. When measuring input impedance, the applied pressure and resulting flow are measured at the airway opening. Alternatively, transfer impedance may be studied by measuring pressure and flow at two different points of the respiratory system, usually with pressure applied to the body surface and flow measured at the airway opening. Since oscillations are imposed on the subject's spontaneous breathing, the forced oscillation technique is non-invasive and does not require active cooperation. However, interpretation of results is limited by the wide range of values

Figure 11.1 Infant whole body plethysmography

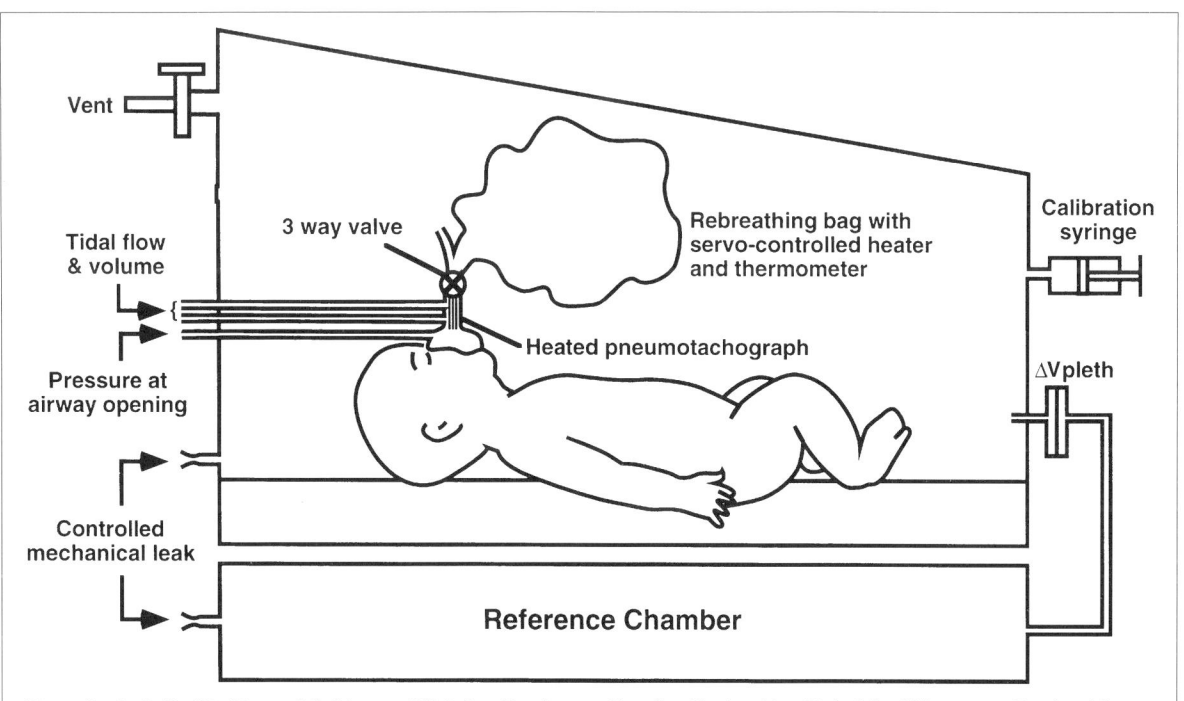

(From Stocks J, Sly PD, Tepper RS, Morgan WJ. Infant Respiratory Function Testing. New York: John Wiley, 1996. Reprinted by permission of Wiley-Liss, Inc., a division of John Wiley & Sons Inc.)

Figure 11.2 Representative pressure-flow and flow-volume curves during rebreathing in infants.

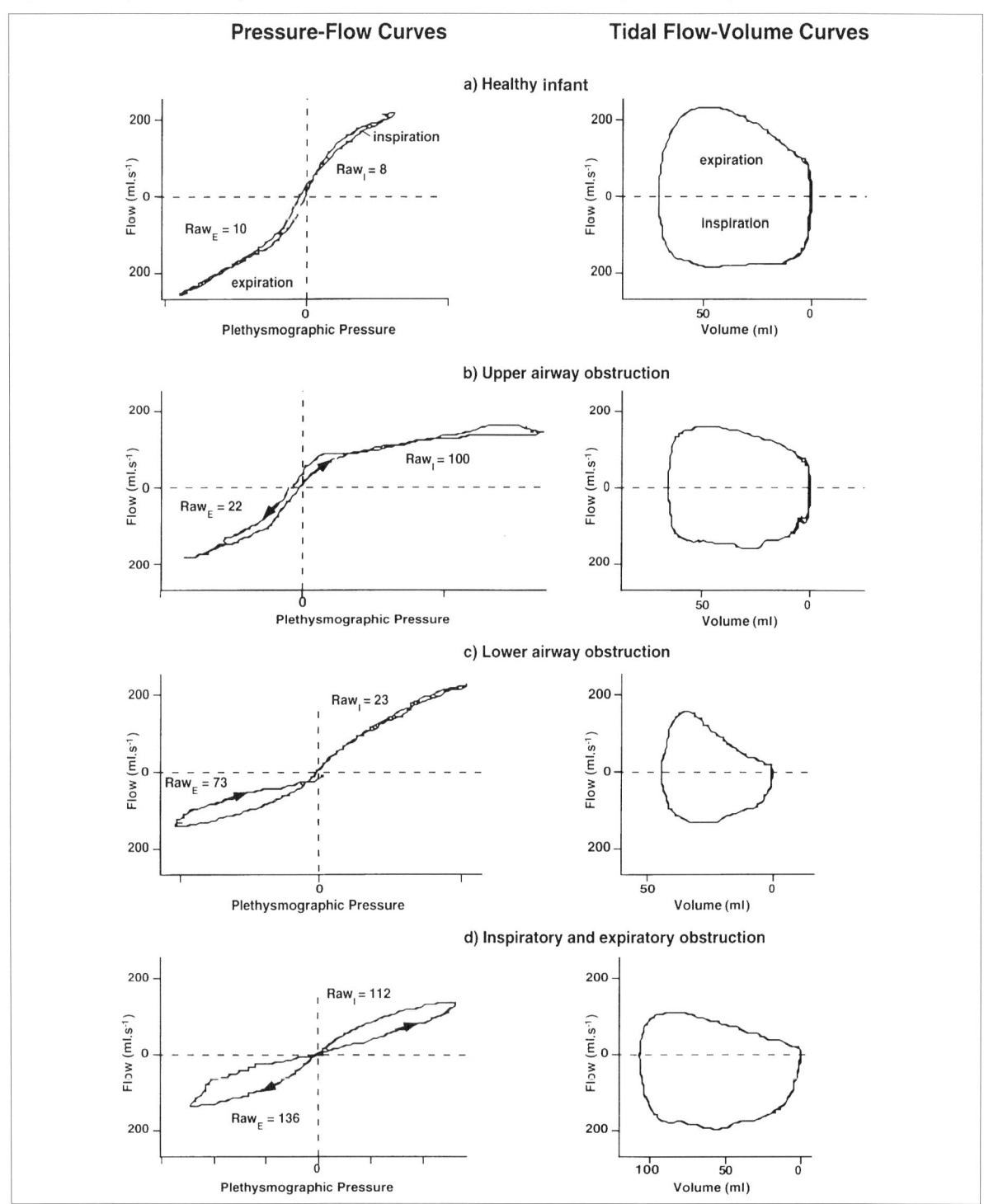

Raw_I and Raw_E = inspiratory and expiratory airways resistance calculated at 50% peak inspiratory and expiratory flow. All values are in $cmH_2O.L^{-1}$ s. Divide by 10 for values in $kPa.L^{-1}$ s. Note variation in scales for some plots.

reported from healthy infants, the domination of upper airway resistance and, when using the simpler technique of input impedance, the compliance of the cheeks and pharynx.

Occlusion techniques

Methods of measuring passive respiratory mechanics are simple and rapid to perform, requiring only a face mask, shutter (or more simply a thumb across the opening of the apparatus), and pneumotachograph (Figure 11.3a), and are being increasingly used in clinical situations. If pressure changes are measured at the airway opening during relaxation against an end-inspiratory airway occlusion, they represent the driving force across the chest wall, tissues, and airways (i.e. the elastic recoil of the respiratory system) and can be used to measure passive respiratory mechanics.[4(pp 283–328)] Currently, the most widely used techniques are the multiple occlusion technique (MOT) and the single-breath technique (SBT), which can be applied to both spontaneously breathing and intubated ventilated infants. Both rely on the assumption that the Hering-Breuer inflation reflex, which has been shown to be present in infants up to at least one year of age,[6] can be elicited during brief airway occlusions. Providing the infant relaxes against the occlusion and complete equilibration of pressure occurs, pressure at the airway opening reflects the static elastic recoil pressure of the respiratory system (Figure 11.3b). *(Note the more elaborate analysis of respiratory mechanics with constant flow ventilation used in the Intensive Care Unit – see Chapter 12)*. The SBT also assumes that, on release of the occlusion, expiration remains entirely passive and that the respiratory system can be represented by a single time constant as shown by exponential decline of flow and volume on a time based trace and a linear portion of the expiratory flow volume curve (Figure 11.3c).

While the assumption that the respiratory system can be regarded as a single compartment model is probably valid in most healthy infants, this is unlikely to be true in the presence of lung or airway disease. There is evidence that the SBT may underestimate resistance in wheezy infants, and overestimate it in the presence of marked laryngeal braking.[4(pp 190–240)]

Figure 11.3 Measurement of compliance (Crs) and resistance (Rrs) of total respiratory system in infants during relaxation of respiratory muscles (single-breath technique)

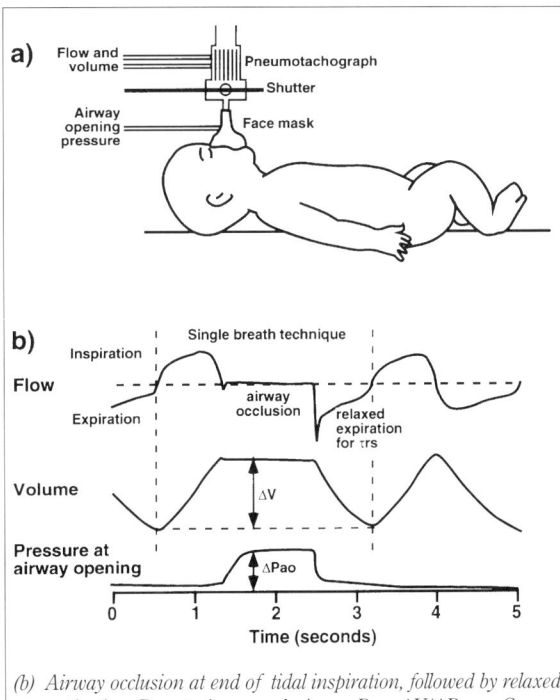

(b) Airway occlusion at end of tidal inspiration, followed by relaxed expiration. Pao at airway occlusion = Prs . ΔV/ΔPao = Crs.

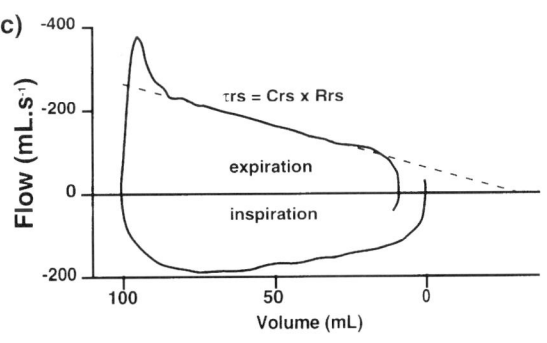

(c) Relaxed expiration plotted as expiratory flow versus expired volume curve. The time constant of the respiratory system (τrs = Crs × Rrs) is obtained from 1/slope of this curve (dotted line). Crs is known from (b), allowing Rrs to be derived.

The latter is common in healthy babies during the neonatal period. Again, nasal resistance is usually included in these measurements.

Indices of forced expiratory flow

Thoraco-abdominal compression technique

Although infants cannot be instructed to perform forced expiratory maneuvers, partial expiratory flow volume (PEFV) curves can be produced by wrapping an inflatable jacket around the child's thorax and abdomen and allowing it to breathe through a pneumotachograph attached to a face mask (Figure 11.4). This technique is usually referred to as the 'squeeze' or rapid thoraco-abdominal compression (RTC) technique.[1(pp 379–410)] The jacket is connected via a tap to a reservoir which contains air at pressures up to 100 cmH$_2$O (10 kPa). At end inspiration, the tap is suddenly turned, causing rapid inflation of the jacket which compresses the chest and forces air out of the infant's lung to produce the PEFV curve. A reproducible end-expiratory level must be established prior to performing the RTC maneuver, and time should be left between each inflation to ensure that the end-expiratory level is re-established. Jacket compression pressure usually commences at 20–30 cmH$_2$O (2–3 kPa) and is increased in 5–10 cmH$_2$O increments to a maximum of 100 cmH$_2$O, or until evidence of flow limitation is achieved, i.e. there is no further increase in flow despite increases in jacket pressure. Measurements are standardized by measuring maximal flow at functional residual capacity (MEF$_{FRC}$ or $\dot{V}_{maxFRC}$) from the PEFV curve (Figure 11.4). The curves obtained from healthy infants usually have a shape convex to the volume axis (Figure 11.4bi) whereas those from infants with airway obstruction, in whom there is

Figure 11.4 Measurement of partial expiratory flow volume curves using the rapid thoraco-abdominal compression (RTC) technique

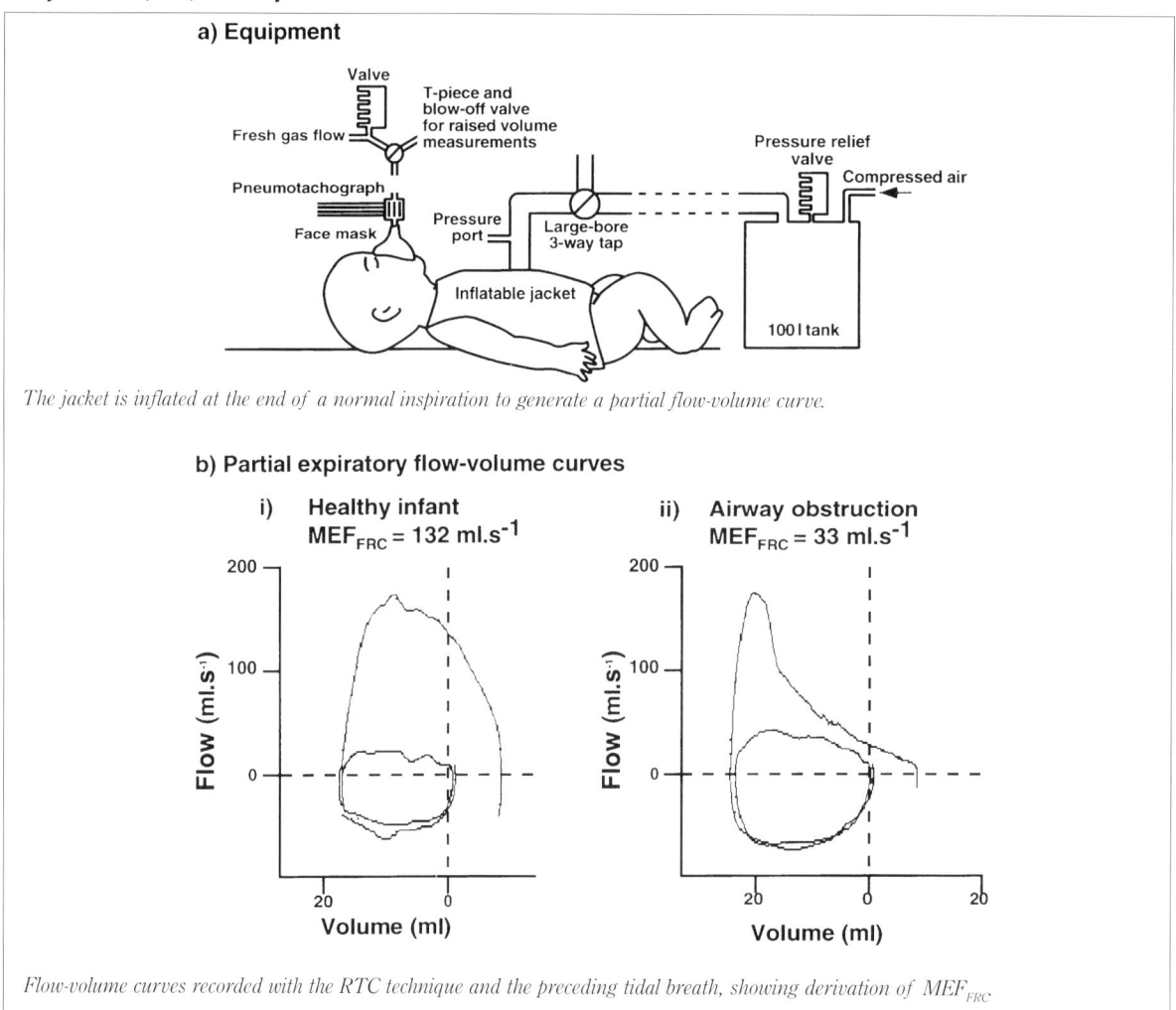

The jacket is inflated at the end of a normal inspiration to generate a partial flow-volume curve.

Flow-volume curves recorded with the RTC technique and the preceding tidal breath, showing derivation of MEF$_{FRC}$.

marked reduction in MEF_{FRC}, are usually associated with concavity of the flow volume curve (Figure 11.4bii). If forced expirations from raised lung volumes are required[4(pp379-410)], circuitry to enable lung inflation prior to jacket inflation must be included. Measurements of MEF_{FRC} have been used to characterize the normal growth and development of the lungs during infancy and the pulmonary abnormalities associated with acute and chronic lung disorders during early childhood.

Interpretation of maximal expiratory flow MEF_{FRC} is thought primarily to reflect airway caliber upstream to the airway segment subjected to flow limitation and therefore to give a measure of peripheral airway function that is relatively uninfluenced by the resistance of the upper airways. This makes it the only measure of intrathoracic airway function in infants, in whom nasal resistance comprises about 50% of total resistance. However, since the caliber of the intrathoracic airways is determined not only by their anatomic dimensions but by the distending pressures surrounding them, full interpretation of results often requires simultaneous measurements of lung volume and elastic recoil of the respiratory system (see Chapter 3). Whether or not flow limitation can be reached in healthy infants using this technique remains controversial.[4] Nevertheless this technique provides a useful forcing function (>100 cmH$_2$O in the jacket at FRC) which can provide a valuable measure of airway function in infants. This technique is the most practical available for assessing response to bronchodilators or bronchial challenge in infants, although interpretation of results may be confounded by numerous factors including changes in lung volume associated with such interventions.

During the last few years adaptations of this technique have been described wherein the infant's lungs are passively inflated towards total lung capacity (TLC) before applying the compression pressure. This enables full forced expiratory maneuvers to be obtained in infants as in adults. It has been suggested that the raised volume technique may be more reproducible and sensitive than the partial flow volume curves and may provide data comparable to FEV_1 in older subjects.[4(pp 379-410)]

Tidal breathing

The observation that the time to peak tidal expiratory flow (t_{PTEF}) as a proportion of total expiratory time ($t_{PTEF}:t_E$) was less in adults with airway obstruction aroused considerable interest in the field of infant lung function testing on account of its simplicity and potential applicability to both clinical and epidemiological studies.[4,7] However, although several studies have demonstrated a diminished ratio of this parameter in infants with airway disease, its relation to other indices of airway function is generally weak and its value may be limited by the marked variability both within and between infants, especially during the first month of life.

Body surface measurements

The possibility of measuring respiratory function without attachments at the airway opening, thereby avoiding problems associated with arousal and increased dead space in infants, has generated considerable interest in the use of body surface measurements such as impedance pneumography, magnetometry, strain gauges, and respiratory inductance plethysmography (RIP). Of the currently available methods, RIP is the most widely used in infants and has been shown to be a valid method of recording respiratory rate and changes in tidal volume, and of assessing the degree of thoraco-abdominal asynchrony, which is usually expressed as a phase angle.[4(pp 139-164, 329-354)] In the presence of upper airway obstruction, there will be paradoxical movements between the rib cage and abdomen (phase lag) making this a valuable monitor for obstructive sleep disorders in infants. Changes in phase lag within children with lower airway disease have also been used to characterize response to therapy. The main advantage of this technique is that it is totally non-invasive and does not require sedation, making it an ideal tool for long-term monitoring. However, interpretation of results is critically dependent on using a properly calibrated system, which may be difficult to achieve in infants. Furthermore, recordings are invalidated by movement error and change in posture, so reliable recordings can only be obtained while the infant is sleeping quietly.

Lung volumes

The only lung volume that can be measured routinely and reliably in infants and young children under three years of age is FRC. Such measurements are obtained using either plethysmography[4(pp 190–240)] or gas dilution (nitrogen wash-out or helium dilution)[4(pp 165–189)] as in adults. Plethysmography requires expensive, complex equipment but provides rapid, reproducible results and can be used for simultaneous measures of both lung volume and airways resistance. By contrast, gas dilution methods are simple, cheaper, and more portable, but are relatively time consuming because of the period of wash-out and wash-in required, especially in the presence of airways obstruction. Accurate measurements are dependent on adequate miniaturization and adaptation of equipment. Plethysmographic measurements are consistently higher (approximately 15%) than those derived by gas dilution, even in healthy infants (the reasons for this are discussed fully elsewhere),[8] making essential the use of different prediction equations for the two techniques. Although other static lung volumes such as TLC or RV cannot be easily measured at the present moment, an inflation technique which allows the lungs of spontaneously breathing infants to be inflated to predefined pressures has been introduced recently and may permit these lung volumes to be measured.[4(pp 379–410)]

Lung volume is not simply a measure of lung growth and development, but a measurement of overall lung size. Except in early infancy, even those children with severely hypoplastic lungs at birth may have apparently normal lung volumes since decrease in alveolar number may be largely compensated for by increase in alveolar size. Lung volume can be reduced by restrictive disorders of the lungs and chest wall, by collapse or consolidation, or in early infancy as a result of impaired fetal lung growth. Hyperinflation can be dynamic (as a result of airway obstruction) or fixed, as in the presence of lung cysts or congenital lobar emphysema.

Lung and chest wall elasticity

Newborn infants have a highly compliant chest wall so that measurements of total respiratory compliance (C_{rs}) generally give a reasonable estimate of lung compliance (C_L), especially in young and preterm infants with lung disease. A wide variety of techniques is available including the occlusion techniques, using single or multiple breath airway occlusions (see Occlusion Techniques), or weighted spirometry for the assessment of C_{rs}, and esophageal manometry for the measurement of dynamic lung compliance (see Esophageal Manometry). The relative advantages and limitations of these techniques are summarized in Table 11.7.

Respiratory diseases causing reductions in lung and respiratory compliance are most commonly encountered during the neonatal period, with airway disease predominating in older infants and young children. Nevertheless, there are certain situations when the assessment of compliance can be very useful in older babies (e.g. prognosis of infants with neuromuscular and skeletal abnormalities and follow-up of those undergoing chemotherapy). In addition, knowledge of the elasticity of the lung and chest wall can be extremely helpful when interpreting measures of lung volume, airway resistance, and MEF_{FRC}.

Non-invasive determination of blood gases

Achieving and maintaining gas exchange is the primary function of the lung; respiratory function testing should therefore include a determination not only of lung mechanics but of blood gases. Ideally, these should be measured non-invasively and continuously – especially in sedated infants and those undergoing therapeutic interventions. Suitable devices include:

- pulse oximetry to measure oxygen saturation, which gives an accurate means of detecting and monitoring hypoxemia
- transcutaneous oxygen and carbon dioxide electrodes which are less accurate, but useful as trend monitors in intensive care situations
- mainstream or sidestream capnographs to assess end-tidal carbon dioxide. Even in rapidly breathing infants, the last can provide a useful reflection of arterial carbon dioxide, as long as there is even distribution of ventilation and no major perfusion abnormality.

A review of the technical aspects related to currently available methods for non-invasive determination of blood gases in infants and young children has recently been published.[4(pp 411–444)]

Table 11.7 Comparison of techniques for assessing lung and chest wall elasticity

Technique	Applicability ICU	Applicability NBI	Applicability Sed	Advantages	Limitations
Esophageal manometry (C_L)	✓	✓	(✓)	• Simultaneous $R_L + C_L$ • Continuous measurements throughout breath with minimal disturbance to infant once catheter in situ	• Esophageal catheter not routinely applicable in older infants • Technically demanding • ΔPes may not represent mean ΔPpl
Weighted spirometry (Crs)	✗	✓	✓	• Simple adaptation of standard spirometer – requires simultaneous measures of FRC • Minimal disturbance	• Assumes passive expiration during applied pressures • Depends on very stable EELV
Multiple occlusion (Crs)	✓	✓	✓	• Simple, cheap, portable equipment • Data collection relatively simple	• Assumes complete relaxation and pressure equilibration during airway occlusions and a stable EELV
Single-breath (Crs)	✓	✓	✓	• Simultaneous measurement of Rrs and Crs • Simple, cheap, portable equipment	• Assumes that (a) respiratory system can be represented by single time constant (b) complete muscle relaxation occurs during and after airway occlusion (c) rapid equilibration during occlusion. These conditions are unlikely to be met in presence of airway disease

Key:
EELV   end-expired lung volume
ICU   Intensive Care Unit, i.e. intubated, ventilated infants
NBI   unsedated newborn infants (< 6 weeks)
Sed   sedated spontaneously breathing infants (> 6 weeks)

The main application of these techniques, in addition to safety monitoring during sedated studies, is for monitoring acute clinical situations and for inpatient and domiciliary recordings during sleep where they are used to assess infants with sleep apnea or obstructed breathing, as part of polygraphic monitoring (see below). Domiciliary measurements by pulse oximetry are valuable in monitoring the efficacy of long-term oxygen therapy in pre-term infants with bronchopulmonary dysplasia and in children with neuromuscular disease or sleep apnea. Single overnight recordings are useful in the identification of hypoxia in children with suspected obstructed sleep apnea syndrome. It should be remembered, however, that sleep can be severely disrupted by airway obstruction without hypoxemia developing (see Chapter 10).

Reference ranges for arterial blood gases in infants above 6 months of age are not significantly different from adult values.[4(pp 411–444)] There are major differences during the first few hours and days after birth as the infant adapts to extra-uterine life. A combination of anatomic shunts through fetal vessels (ductus arteriosus and foramen ovale) and non-alveolarized vessels, together with physiological shunts through areas with low ventilation-perfusion ratios, contribute to the relatively large A–aPO$_2$ found even in healthy infants during the first weeks of life. PaO$_2$ rises from approximately 50 mmHg (6.7 kPa) 10 minutes after birth, to 60 mmHg (8.0 kPa) at 1 hour, 75 mmHg (10 kPa) by 5 hours, and 60–80 mmHg (8–10.7 kPa) by 1–3 weeks of age. These changes are accompanied by relative hyperventilation (compared to adults), with PaCO$_2$ being in the range 33–38 mmHg (4.4–5.1 kPa) during this period.

Distribution of ventilation

As in older subjects, regional lung function and ventilation–perfusion abnormalities can be assessed in infants and children when clinically indicated using radioisotopes such as krypton-81m and technetium-99m (Chapter 5). Increasing use is also being made of computerized tomography and MRI scans in the detection and diagnosis of respiratory disease in this age group. In recent years there has also been a resurgence of interest in the assessment of indices of gas exchange and mixing using computerized analysis of wash-in and wash-out curves.

Gas distribution can be adversely affected by any focal or generalized disorder of the lungs. Little use has been made of these techniques in studying infant lung function. Most tests are based on an assessment of the efficiency with which a tracer gas can be removed from or equilibrated with the lungs. Nitrogen clearance during oxygen breathing is the usual basis, providing indices of efficiency such as pulmonary clearance delay, gas distribution index, or distribution of moments. Techniques which can be applied to oxygen-dependent infants and which treat the lungs as a multi-compartmental system have recently been described. The multiple inert gas methods, which have provided a wealth of data on ventilation–perfusion relationships in adult lung disease await adaptation for use in the newborn.

Cardiorespiratory polygraphic monitoring

Isolated measurements of respiratory function may be of limited value if viewed as brief snapshots without some knowledge of background cardiorespiratory patterns and infant behavior. The pathophysiology of many respiratory disorders in infancy and early childhood is sleep related, thereby necessitating appropriate methods of monitoring. Prolonged polygraphic measurements which include recordings of sleep state, body movement, non-invasive blood gases, and chest and abdominal movements can provide vital information regarding circadian rhythm, control of breathing, and intermittent events such as apnea, upper airway obstruction, and cardiac dysrhythmias[4,(pp 485–520)] particularly if combined with audio-visual recordings. There is increasing use of portable non-invasive techniques for monitoring high risk infants (persistent apnea, apparent life threatening events, etc.) at home. However, it should be noted that these investigations should only be used under close clinical supervision and are not 'apnea monitors'.

Control of breathing

Despite the huge number of publications describing studies designed to assess control of breathing in infants, this remains a highly controversial area – reflecting the difficulties in applying and interpreting such tests in babies. Nevertheless, tests of both chemo-

and mechano-sensitivity have been well described[6,9,10] and it has been established that breathing and arousal responses of the newborn to inhaled CO_2 are brisk and sustained, whereas responses to hypoxia vary from a decrease in ventilation during the early neonatal period to modest increases with advancing age. Vagally mediated mechano-reflexes (Hering–Breuer Inflation Reflex) remain active over the tidal range throughout at least the first year of life.[6]

ASSESSMENT OF RESPIRATORY FUNCTION IN UNSEDATED PRE-SCHOOL CHILDREN

Background

The 'Dark Ages' of pediatric pulmonary function measurement extend from about 18 months to 4 or 5 years. The lower limit is defined by the age below which it is reasonable to sedate a child in order to measure lung function, and the upper by the child's competence in performing lung function tests of the type which are used in school children and adults. In general, little girls are a good deal more competent than their male colleagues at this age. It has been so difficult to measure lung function in this age group that there are virtually no routine clinical applications for most measurements and very few reference values. The techniques described have almost all been used in research protocols. The advent of new computer techniques with which young children are able to cooperate may allow simpler measurements to become commonplace over the next few years.

The sorts of clinical problem for which lung function may provide an answer are listed in Table 11.3. It is clear from the table that relatively few of the problems of pre-school children are amenable to lung function measurements. Management is usually based on symptom modification alone, and diagnostic procedures rely heavily on imaging (often under general anesthetic). Although it would be possible to measure lung function under anesthesia for the most common airway problems, this snapshot of the lungs would be of little relevance to the management of a chronic illness during waking life.

The main differences between lung function measurement in toddlers and pre-school children and in their older counterparts lie in the skills of the technical staff in coping with the unpredictability of young children and their parents. It is wise to prepare families for a visit to the laboratory by means of a preliminary visit and by involving play specialists wherever possible to allow children to feel comfortable and confident in the environment. Parents should be encouraged to be positive about the experience and certainly to avoid threatening children with some unspecified punishment from the laboratory staff for failing to cooperate.

Laboratory conditions

Minor modifications to equipment may be required to make it more adaptable to young children. For instance, smaller mouthpieces and, wherever possible, the avoidance of nose clips should be considered. A face mask incorporating a mouthpiece has been devised by Klug and Bisgaard.[11] It may be necessary to allow children to play on the floor or sit on their parent's lap while performing tests. Adaptability is critical. It is almost impossible to persuade a toddler to do anything against his will and, in fact, it might be counter-productive to try to do so. Plenty of toys should be available and it is wise to discuss facilities in the lab and techniques for dealing with young children with local play specialists from the Pediatric Department.

Quality control is a major concern since the level of cooperation and, hence, repeatability for young children is limited. It is important to have a visual display of raw data rather than simply a highly processed result unless the processing is of a sophisticated nature which allows artifacts to be identified.

Techniques available

Airway function

Plethysmographic techniques can be used in pre-school children.[11] It is possible to seat a child on a parent's or technician's lap inside an adult whole body plethysmograph. While the adult exhales slowly and steadily, producing a correctable background drift, the usual procedures can be carried out by the child breathing through a mouthpiece attached to the apparatus. This procedure requires experience and dedication.

The measurement of specific resistance does not need a period of occluded breathing and in some cases provides a very sensitive measure of airway function.[11]

Forced expiratory maneuvers can be carried out by many pre-school children. About 30% of 5 year olds could be expected to perform an FEV_1 maneuver reliably[12] and a greater proportion a peak flow maneuver. Practice sessions should emphasize the importance of reaching TLC as the starting point since this is critical for all maneuvers. It is almost impossible to obtain a satisfactory vital capacity in pre-school children, and this precludes the accurate measurement of indices from the forced expiratory flow-volume curve, such as MEF_{50} or MEF_{25-75}. As a surrogate, MEF_{FRC} can be measured in pre-school children by encouraging them to blow out hard through a pneumotachograph after a period of quiet breathing.[13] This index is comparable to the maximum flow obtained by the RTC technique in infants but has very poor repeatability and a sensitivity of little value for individual subjects. It has been used as an epidemiological tool.[14]

Impedance methods hold the most promise for the future. The forced oscillation technique (input impedance) is seductively easy but, in this age group, has a low success rate and is highly insensitive to changes in lower airway function, probably because of the effect of upper airway shunt on the sensitivity of the technique.[15] It has been used to measure bronchial responsiveness in young children but is more sensitive to bronchodilator effects (reduction in airway resistance) than in detecting bronchoconstriction in response to a challenge test.[16] Interrupter techniques have similar defects but have the advantage of being easier to administer, using hand-held equipment which is highly mobile.[17] Techniques for measuring high-frequency input or transfer impedance in conjunction with sophisticated computer modeling, may combine the advantages of miniaturized equipment with the sophistication of detailed information about the mechanical properties of the lungs and relative immunity to the effects of upper airway compliance.

Indirect methods of measuring an airway response to bronchodilator or bronchoconstrictor challenge may be valuable in pre-school children. Tracheal auscultation and $tcPO_2$ measurements have both been used to measure bronchial responsiveness in clinical studies.[16]

The results of these tests are largely in the domain of clinical research. Owing to the high degree of stability of the transcutaneous PO_2 electrode, this method is particularly sensitive in comparison with other techniques for children of this age.[16]

Other lung function techniques

Compliance of the respiratory system can be measured in young children by means of the weighted spirometer technique, or by a variant of the multiple occlusion technique described above for infants (see Occlusion Techniques). The measurement of dynamic lung compliance and pulmonary resistance using esophageal manometry can be performed in young children, but is not to be undertaken lightly.[4(pp 241–281)] These are research tools. Similarly, measurement of **lung volume** by helium dilution technique has also been successfully achieved in children down to the age of 2 years but, again, there are few standards, a low success rate, and poor repeatability, so that this is also only valuable in the research domain.[4,8]

Polygraphic monitoring, including indirect (transcutaneous) blood gas and arterial saturation measurement, is useful in the assessment of children with sleep disordered breathing or neuromuscular diseases. Non-invasive techniques are essential and may be combined with video-recording in order to determine the relationship between disordered breathing, body movement, and snoring. This type of study is best carried out either at home or in a specifically designed sleep laboratory/cubicle. Overnight studies in hospital should be carried out in the clinical area. The full value of tidal breathing analysis has yet to be explored in this age group.

MEASUREMENTS IN SCHOOL CHILDREN

With a sensitive approach to the concerns of school children, it is possible to carry out the full range of lung function tests. The youngest children require careful, sensitive handling, together with plenty of opportunities for practice. Positive encouragement and absence of criticism are important as even quite young children are self-conscious and should not be 'put on show'. When children are expected to remain in the laboratory for several hours or a whole day, appropriate diversions should be provided. It helps to have two or three children of a similar age together rather than to deal with children in isolation. Teenagers have different needs and may be particularly worried about 'looking silly' while performing measurements.

Children with neuromuscular disease may have difficulty using mouthpieces. In those with scoliosis, the appropriate reference values should be determined from arm-span, which is normally equal to height.

Reference values should be up-to-date and appropriate for the relevant sex and ethnic group.[4(pp 521–550),8,18–20] It is unclear whether pubertal stage has a significant influence on lung function[5] independent of height. At the moment, almost all reference data ignore puberty, but recent UK reference ranges[19,20] use different regression equations for children below and above 152.5 cm (for girls) and 162.5 cm (for boys) to take into account changes around puberty.

Clinical situations in schoolchildren

(Table 11.3)

Asthma

Most requests for lung function testing relate to asthma. For diagnosis, domiciliary recordings allow PEF variability to be assessed. Their graphical display provides objective evidence of the pattern and severity of disease as well as the level of control achieved in response to changes in treatment. Domiciliary spirometry using miniature electronic data storage services is possible. However, issues of quality control for younger children have not been adequately addressed; for instance, it may be impossible to ensure adequate maximal effort away from the laboratory environment.

For routine evaluation, spirometry is by far the most useful investigation in childhood asthma. Full flow-volume loops allow children with alternative diagnoses ('treatment failures') to be diagnosed. Examples include: blunted expiratory loop in fixed large airway disease; flattened inspiratory loop in fixed upper airway disease; very variable inspiratory pattern with laryngeal dysfunction syndrome; scooped (convex to origin) expiratory flow-volume curve with no bronchodilator response in widespread peripheral airway obstruction, such as bronchomalacia or bronchiectasis.

With the onset of respiratory failure in severe asthma, as PEF and FEV fall below 25–30% of optimum, progressive hypoxemia is accompanied by a rise in arterial PCO_2.

Cystic fibrosis

Intrathoracic airway obstruction together with hyperinflation (increased EELV [FRC]) are the main features. There is short-term variation, associated with respiratory tract infection, against a background of deterioration, especially during teenage and early adult life. Bronchodilator responsiveness is present in most cases, but to a lesser degree than in asthma. Bronchomalacia may develop as destructive changes occur associated with widespread bronchiectasis. Hypoxemia is a late feature of declining lung function, sometimes associated with pulmonary hypertension.

Upper airway obstruction (nasal polyps) may lead to obstructive sleep disruption and hypoxemia during sleep.

Chest wall disorders

Both kyphoscoliosis and neuromuscular causes of chest wall disease lead to a reduction in the efficiency of muscle action. The decline in FRC and vital capacity (hence TLC) have secondary effects on lung elasticity, leading to a further fall in lung compliance. This vicious circle may lead initially to a reduction in exercise capacity and later to chronic respiratory failure with hypoxic pulmonary hypertension. Vital capacity is the single most important means of monitoring change in function. In the presence of diaphragmatic weakness, lying vital capacity is especially reduced (by more than 10% of standing VC) and, indeed, the supine posture may be extremely uncomfortable. The maximum mouth pressures generated during inspiration and expiration (P_{IMAX} and P_{EMAX} respectively) can be a guide to the strength of chest wall musculature, but individuals with weak facial muscles may have difficulty forming a seal with the mouthpiece.

Nocturnal hypoxemia is common in these conditions and, with it, sleep disruption.

Obstructive sleep apnea (OSA)

OSA is common in childhood, in association with tonsillar hypertrophy. Other causes include floppy pharyngeal musculature (neuromuscular disease), small pharynx (Down's syndrome), large tongue, and obesity. It is most prevalent in pre-school children. Sleep studies which use only oximetry will miss a significant proportion of OSA since arousal is so rapid in some children (and adults) that hypoxemia does not develop. A video-recording or sensitive sound/movement detector is also required.

GUIDANCE TO INTERPRETATION OF RESULTS

Poor specificity and sensitivity of most tests of pulmonary physiology currently limit their use in diagnosis, although they may still provide valuable information regarding the type and severity of functional disorders. Reference values are needed for several reasons, one of the most important being their value as standards of comparison between different laboratories. Deviation from normality and determination of pathophysiology are based on reference data. While the response to treatment can be determined by internal reference, completeness of recovery requires data from a reference population. Longitudinal reference data are important in the evaluation of the growth of lung function and for epidemiological studies.

However, in any of these situations, without complete data, false interpretations are likely. For instance, a low FRC in infancy may be due to a genuine reduction in alveolar number (pulmonary hypoplasia) but is far more likely to be the result of abnormal surface forces (in hyaline membrane disease) leading to atelectasis, interstitial disease (alveolitis), or an abnormal chest wall (spinal muscular atrophy). Similarly the use of airway function tests such as airway resistance or partial expiratory flow-volume curves in infants by the rapid thoracic compression technique have drawbacks. Short-term changes in lung function have been used as a measure of response in single dose bronchodilator studies but may be misleading. An appropriate measure of bronchodilator response may require several doses given over many hours and assessed by clinically relevant observations including non-invasive oxygen monitoring combined with lung function measurement.

In the clinical realm, qualitative rather than quantitative measurements may have an important role in monitoring lung function in infants and young children. Most importantly, clinical reasoning and an understanding of the clinical questions being posed, rather than simply availability of equipment and expertise, should determine the choice of technique. Similarly, the integration of results and the actions arising from lung function measurement in children requires close communication between those requesting and those performing the measurements.

From what has been written, it will be clear that technical and subjective limitations are particularly important in pediatric lung function testing. In reporting results, it is therefore important to provide not only a numerical summary but a careful description of the quality of the data. This will depend on an interpretation of the level of cooperation or quality of sleep of the child, together with any other technical problems. Reference ranges should always be provided and, wherever possible, instead of expressing results as '% predicted', a standard deviation score should be given.

CONCLUSIONS

Lung function measurements in infants and young children always present a challenge. It is therefore particularly important that the purpose of any test session is clearly defined before starting. As is the case for physical examination in young children, there is not necessarily a 'routine' approach to lung function testing in children. Opportunities must be taken whenever they present themselves.

It is often necessary to go back to basics in analyzing the results of lung function measurements in young children, and many whose experience is with automated equipment for older subjects find that they gain professionally from the experience as well as having a lot of fun!

References

1   Chernick V & Mellins RB. Basic mechanisms of pediatric respiratory disease: cellular and integrative. Philadelphia: Marcel Dekker 1991.
2   Hislop A. Developmental anatomy and cell biology. In: Silverman M (ed) *Childhood Asthma and Other Wheezing Disorders*. London: Chapman & Hall 1995: 35–54.
3   Silverman M & Taussig LM. Early childhood asthma: what are the questions? *Am J Respir Crit Care Med* 1995; **151**: S1-S42.
4   Stocks J, Sly PD, Tepper RS, Morgan WJ. *Infant Respiratory Function Testing*. New York: John Wiley 1996.

5. Borsboom GJJM, Van Pelt W & Quanjer PH. Interindividual variation in pubertal growth patterns of ventilatory function, standing height, and weight. *Am J Respir Crit Care Med* 1996; **153**: 1182–6.
6. Rabbette PS, Fletcher ME, Dezateux CA, Soriano-Brucher H, Stocks J. Hering-Breuer reflex and respiratory system compliance in the first year of life: a longitudinal study. *J Appl Physiol* 1994; **76**: 650–6.
7. Clarke J & Silverman M. Infant lung function and tidal breathing patterns. *Pediatr Pulmonol* 1995; **20**: 135–6.
8. Stocks J & Quanjer PH. Reference values for residual volume, functional residual capacity and total lung capacity. ATS Workshop on Lung Volume Measurements. Official Statement of the European Respiratory Society. *Eur Resp J* 1995; 8: 492–506
9. Gaultier C. Cardiorespiratory adaptation during sleep in infants and children. *Pediatr Pulmonol* 1995; **19**: 105–17.
10. Hanson MA, Spencer JAD, Rodeck CH, Walters D. *Fetus and Neonate: Physiology and Clinical Applications*. Cambridge: Cambridge University Press 1994: 3–400.
11. Klug B & Bisgaard H. Measurement of lung function in awake 2–4 year old asthmatic children during methacholine challenge and acute asthma. *Pediatr Pulmonol* 1996; **21**: 290–300.
12. Kanengiser S & Dozor AS. Forced expiratory maneuvers in children aged 3–5 years. *Pediatr Pulmonol* 1994; **18**: 144–9.
13. Buist AS, Adams BE, Sexton GJ, Azzam AH. Reference values for functional residual capacity and maximal expiratory flow in young children. *Am Rev Resp Dis* 1980; **122**: 983–8.
14. Martinez FD, Wright AL, Taussig LM, Holberg CJ, Halonen M, Morgan WJ, and Group Health Medical Associates. Asthma and wheezing in the first six years of life. *New Engl J Med* 1995; **332**: 173–8.
15. Solymar L, Aronsson P-H, Bake B, Bjure J. Respiratory resistance and impedance magnitude in healthy children aged 2–18 years. *Pediatr Pulmonol* 1985; **1**: 135–40.
16. Wilson NM, Bridge P, Phagoo SB, Silverman M. The measurement of methacholine responsiveness in 5 year old children: three methods compared. *Eur Resp J* 1995; **8**: 364–70.
17. Phagoo SB, Wilson NM & Silverman M. Evaluation of the interrupter technique for measuring change in airway resistance in 5 year old asthmatic children. *Pediatr Pulmonol* 1995; **20**: 387–95.
18. Quanjer PH, Stocks J, Polgar G, Wise M, Karlberg J, Borsboom G. Compilation of reference values for lung function measurements in children. *Eur Resp J* 1989; **2**(suppl 4): 184s-261s.
19. Rosenthal M, Bain SH, Cramer D *et al.* Lung function in white children aged 4 to 19 years. I Spirometry. *Thorax* 1993; **48**: 794–802.
20. Rosenthal M, Cramer D, Bain SH *et al.* Lung function in white children aged 4 to 19 years. II Single breath analysis and plethysmography. *Thorax* 1993; **48**: 803–8.

12 Pulmonary Function in the Intensive Care Unit

P D MacNaughton and T W Evans

- **INTRODUCTION**
- **ASSESSMENT OF GAS EXCHANGE**
  Arterial blood gas tensions
    Effect of increasing F_IO_2
  Venous admixture/shunt
    Cardiac output and shunt
  Oxygen delivery
  Other factors
    Posture
    Applied PEEP
  Carbon monoxide transfer factor
- **PULMONARY MECHANICS**
  Lung volumes
    Vital capacity
    Functional residual capacity
  Compliance
  Intrinsic PEEP
  Airway resistance
- **ASSESSMENT OF THE RESPIRATORY MUSCLES**
  Respiratory drive
  Maximal airway pressures
  Respiratory muscle fatigue
- **LUNG PARENCHYMA**
  Extravascular lung water
    Thermal dye technique
    Other techniques
  Endothelial permeability
  Epithelial barrier integrity
- **CONCLUSIONS**

INTRODUCTION

The most common reason for a patient to require admission to an intensive care unit (ICU) is to receive mechanical ventilatory support using positive pressure ventilation. This is used to treat acute respiratory failure which may result in either hypercapnia (ventilatory failure) and/or severe hypoxemia. Common causes of ventilatory failure (respiratory muscles unable to meet the demand) include acute exacerbations of chronic obstructive pulmonary disease, acute severe asthma, and neuromuscular diseases affecting the respiratory muscles such as the Guillain-Barré syndrome. Conditions which may cause severe and progressive hypoxemia requiring ventilatory assistance to maintain a reasonable arterial PO_2 level include acute left ventricular failure, pneumonia, and the adult respiratory distress syndrome (ARDS).

ARDS is a clinical syndrome of acute onset which is characterized by refractory hypoxemia, reduced pulmonary compliance, and widespread airspace shadowing on the chest radiograph. It arises from an abnormal increase in pulmonary endothelial permeability which causes pulmonary edema in the absence of fluid overload or heart failure. A wide range of conditions may precipitate ARDS, including generalized sepsis, severe trauma, acute pancreatitis, pulmonary aspiration of gastric contents, and smoke inhalation injury.

A number of factors should be considered when performing lung function tests in patients in the ICU. Such patients are often dependent upon the complex equipment within the ICU such that they cannot be easily moved. Critically ill patients are invariably sedated and may be unable to undertake volitional maneuvers. Furthermore they may be dependent upon high inspired oxygen concentrations and will not tolerate brief periods of breathing lower inspired oxygen tensions. To apply mechanical ventilatory support, patients will have an artificial airway in place in the form of an endotracheal tube or a tracheostomy. This allows ready access to the airway and simplifies certain measurements including lung volumes and pressure-volume relationships. The mode of ventilation that a patient receives can range from complete ventilatory support, such as continuous mandatory ventilation (CMV), to spontaneous breathing with the aid of continuous positive airways pressure (CPAP). The mode of ventilation has an important influence upon the ability to perform certain tests. Thus a patient receiving CMV may be unable to perform a vital capacity measurement although a complete passive pressure-volume curve may be readily undertaken.

This chapter outlines how standard tests may be modified for application in the Intensive Care Unit and describes in detail some tests which are performed almost exclusively in the ICU. Further details of measurements of gas exchange and mechanical properties can be found in earlier chapters.

- ICU patients are sedated, have an artificial airway (intubated), and cannot be moved easily.
- ARDS is caused by pulmonary edema secondary to increased capillary permeability and results in refractory hypoxemia.

ASSESSMENT OF GAS EXCHANGE

Arterial blood gas tensions

Measurement of arterial blood gas tensions in critically ill patients is simplified by the widespread use of indwelling arterial catheters. Patients may receive a wide range of inspired oxygen concentrations, and a number of indices of gas exchange efficiency have been proposed so that PaO_2 can be assessed at different inspired oxygen concentrations. Of these the $PaO_2:FIO_2$ ratio is the simplest and most widely used. Although it does not correct for changes in $PaCO_2$, this empirical index is a useful method of quantifying the impairment of pulmonary gas exchange and is relatively independent of changes in FIO_2, particularly in the 21–40% inspired oxygen range (see Chapter 5). The $PaO_2:FIO_2$ ratio is one of the criteria used to define the adult respiratory distress syndrome (ARDS) ($PaO_2:FIO_2 < 200$ mmHg or 26 kPa).

Effect of increasing inspired oxygen fraction (FIO_2)

The change in arterial oxygen tension which occurs following an increase in FIO_2 depends upon the underlying mechanism(s) of hypoxemia. Thus a modest increase in FiO_2 results in a marked increase in PaO_2 in patients with hypoxemia secondary to hypoventilation or ventilation-perfusion mismatch. The hypoxemia which characterizes ARDS is caused by intrapulmonary shunt or lung units with very low ventilation-perfusion ratios and the response to increasing FiO_2 depends upon the level of shunt (Figure 12.1). With a shunt fraction of 50% there is a very little change in PaO_2, even with an FiO_2 of 1.0 (Figure 12.1a). On the other hand, the increase in oxygen *content* as FiO_2 increases from 30% to 100% is constant and linear at levels of shunt from 10–50% (Figure 12.1b), which is equivalent (at normal hemoglobin levels [14.0 g.dL^{-1}] to 0.22 ml.dL^{-1} of oxygen entering arterial blood for each 10% increase in FiO_2. Thus, independent of the level of shunt, *oxygen delivery* can be increased quite reliably, simply by raising FiO_2 (see Chapter 5 for further discussion).

Venous admixture/shunt

In a lung with abnormal gas exchange, regions with little or no ventilation (collapse or consolidation) act as shunts and the oxygen tension of mixed venous blood (which is added almost unchanged to the arterial blood) is an important determinant of PaO_2. Mixed venous PO_2 reflects peripheral oxygen delivery and consumption, and these non-pulmonary factors can be taken into account by estimating the venous admixture or shunt like effect. This quantifies the difference in arterial and pulmonary capillary oxygen content in terms of the admixture of mixed venous with pul-

Figure 12.1 PaO_2 and CaO_2 at different levels of shunt

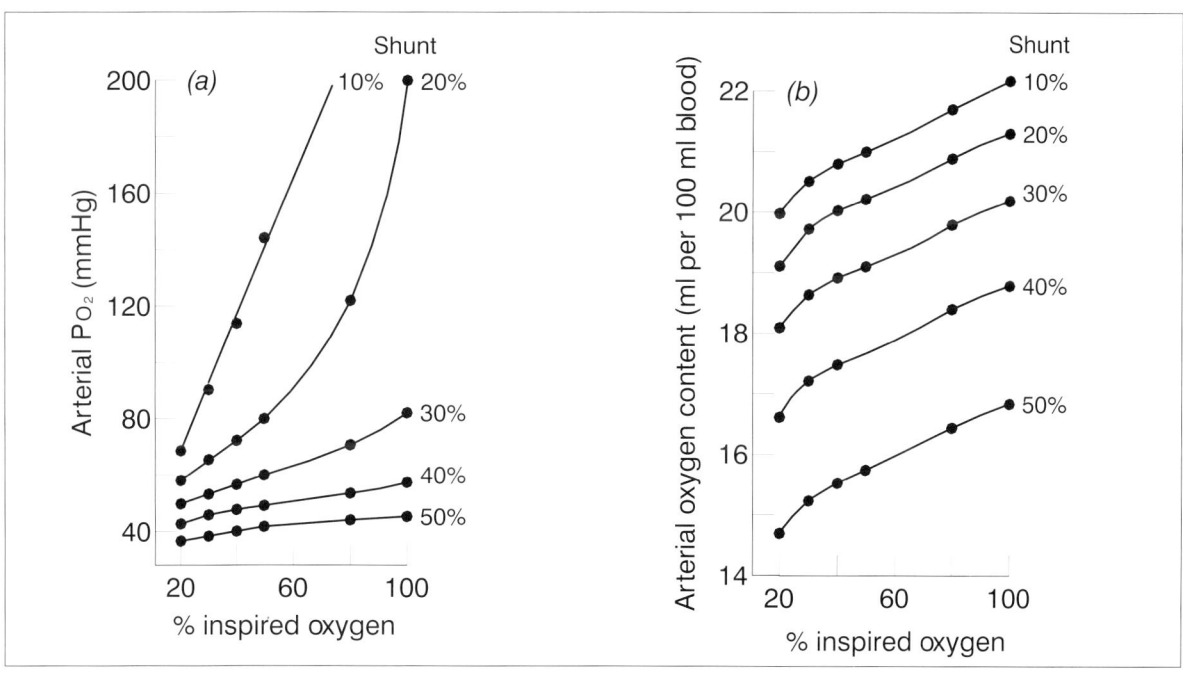

The increase in PaO_2 with FiO_2 increase is very dependent on the shape of the oxygen dissociation curve (ODC) and is small with shunts ≥ 30% because of the steepness of the ODC at that PaO_2.

*On the other hand, the increase in arterial oxygen **content** is linear and constant at all levels of shunt in the FiO_2 range 30–100%.*
*(Reproduced with permission, Dantzker DR. Gas exchange in the adult respiratory distress syndrome. Clin Chest Med 1982; **3**: 57–67.)*

monary capillary blood.[1] A simultaneous measurement of arterial and mixed venous gas tensions enables venous admixture to be estimated from the following equation:

$$\dot{Q}_S/\dot{Q}_T = (Cc'O_2 - CaO_2)/(Cc'O_2 - C\bar{v}O_2)$$

where $\dot{Q}_S/\dot{Q}_T$ is the ratio of shunted blood flow to total blood flow and CaO_2 and $C\bar{v}O_2$ are the oxygen content of arterial and mixed venous blood respectively. The oxygen content of pulmonary end-capillary blood, $Cc'O_2$ (the 'ideal' value in the three compartment model; see Chapter 5), cannot be measured directly but is derived from the calculated 'ideal' alveolar PO_2 which is considered to equal end-capillary oxygen tension ($Pc'O_2$). Estimating venous admixture from the isoshunt plots assumes a normal value for mixed venous PO_2 and is invalid in the critically ill in whom samples of mixed venous blood must be obtained via a pulmonary artery catheter.

The calculated venous admixture will vary according to the FiO_2. If PaO_2 is measured with the patient breathing 100% oxygen, an 'anatomic' or 'pure' shunt will be obtained which is independent of poorly ventilated units with $\dot{V}_A/\dot{Q}$ ratios down to 0.001, provided that nitrogen has been efficiently 'washed-out'. In ARDS, for example, the 100% oxygen shunt is due to blood flow to large areas of consolidated or edematous lung, inaccessible to inspired oxygen even by molecular diffusion from neighboring ventilated regions. Measurements of shunt or venous admixture at lower FiO_2 include a contribution from units with low $\dot{V}_A/\dot{Q}$ ratios. Shunt is a better measure of gas exchange efficiency than indices derived from PaO_2, though all are dependent on the level of FiO_2. In day to day practice, the PaO_2 and the PaO_2:FiO_2 ratio suffices, and the placement of pulmonary artery catheters for shunt estimations is not free from hazard.

Cardiac output and shunt

Arterial oxygen tension is influenced by changes in mixed venous oxygen content, which in turn is affected by the cardiac output and peripheral oxygen utilization ($\dot{V}O_2$). If mixed venous oxygen content falls but shunt fraction remains unaltered, the PaO_2 will also fall with the magnitude of change in PaO_2 depending upon the level of shunt. Thus, at high levels of shunt the PaO_2 is greatly influenced by changes in $P\bar{v}O_2$. However, the relationship between cardiac output and shunt needs to be considered. Whenever a fall in cardiac output occurs there is a parallel *decrease* in shunt. The result is that PaO_2 does not usually fall significantly when cardiac output drops, although total oxygen delivery is reduced (see below).

Oxygen delivery

The most important function of the cardiac and respiratory systems is to deliver oxygen to the cells of the body. The total global oxygen delivery or flux in ml per minute (DO_2) can be calculated from the product of cardiac output ($\dot{Q}$ [L.min^{-1}]) and arterial oxygen content (CaO_2 [ml.L^{-1}]):

$$DO_2 = \dot{Q} \times CaO_2$$
$$CaO_2 = SaO_2 \times Hb \times 1.39$$

where SaO_2 = saturation of arterial blood and Hb = hemoglobin concentration in g.L^{-1}. The constant 1.39 represents the volume of oxygen in ml which combines with 1 g of fully saturated hemoglobin. Cardiac output is usually measured by the thermodilution technique which requires the insertion of a pulmonary artery catheter. Inadequate oxygen delivery is associated with a poor outcome in the critically ill, and the use of pulmonary artery catheters permits oxygen delivery to be monitored and optimized.

Other factors

Posture

Critically ill patients may be nursed in a variety of postures including supine, semi-recumbent (45°), lateral, and prone. Changes in posture can have profound effects on PaO_2, attributable to changes in shunt and $\dot{V}_A/\dot{Q}$ matching. On adopting the semi-recumbent or erect posture from supine, gas exchange may improve dramatically due to a number of factors including an increase in functional residual capacity (FRC), reduced airway closure during tidal ventilation, and improved $\dot{V}_A/\dot{Q}$ matching. In patients with unilateral lung disease such as consolidation or atelectasis, a significant reduction in PaO_2 may occur when the patient lies with the affected lung in the dependent position. The effect of gravity is to increase blood flow through the dependent and poorly ventilated abnormal lung, resulting in an increase in $\dot{V}_A/\dot{Q}$ mismatch. The prone posture may result in a dramatic improvement of gas exchange in ARDS and has been used therapeutically in this condition. A number of mechanisms may be involved including increased FRC and altered distribution of perfusion and ventilation resulting in reduced shunt and improved $\dot{V}_A/\dot{Q}$ matching.

Applied PEEP

Positive end-expiratory pressure (PEEP) is commonly applied to patients undergoing ventilation. It acts to increase end-expiratory lung volume above closing volume and promotes the re-expansion of atelectatic regions. The net result is a reduction in shunt and improved $\dot{V}_A/\dot{Q}$ matching with an improvement in PaO_2. However the associated increase in mean intrathoracic pressure may reduce cardiac output, and therefore oxygen delivery may not be significantly improved.

- $PaO_2:FiO_2$ ratio is a commonly used index of oxygenation and corrects for changes in FiO_2.
- Ventilation in the prone position can increase PaO_2 in ARDS.
- Applied PEEP re-expands collapsed lung, increases FRC, and improves $\dot{V}_A/\dot{Q}$ matching.
- Applied PEEP increases PaO_2 but may reduce cardiac output.

Carbon monoxide gas transfer

The rebreathing technique is the most suitable method for making measurements of D_{LCO} (T_{LCO}) at the bedside. A simplified technique has been described for use in the ICU in which the patient rebreathes from a one liter bag containing a helium/carbon monoxide mixture (He 14%, CO 0.3%, O_2 35% or 70%) for a period of six respiratory cycles.[2] Estimates of D_{LCO}, FRC, and K_{CO} are obtained from standard equations. The values of D_{LCO} measured with this technique are approximately 50% of those obtained using conventional methods, although the values of K_{CO} are similar. D_{LCO} is influenced by many factors including the FiO_2, posture, mode of ventilation, and the inhaled volume. This prevents comparison of the results obtained with the simplified rebreathing technique and the normal predicted values. However, if serial measurements are undertaken in the same individual, the technique provides a sensitive method of investigating changes in the efficiency of gas exchange independent of cardiac output. Serial measurements showing a rise and fall in K_{CO} can be used to detect alveolar hemorrhage (chapter 16).

PULMONARY MECHANICS

Lung volumes

Vital capacity

Portable spirometers permit the bedside measurement of vital capacity (VC) and forced expiratory volume (FEV_1) in extubated, spontaneously breathing subjects. In intubated subjects a moving vane spirometer (e.g. Wright's respirometer) or a pneumotachograph (with integration of flow) are favored methods for measuring VC. Accurate VC measurements require patient cooperation and effort and are difficult to undertake in the ICU where many of the subjects may be confused or sedated. A reduced value may reflect underlying lung disease, respiratory muscle weakness, or inadequate patient effort. A VC > 10 ml.kg^{-1} appears to be required to sustain spontaneous ventilation; a lower value is a sensitive indicator of the need for positive pressure ventilation in neuromuscular disease, such as the Guillian-Barré syndrome. VC measurements are less useful in indicating the need for ventilatory support or in predicting successful weaning in other causes of ventilatory failure.

Functional residual capacity

A number of methods have been described to measure FRC in the ICU. A simple helium dilution technique uses a short period of rebreathing (6 breaths) from a 1 L bag within a bag in bottle system to ensure that the set ventilatory parameters such as PEEP are unaltered. This method underestimates FRC in patients with airway obstruction, but can produce consistent results in restrictive lung disease where there is rapid equilibration of the helium. Other techniques occasionally used in the ICU include nitrogen wash-out or prolonged inert gas (He or SF_6) dilution.

FRC (normally between 2.0 and 3.0 L) is often considerably reduced in ventilated subjects and values less than 1.0 L are common. Factors reducing FRC include underlying lung disease (pulmonary edema, atelectasis, pneumonia), supine posture, sedative and neuromuscular blocking drugs, and abdominal distension. A goal of many of the ventilatory modes utilized in acute respiratory failure is to re-expand or 'recruit' collapsed alveoli by applying positive end-expiratory pressure (PEEP) and therefore to increase FRC and reduce shunt. Chest physiotherapy is also used to re-expand atelectatic lung. Measurement of FRC can be used to assess the effectiveness of these techniques.

> - Vital capacity (VC) measurements require patient cooperation and effort.
> - VC < 10 ml.kg^{-1} predicts the need for ventilatory support in the Guillian-Barré syndrome.
> - Lung volumes are reduced in ARDS, and mechanical ventilation aims to increase FRC.

Compliance (see also Chapter 3)

The presence of an endotracheal tube in a well sedated patient allows measurements of total respiratory compliance (Crs) to be made in the ICU. Pressures measured within the airway will be identical to alveolar pressures when airflow has ceased. Airway pressure is usually measured at the proximal (ventilator) end of the endotracheal tube and is termed pressure at the airway opening (Pao). When a constant flow inspiration followed by a post-inspiratory pause is imposed by a ventilator, analysis of the detailed trace of Pao versus time enables total respiratory compliance (Crs) and resistance (Rrs) in the tidal range to be measured (Figure 12.3).

These measurements can readily be obtained from most ventilators. Accurate measurement of Crs requires that the patient is not making any spontaneous respiratory efforts which alter airway pressures. This may necessitate the use of sedatives or neuromuscular blocking agents. A sealed respiratory circuit free of any leaks is essential and a cuffed endotracheal tube must be in place. The compliance of distensible ventilator tubing contributes significantly to the total compliance in patients with abnormally stiff lungs and should be taken into account.

Values of compliance are influenced by the tidal volume at which the measurements are made. With large tidal volumes, the volume impinges upon the flat, less compliant part of the lung pressure-volume curve, thereby reducing the value obtained.

Consequently, measurements are usually made between FRC and a volume of 500 ml above FRC.

The complete inspiratory pressure-volume curve of the respiratory system can be recorded by measuring the changes in airway pressure following a series of progressive 100 ml increases in lung volume introduced with a large calibrated syringe during a prolonged apnea. After each increment in volume the static change in airway pressure is recorded. Inflation is continued until the airway pressure reaches 40 cmH$_2$O, representing TLC (Figure 12.2). An alternative method is to measure the individual inspiratory plateau pressures which are obtained after a series of step changes in tidal volume set on the ventilator between FRC and TLC.

Low values of Crs are found in many critically ill subjects; values of Crs < 50 ml.cmH$_2$O^{-1} are common while patients with severe ARDS may have values < 20 ml.cmH$_2$O^{-1}. Measurements of compliance are useful in assessing the response to various ventilatory techniques aiming to re-expand atelectatic lung. Optimal applied PEEP has been described as that value which results in the largest improvement in Crs and may be obtained from the complete pressure-volume curve in patients with ARDS (Figure 12.2). As airway pressure is increased, an inflection point occurs where compliance starts to increase, reflecting airway opening. As pressure is increased a point is reached

Figure 12.2 Inspiratory pressure-volume curve of total respiratory system in a patient with acute lung injury

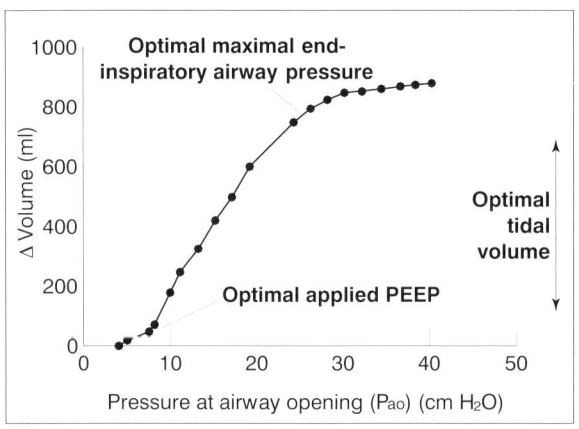

Volume change plotted against pressure at airway opening (Pao) in a relaxed subject on mechanical ventilation (temporarily discontinued). Lead lines indicate upper and lower inflection points. Tidal volume should be over this part of the curve. Slope [Crs] = 46 ml.cmH$_2$O^{-1} between 10 and 20 cmH$_2$O (normal > 100).

Figure 12.3 Measurements and analysis of respiratory mechanics in sedated patients during constant flow inflation by a ventilator in ICU

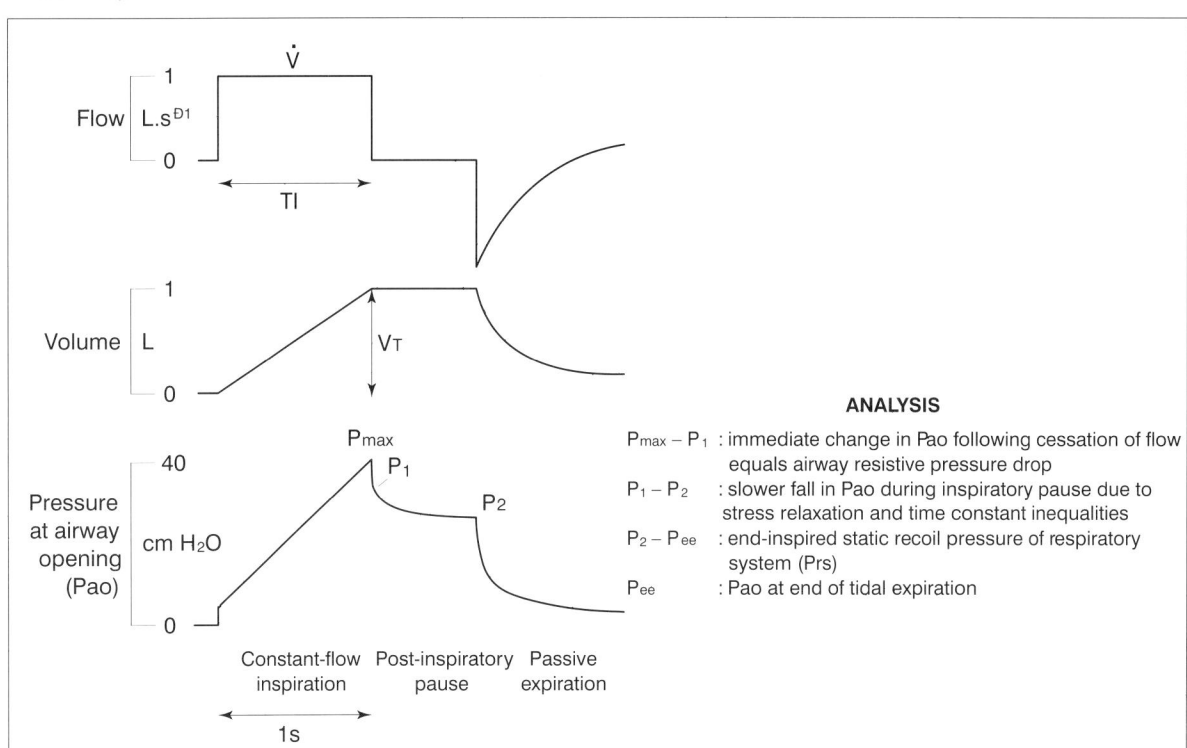

ANALYSIS OF RESPIRATORY MECHANICS[5]

Total respiratory impedance
Impedance to mechanical ventilation is indicated by Pmax but this includes the pressure to overcome resistance (Pres) as well as elastic recoil (Prs) and is influenced by the presence of PEEP.

Compliance of the total respiratory system (Crs)
To measure Crs over the tidal range, the difference between alveolar pressure (Palv) at points of no flow at end expiration and end-inspiration needs to be known. At end inspiration cessation of flow leads to a rapid fall from Pmax to P1 and a slower fall to P2. At end-expiration, if there is no intrinsic or applied PEEP, Palv and Pao are both 0 (atmospheric pressure). If there is intrinsic PEEP, end-expiratory [ee] Palv will be > Pao; the value of intrinsic PEEP may be obtained by measuring Pao after occluding the airway at end expiration to obtain true Palv[ee] (Figure 12.4).

$$\text{Dynamic Crs} = V_T/(P_1 - Palv[ee])$$
$$\text{Static Crs} = V_T/(P_2 - Palv[ee])$$

If Pao at end expiration is used to indicate Palv[ee] this will reduce the apparent value of Crs when intrinsic PEEP is present. Crs can also be measured by interruption during expiration using the plateau value of Pao.

Airflow resistance
During constant flow inspiration, the rise in Pao reflects the pressure needed to overcome Crs, dyn and an additional pressure (Pres) to overcome flow resistance; Pres with a constant flow (usually 1 L.s^{-1}) is assumed to be constant through the breath. When flow ceases at the onset of the post-inspiratory pause, the immediate change in pressure (Pmax – P1), where P1 is determined by the inflection on the Pao versus time curve, is used to calculate resistance of the conducting airways (Raw). The slower change in pressure (P1–P2) is used to calculate the additional non-ohmic resistance due to stress relaxation and the time constant inequalities (ΔRrs).

$$Raw = (Pmax - P_1)/\dot{V}$$
$$\Delta Rrs = (P_1 - P_2)/\dot{V}$$

Total respiratory resistance can also be measured by interruption during expiration if a pneumotachograph is included in the circuit to measure flow immediately before each interruption.

where compliance starts to fall, reflecting the onset of over-inflation. The optimal airway pressures fall between these two points. Use of these measurements to adjust the tidal volume and pressures imposed during positive pressure ventilation may improve gas exchange and reduce ventilator induced lung damage.[3]

When measuring compliance it is essential that the total value of PEEP is recorded. PEEP can be applied externally via the ventilator and is readily recorded (applied PEEP). In the presence of airflow obstruction, however, intrinsic PEEP may arise (see below) and total PEEP (applied PEEP + intrinsic PEEP) will be greater than applied PEEP. If intrinsic PEEP is ignored then the value of compliance will be underestimated.

Most measurements made in the ICU rely on measuring Pao and so measure total Crs, which reflects the combined influence of compliance of the chest wall (Ccw) and the compliance of the lungs (C_L). In practice, most reductions in Crs in acutely ill patients reflect changes in the lungs (usually edema, consolidation, atelectasis, or pre-existing lung disease) rather than in Ccw. However Ccw can be reduced by increased respiratory muscle tone, abdominal distension, or rib cage abnormalities (for instance kyphoscoliosis or thoracoplasty). The two components of Crs can be separated by estimating pleural pressure using an esophageal balloon catheter. The analysis of compliance (and resistance) made during tidal breathing or over an extended volume range can then be made by using the difference between Pao and esophageal pressure (Pes) to measure lung mechanics and the changes in absolute Pes to measure chest wall mechanics (see Chapter 3 for further information on Ccw and Crs).

- Total respiratory compliance (Crs) is usually reduced in acute respiratory failure and can be readily measured in intubated patients.
- Lung compliance is markedly reduced in ARDS.
- Re-expansion of lung units will result in an increase in compliance.
- 'Optimal' PEEP is the PEEP level resulting in the largest increase in Crs.

Intrinsic PEEP

Intrinsic or auto PEEP (PEEPi) describes the increase in end-tidal alveolar pressure that occurs whenever the expiratory time is inadequate to allow the lung to deflate to its relaxation volume.[4] Under these conditions expiratory flow has not stopped before the next inspiration occurs in either spontaneous or positive pressure respiration. Intrinsic PEEP will occur if expiratory resistance is increased (e.g. airway obstruction) or if expiratory time is reduced. The dynamic increase in end-expiratory volume (FRC) results in hyperinflation and a positive alveolar pressure at end expiration.

The presence of PEEPi has a number of important clinical consequences:

- increased inspiratory work of breathing during spontaneous ventilation
- reduced ability to trigger the ventilator during assisted modes of ventilation
- hemodynamic effects of increased intrathoracic pressure
- increased risk of barotrauma
- errors in calculation of compliance.

Figure 12.4 Measurement of intrinsic PEEP by end-expiratory occlusion. Positive alveolar pressure at end-expiration (at onset of inspiration) caused by airflow obstruction and slowed expiration

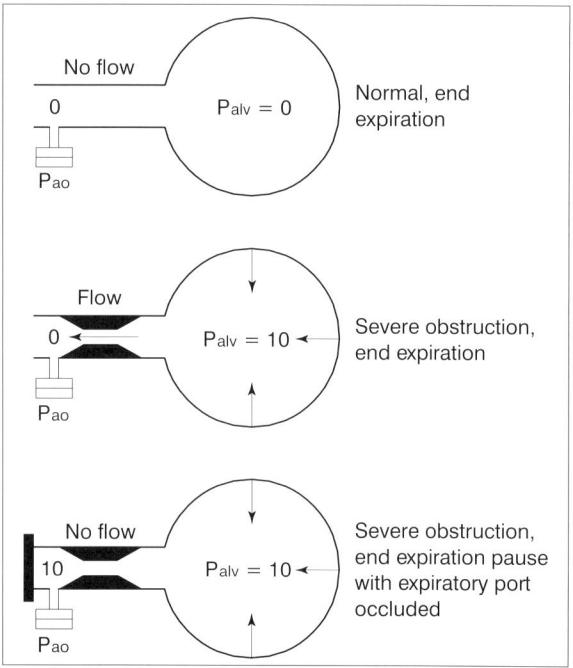

When expiratory resistance is increased, alveolar pressure (Palv) is greater than pressure at the airway opening (Pao) at end of normal expiration. This is intrinsic PEEP which can be measured from the airway pressure during an end-expiratory pause with expiratory port occluded when Pao = Palv.

PEEPi should be monitored in all patients at risk during mechanical ventilation. The static PEEPi can be measured by occluding the airway at the end of expiration with the resulting plateau pressure representing the average PEEPi present within the non-homogenous lung (Figure 12.4). A dynamic measurement of PEEPi can be obtained by recording the airway pressure at which inspiratory flow commences during inspiration. Inspiratory flow commences only after airway pressure has exceeded the value of PEEPi. This dynamic measurement reflects the lowest regional value of PEEPi and may be considerably less than static PEEPi in patients with airflow limitation and significant pulmonary inhomogeneity. Measurements of PEEPi should be made without any external PEEP applied. The value of static PEEPi observed in patients with COPD during mechanical ventilation depends upon the airway resistance and on the imposed ventilatory parameters (tidal volume, expiratory time). Values up to 20 cmH_2O are not uncommon and measurements of PEEPi may be used to assess the response to bronchodilators and to titrate ventilator settings. The increased inspiratory work of breathing caused by PEEPi is reduced by the application of external PEEP which may be beneficial during spontaneous breathing.

- Intrinsic PEEP may occur if expiratory resistance is increased or expiratory time is short.
- Intrinsic PEEP is measured from airway pressure recorded after end-expiratory occlusion of ventilator tubing.
- Level of intrinsic PEEP reflects degree of airway obstruction.

Airway resistance

Inspiratory airflow resistance can be calculated from the airway pressure changes that occur following an airway occlusion during a constant inspiratory flow (usually at 1 $L.s^{-1}$) (Figure 12.3). Following occlusion, the immediate fall in airway pressure is an indication of conventional resistance of the conducting airways (Raw) similar to that measured by body plethysmography. If the plateau pressure during the inspiratory pause is recorded, then the additional resistance due to stress relaxation and time constant inequalities can be measured. When Pao only is measured, these values indicate total respiratory resistance (Rrs – the flow resistance of the lungs and chest wall), but in practice differ little from those of the lungs alone. Expiratory resistance can also be calculated if a series of brief interruptions to flow are performed during a complete passive expiration. During each interruption Pao increases to the elastic recoil pressure (Prs) for the particular volume remaining in the lung. If the flow immediately prior to each occlusion is recorded by a pneumotachograph, then a range of expiratory resistances can be calculated.

Calculating airway resistance is useful in assessing the causes of increased airway pressures during mechanical ventilation (Table 12.1). Increased airway resistance commonly occurs due to airway obstruction from bronchospasm or chronic airways disease, or from secretions within the airway lumen. Regular monitoring of airway resistance is the most accurate method of assessing responses to bronchodilator therapy in ventilated patients.

Airway resistance is also increased in many patients undergoing positive pressure ventilation[5] for ARDS or cardiogenic pulmonary edema; this may reflect edema in the airway wall and the presence of fluid or secretions within the airway lumen. An additional factor may be a reduction in the number of patent airways due to the marked loss of functional lung volume.

Table 12.1 Typical values of airway resistance ($cmH_2O.L^{-1}s$) during mechanical ventilation in different clinical conditions[5] (mean ± SD)

Normal ventilated	4.2 ± 1.6
Cardiogenic pulmonary edema	12.1 ± 5.5
ARDS	15.5 ± 4.6
COPD	26.4 ± 13.4
[Normal spontaneously breathing	2.5]

ASSESSMENT OF THE RESPIRATORY MUSCLES

Bedside assessment of the respiratory muscles in the ICU has an important role in assessing the need for mechanical ventilation and in predicting the likely success of weaning from ventilation.[6] The ability to sustain spontaneous breathing depends upon respiratory drive, respiratory muscle strength and endurance, and respiratory muscle load (resistance and compliance together with PEEPi if present). Respiratory muscle weakness is common in critically ill patients and is either due to a primary neuromuscular disorder or is more commonly a consequence of serious illness. Factors which may contribute include muscle wasting following prolonged mechanical ventilation, metabolic disorders, malnutrition, and critical illness polyneuropathy which is a common complication of multiple organ failure.

Respiratory drive (see Chapter 7)

Respiratory drive can be assessed by measuring the airway pressure 0.1 s after initiating an inspiratory effort against a closed airway ($P_{0.1}$). Some ventilators include the facility to undertake this measurement. The mean of a number of measurements should be recorded. $P_{0.1}$ reflects the neuromuscular activation of the respiratory system and correlates with the work of breathing. High $P_{0.1}$ (>6 cm H_2O) implies an excessive and unsustainable work of breathing. Very low values of $P_{0.1}$, reflecting inadequate respiratory drive, are also associated with failure to wean.

Maximal airway pressures

A global assessment of respiratory muscle strength can be made by measuring Pao (at the mouth or at the proximal end of the endotracheal tube), while the patient makes either a maximal inspiratory ($P_{I}max$) or expiratory ($P_{E}max$) effort against a closed airway.* Both measurements are effort and technique dependent and require patient cooperation. In uncooperative patients, a unidirectional valve can be placed temporarily in the respiratory circuit, allowing exhalation but not inhalation; the patient will then make increasing inspiratory efforts against a closed airway and $P_{I}max$ can be recorded over a 20 second period. Such measurements do not assess respiratory muscle endurance, which may be the more important factor for successful weaning.

Respiratory muscle fatigue

Muscle fatigue occurs when the work expended reaches a level which is not sustainable and muscle contraction fails. Respiratory muscle fatigue is likely to be a common cause of failure to wean from positive pressure ventilation. A number of measurements have been used to predict successful weaning[7].

Table 12.2 Predictors of successful weaning[7]

PaO_2 #	> 75 mmHg (10 kPa) at FiO_2 ≤ 0.5
Respiratory pattern	No diaphragm-rib cage discoordination or inspiratory abdominal paradox
Minute ventilation	≤ 10 L.min⁻¹ and can be doubled voluntarily
Respiratory freq (f)	< 35 min⁻¹
Tidal volume (V_T)	> 5 ml.kg⁻¹
Frequency/V_T	≤ 80 min⁻¹/L
Occlusion press ($P_{0.1}$)	< 6 cmH_2O
Vital capacity*	> 10 ml.kg⁻¹
$P_{I}max$*	< −20 cmH_2O

\# The patient should not be dependent on a high FiO_2
* Effort dependent

A particularly useful test is to discontinue mechanical ventilation and study spontaneous breathing when still attached to the ventilator. More elaborate methods such as the diaphragm pressure-time index require a cooperative patient and gastric and esophageal balloons, and are rarely practical.

- Maximal inspiratory pressures measure muscle strength and not endurance.
- Failure of weaning from ventilation occurs due to respiratory muscle fatigue.
- A respiratory frequency:tidal volume ratio (min⁻¹/L) of less than 80 is a sensitive predictor of successful weaning.

---

* In the future it may be possible to measure non-volitional twitch Pao after magnetic stimulation of the phrenic nerves (see Chapter 4).

LUNG PARENCHYMA

Extravascular lung water

Pulmonary edema is a common cause of respiratory failure and arises secondary to endothelial damage (acute lung injury or ARDS) or from increased pulmonary capillary pressures (heart failure or fluid overload). The manipulation of total body fluid balance may result in a reduction of lung water (both intravascular and extravascular) and an improvement in lung function. Extravascular lung water (EVLW) can be estimated by a number of techniques including thermal dye dilution, soluble inert gas uptake, and transthoracic impedance measurements.

Thermal dye technique

Method

This method for measuring EVLW uses two indicators – ice cold saline and indocyanine green. These two indicators are injected together rapidly into a central vein and temperature and indocyanine green concentrations are monitored downstream in the femoral artery with a special catheter which has a fiberoptic sensor and a thermistor (Figure 12.5a). Heat acts as a diffusible indicator as the 'cold' bolus passes through the pulmonary capillary bed, and the temperature exchange between the blood and the surrounding extravascular lung water is instantaneous. This heating effect of lung tissue and edema fluid in contact with the pulmonary microvascular bed is 'seen' by the intrathoracic blood volume. (The amount of heat gained in the right heart or large vessels from pulmonary artery to femoral artery is negligible because of the restricted surface:volume ratio for fluid exchange.) Indocyanine green is non-diffusible and remains within the intravascular space. Its volume of distribution from injection to sampling site (central vein to femoral artery) is less than that of the heat-diffusing cold indicator, so its mean transit time (MTT) is shorter. The *difference* in mean transit times reflects the difference between the [*vascular plus extravascular*] pool and the *vascular* pool, i.e. the **extravascular** pool. (Fig 12.5b).

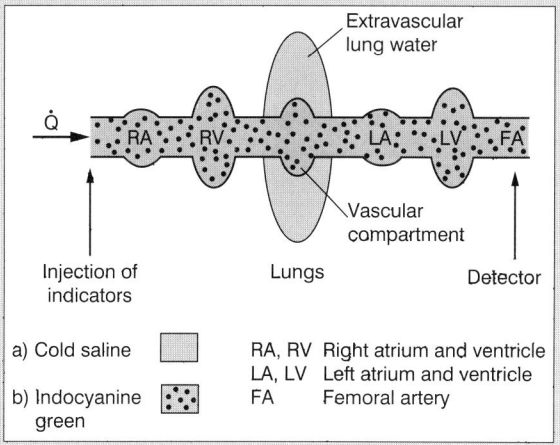

Figure 12.5 (a) Dual indicator technique for EVLW

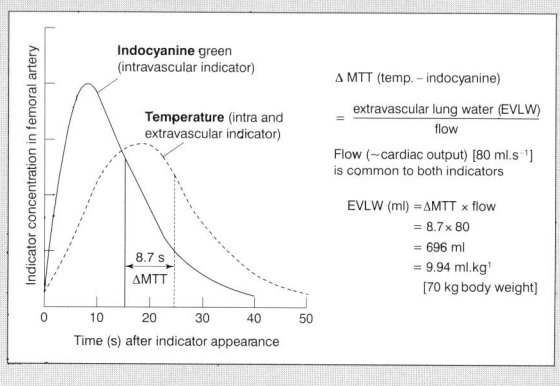

(b) Indicator dilution curves from femoral artery catheter in cardiogenic edema

Typical values	Mean EVLW ± SD
No edema	5.5 ± 1.1 ml.kg^{-1}
Cardiogenic edema	10.2 ± 3.1 ml.kg^{-1}
Permeability edema	15.8 ± 4.6 ml.kg^{-1}

Reliability and clinical utility There are two main problems with this technique. First, recirculation of the indicators, if rapid, distorts the downslope of the indicator dilution curves and increases the amount of 'extrapolation' which necessarily has to be imposed; this leads to an underestimation of EVLW. A slow injection also leads to loss of definition of the downslope. (There are mathematical techniques of 'deconvolution' which can adjust the input curve to the lung to the ideal 'spike' function, but only if a sensor catheter is placed in the pulmonary artery.) Secondly, EVLW can only be measured in perfused areas of the lung and so this method underestimates extravascular lung water in regions where blood flow is low or absent. Applied PEEP may improve the distribution of pulmonary blood flow, by opening up atelectatic regions (thus lowering their high pulmonary vascular resistance), and paradoxically *increase* the measured value of EVLW.

The clinical utility of EVLW measurements is unclear at present. The more edematous the lung, the less accurate the measurement; its inherent 'underestimation' in this context may give a false sense of security. An EVLW measurement of less than 7 ml.kg^{-1} has been used as a therapeutic target in patients with pulmonary edema treated with fluid restriction and diuretic therapy. Further studies are required which compare EVLW measurements with more conventional assessments (chest radiograph and fluid balance).

Other techniques

The soluble inert gas technique derives lung water from the differences in the *initial* volumes of distribution following the inhalation of a mixture of soluble (e.g. freon) and insoluble (e.g. argon) gases. Unlike the thermal dye technique, there is no intravascular indicator so the volume of distribution includes the pulmonary microvascular volume, though this is only ≤ 100 ml. Although the technique is non-invasive it has not been extensively evaluated in the ICU as it requires a sensitive method of gas measurement such as a respiratory mass spectrometer. Typical values in normal subjects are 5.0–6.0 ml.kg^{-1} (similar to EVLW with thermal dye) but the reproducibility of the method is likely to be poor in ventilated patients.

Changes in total lung water can be inferred from alterations in transthoracic impedance, measured from skin electrodes applied to the chest wall. The technique is totally non-specific, however, not distinguishing vascular from extravascular volumes and being affected by the ratio of air to water, i.e. by the expansion of the lung. Thus, atelectasis, ventilatory mode, level of PEEP, and fluid volume (e.g. cardiac size, pleural fluid) all affect the measurement. Furthermore, it does not produce an actual lung water value, but it could reflect short-term changes.

Endothelial permeability

Pulmonary endothelial permeability can be quantified with a radioisotope double indicator technique.[9]

Method

Detection is via scintillation counters placed over the lung periphery and the heart. Transferrin (a plasma protein similar in size to albumin) and red blood cells (RBC) are labeled in vivo after intravenous injection of indium-113m and technetium-99m respectively. Transferrin should not normally leak out of the pulmonary circulation in detectable amounts. For the measurement, one counter is placed over the lung (usually the right upper zone) and another over the heart.

Figure 12.6 (a) Double indicator method with external counting to detect protein accumulation in permeability edema

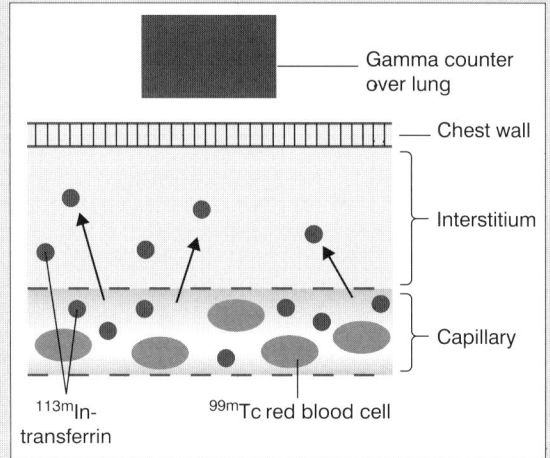

The intravascular marker (^{99m}Tc-RBC) acts as a check on pulmonary blood volume, because changes in vascular volume over the 50–60 minute observation period would be a confounding factor. The heart counter (a vascular pool where ^{113m}In/^{99m}Tc ratio should remain relatively constant during the observation period) corrects for the counting efficiencies of the external detectors for the different γ-energies of In^{113m} and ^{99m}Tc. The protein accumulation index (PAI) is derived from the relative accumulation within the lungs of transferrin compared to red blood cells (Figure 12.6b).

Figure 12.6 (b) Analysis of ^{113m}In-transferrin and ^{99m}Tc-RBC counts for derivation of protein accumulation index (PAI) into the lung

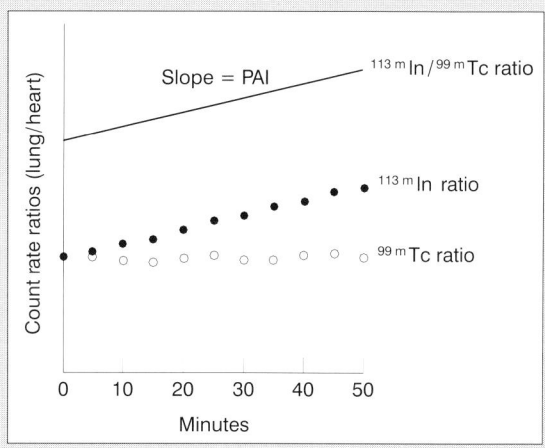

Lung/heart (L/H) ratios for ^{113m}In and ^{99m}Tc and the derived ^{113m}In/^{99m}Tc ratio – [^{113m}In(L/H)/^{99m}Tc(L/H)] – plotted on semi-log against time after i.v. injection of both tracers. PAI is the gradient of the regression line for the ^{113m}In/^{99m}Tc slope in min^{-1} divided by the intercept of its slope with the y-axis (values for intercept are usually between 0.9 and 1.1). Positive slope in this instance represents increased capillary permeability to protein.

Reliability and clinical utility The technique appears highly sensitive and specific; PAI has a positive slope in permeability edema, but no significant slope (i.e. no protein leak) in cardiogenic (hydrostatic) edema. PAI remains a research tool. Although an abnormal increase in PAI may precede the development of clinical acute lung injury, there appears to be a considerable overlap in the PAI values obtained in patients with severe acute lung injury (with gross edema) and other critically ill patients with minimal edema (e.g. following major surgery such as esophagectomy). PAI is not a reliable predictor of which patients are likely to develop clinically significant lung injury. PAI and, by implication, endothelial function may remain abnormal during the recovery phase of acute lung injury, suggesting that other factors play a part in the resolution of permeability edema.

Epithelial barrier integrity

Radiolabelled aerosols carrying molecules of small particle size, such as DTPA (diethylenetriamine pentacetate) (molecular weight of DTPA is about 500 daltons (albumin is about 40 000 daltons)), when inhaled in solution from a nebuliser, deposit on the walls of bronchi and alveoli. From the peripheral airways and alveoli labelled DTPA diffuses passively into the blood compartment with a half-time (t ½) of clearance of about 60 min (20 min in smokers). The rate-limiting step for clearance is considered to be the outer or epithelial cell barrier. If clearance is faster (shorter t ½) as in cigarette smokers and in patients suffering from a variety of lung diseases, including ARDS, the epithelial cell barrier is considered to be 'damaged'.

Method

The technique can be performed in ventilated subjects by connecting a nebulizer containing ^{99m}Tc-DTPA to a conventional anesthetic circuit.

Figure 12.7 (a) Circuit for giving inhaled ^{99m}Tc-DTPA aerosol

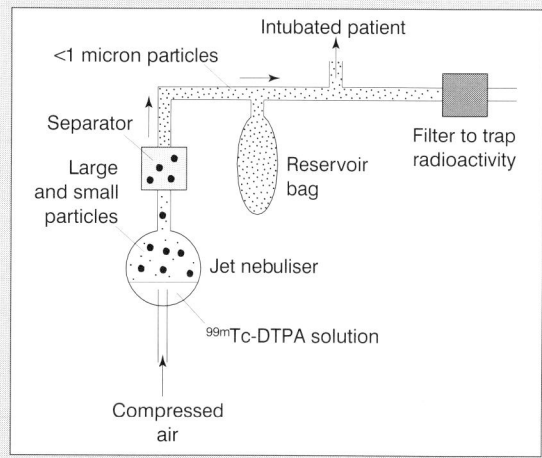

After the patient has inhaled ^{99m}Tc-DTPA for up to 3 minutes, disappearance from the lungs is measured using a gamma camera or scintillation counters applied to the chest wall (usually the right upper zone) with a separate counter over the thigh to measure background tissue activity, which after calibration is subtracted from the chest counts (Figure 12.7b) to give the clearance from the right upper lung zone. ^{99m}Tc-DTPA clearance occurs in an exponential fashion which can be expressed as a half life (t½) in minutes.

Figure 12.7 (b) Counts from scintillation detectors over right upper chest and thigh

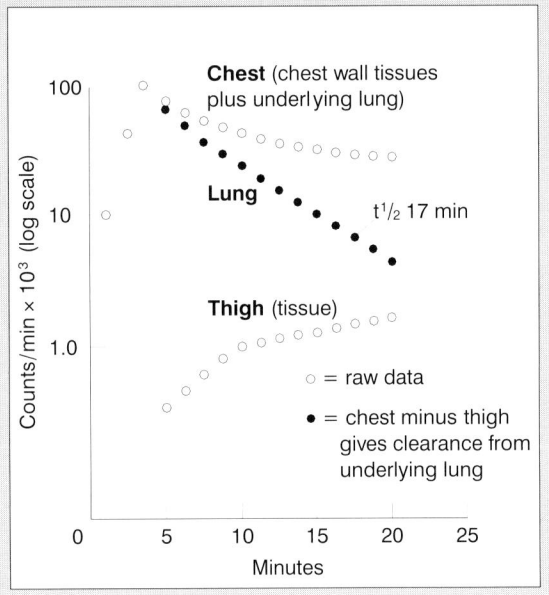

Reliability A wide range of physiological and pathological states influence ^{99m}Tc-DTPA clearance, which is very sensitive but very non-specific. For example, accelerated clearance is observed following an increase in end-expiratory volume, either voluntarily achieved in healthy subjects or occurring after the application of PEEP in mechanically ventilated patients. Serial measurements corrected for lung volume in individual patients could be used to assess changes in epithelial function.

Clinical utility

Normal, non-smoking subjects have a value of approximately 60 minutes, but in current cigarette smokers without respiratory symptoms the t½ is much shorter (10–30 minutes). The half life of ^{99m}Tc-DTPA clearance is less than 20 minutes in patients with ARDS although there is still overlap with the t½ obtained in normal smoking subjects. But, in ARDS, the disappearance of ^{99m}Tc-DTPA is bi-exponential and this is thought to represent more significant lung injury than that seen in asymptomatic smokers (Figure 12.7c).

CONCLUSIONS

Lung function tests are arguably most needed in the critically ill in the ICU. Simple tests can be applied even to individuals receiving mechanical ventilatory support that can significantly influence the diagnosis and aid the selection of appropriate treatment.

Figure 12.7 (c) Bi-exponential lung clearance of inhaled ^{99m}Tc-DTPA aerosol in a patient with acute lung injury

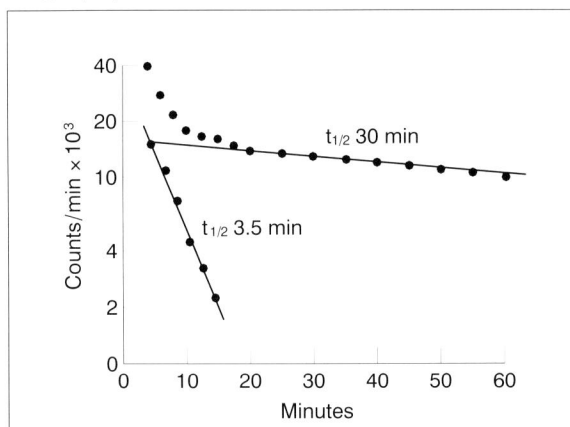

(From Hunter DN, Morgan CJ & Evans TW. The use of radionuclide techniques in the assessment of alveolar capillary membrane permeability on the intensive care unit. Int Care Med 1990; 16:363–71, reproduced with permission from Springer-Verlag GmbH & Co. KG)

References

1. Nunn JF. Distribution of pulmonary ventilation and perfusion. In: Nunn JF *Applied Respiratory Physiology*, 3rd edn. London: Butterworths 1987: 167-76.
2. PD Macnaughton, CJ Morgan, DM Denison, TW Evans. Measurement of carbon monoxide transfer and lung volume in ventilated subjects. *Eur Respir J* 1993; **6**: 231-6.
3. Roupie E, Dambrosio M, Servillo G et al. Titration of tidal volume and induced hypercapnia in acute respiratory distress syndrome. *Am J Respir Crit Care Med* 1995; **152**: 121-8.
4. Rossi A, Polese G, Brandi G, Conti G. Intrinsic positive end expiratory pressure (PEEPi). *Int Care Med* 1995; **21**: 522-36.
5. Broseghini C, Brandolese R, Poggi R, Polese G, Manzin E, Milic-Emili J, Rossi A. Respiratory mechanics during the first day of mechanical ventilation in patients with pulmonary edema and chronic airflow obstruction. *Am Rev Respir Dis* 1988; **138**: 355-61.
6. Moxham J & Goldstone J. Assessment of respiratory muscle strength in the intensive care unit. *Eur Respir J* 1994; **7**: 2057-61.
7. Yang KL & Tobin MJ. A prospective study of indexes predicting the outcome of trials of weaning from mechanical ventilation. *N Engl J Med* 1991; **324**: 1445-50.
8. Sibbald WJ, Warshawski FJ, Short AK et al. Clinical studies of measuring extravascular lung water by the thermal dye technique in critically ill patients. *Chest* 1983; **83**: 725-31.
9. Hunter DN, Morgan CJ & Evans TW. The use of radionuclide techniques in the assessment of alveolar capillary membrane permeability on the intensive care unit. *Int Care Med* 1990; **16**: 363-71.

13 Domiciliary Oxygenation and Assisted Ventilation

A K Simonds

- **INTRODUCTION**
- **ACUTE OXYGEN THERAPY**
- **LONG-TERM OXYGEN THERAPY (LTOT)**
  Effects of long-term home oxygen therapy in COPD
  - *Survival and mortality*
  - *Pulmonary hemodynamics*
  - *Lung function*
  - *Polycythemia*
  - *Sleep and neuropsychological effects*
  - *Quality of life/hospital admissions*

  Assessment of patients
  - *Indications for domiciliary long-term oxygen therapy*
  - *Non-COPD disorders*
  - *Laboratory assessment for domiciliary LTOT*
  - *Oxygen therapy solely at night*

- **DELIVERY OF HOME OXYGEN**
  Oxygen supply
  - *Oxygen concentrators*
  - *Portable oxygen cylinders*
  - *Liquid oxygen*

  Oxygen delivery
  - *Face masks*
  - *Nasal cannulae*
  - *Transtracheal O_2*

  Problems and limitations of domiciliary oxygen therapy
  Air travel
  Conclusions

- **ASSISTED VENTILATION**
  Modes of assisted ventilation for domiciliary use
  - *Nasal intermittent positive pressure ventilation (NIPPV)*
  - *Mouthpiece ventilation*
  - *Negative pressure ventilation*
  - *Tracheostomy-intermittent positive pressure ventilation*
  - *Diaphragm pacing*

Assessment of patients for assisted ventilation
  Acute NIPPV
  Domiciliary ventilation
  Outcome of domiciliary ventilation
  Mechanism of action of nocturnal non-invasive ventilatory support
  Maintenance of ventilatory support equipment
Conclusions
APPENDIX 13.I
Guidelines for institution of NIPPV for acute exacerbations
Problems with NIPPV

INTRODUCTION

Worldwide, the most common cause of respiratory failure in adults is chronic obstructive pulmonary disease (COPD). In the United Kingdom around 0.3% of individuals over the age of 45 years have a chronic arterial oxygen pressure of less than 55 mmHg (7.3 kPa).[1] Primary lung diseases which affect gas exchange and diffusing capacity (emphysema, interstitial lung disease, cystic fibrosis) usually result in hypoxemia in the presence of a low or normal arterial carbon dioxide level. Conditions which reduce the efficiency of the ventilatory apparatus (scoliosis, respiratory muscle weakness, cervical cord lesions) or impair central drive (e.g. primary alveolar hypoventilation or narcotic drugs) lead to hypercapnic respiratory failure. The 'blue and bloated' form of chronic bronchitis is the commonest cause of hypercapnia.

Hypoxemia has a deleterious effect on all organ systems. In response to chronic hypoxemia, the following cardiorespiratory adaptations occur in an attempt to restore ventilation-perfusion matching and oxygen delivery.

Adaptations to chronic hypoxemia
- Increase in ventilation.
- Increase in heart rate and stroke volume.
- Stimulation of erythropoietin production.
- Polycythemia.

The adverse consequences of these responses include an increase in ventilatory workload, rise in pulmonary artery pressure, and increase in myocardial stress.[2] Ultimately progression to cor pulmonale* can occur. The outlook for COPD patients who develop cor pulmonale is poor, with only 30% surviving for 5 years, if untreated.

ACUTE OXYGEN THERAPY

In many patients respiratory decompensation with the development of hypoxemia, with or without hypercapnia, is seen for the first time during a chest infection or following an intercurrent event such as surgery. For patients with COPD, morbidity during an acute exacerbation is related to the degree of acidosis, with a pH of less than 7.26 ([H$^+$] ion concentration more than 55 μmol/L) indicating a poor prognosis. Increasing age and uremia are also adverse features.[3] The greatest risk to patients with respiratory failure is uncontrolled acidosis and tissue hypoxia, so oxygen therapy should be administered promptly to patients with acute hypoxemic respiratory failure due to asthma, acute pneumonia, and pulmonary edema, with the aim of achieving an arterial oxygen saturation level of

---

* Cor pulmonale describes the combination of low PaO_2, high $PaCO_2$, pulmonary hypertension, peripheral edema and polycythemia due to diseases of the lung e.g. (COPD, bronchiectasis), chest wall, respiratory muscles or CNS respiratory control.

90%. High flow oxygen, e.g. 35% or 60%, can be delivered safely as $PaCO_2$ in these situations is usually normal or low. In individuals with a chronic high $PaCO_2$ (e.g. due to blue bloater type COPD, scoliosis, and neuromuscular disease) in whom hypercapnic ventilatory drive is depressed, high flow oxygen therapy may worsen CO_2 retention and so controlled oxygen therapy at 24% or 28% is indicated. However, if adequate oxygenation cannot be achieved without a rise in $PaCO_2$, non-invasive or conventional assisted ventilation should be considered (see below).

During acute exacerbations nebulizers can be driven by high flow oxygen which may reduce the effects of an acute mismatch in ventilation and perfusion precipitated by bronchodilator therapy. For a small proportion of hypercapnic patients oxygen-driven nebulizers worsen CO_2 retention – here the use of an air compressor is preferable.

LONG-TERM OXYGEN THERAPY (LTOT)

Effects of long-term home oxygen therapy in COPD

Survival and mortality

In view of the high morbidity and mortality associated with chronic hypoxemia, several large randomised controlled trials of domiciliary oxygen therapy have been carried out. Both the Medical Research Council (MRC)[4] and Nocturnal Oxygen Therapy Trial (NOTT)[5] showed that long-term oxygen therapy (LTOT) improved survival in hypoxemic COPD, with mortality halved in oxygen recipients (Figure 13.1). The NOTT study[5] compared O_2 24 hours/day (in effect, 19 hours) with overnight (about 8 hours) use of oxygen, whereas the MRC study[4] compared 15 hours a day oxygen with a control group (no O_2). In both studies, oxygen was given with nasal prongs at the lowest flow rate (range 1–4 L.min^{-1}) necessary to achieve a PaO_2 of 60 mmHg (8 kPa) (~ SaO_2 90%) or sufficient to increase PaO_2 by 6 mmHg (0.8 kPa). In the NOTT study,[5] flow rates were increased by 1 L.min^{-1} during the night. All patients had severe COPD with a mean PaO_2 of 51 mmHg (6.8 kPa). The greatest reduction in mortality was seen in the continuous oxygen group with corresponding dose dependent effects on those using 15 hours/day and overnight therapy. In the MRC study, elevation in $PaCO_2$ and red blood cell mass (~polycythemia) predicted early death. Results from a Swedish national database[6] have shown that increasing age, poor performance status, $PaCO_2$, and the use of oral steroid medication (in women) are predictors of poor survival. Most recently, a Polish trial has examined the outcome of LTOT in moderately hypoxemic COPD patients (i.e. mean arterial PaO_2 60 mmHg [8 kPa]).[7] This study showed no beneficial effect on mortality in this less severely affected group (mean FEV_1 0.83L), confirming that there is no indication, as yet, to extend LTOT beyond the existing guidelines given on page 205.

Pulmonary hemodynamics

Oxygen therapy lowers pulmonary artery pressure (Ppa) acutely in COPD by reducing hypoxic vasoconstriction. In the MRC[4] and NOTT[5] studies only small changes in pulmonary vascular resistance were found breathing air. It has been suggested that an early fall in Ppa is predictive of a good response to long-term oxygen therapy, but this has not been widely confirmed. It seems likely that long-term oxygen therapy may prevent a progressive rise in Ppa in some patients, but cannot reverse established structural changes in the pulmonary vascular bed.

Lung function

Mortality in COPD is strongly correlated with FEV_1. Despite the fact that long-term oxygen therapy improves survival, and some short-term studies show a minor improvement in spirometry, a continued fall in FEV_1 is seen in most COPD patients receiving LTOT.

Polycythemia

The MRC study[4] showed no reduction in packed cell volume (PCV) as a result of receiving LTOT, whereas in the NOTT study[5] a greater decrease in polycythemia was seen in those receiving continuous O_2 compared to those getting nocturnal O_2 only. Additional factors such as a carboxyhemoglobin-induced rise in PCV due to smoking are important. It is clear that all patients receiving LTOT must stop smoking – not only to avoid

Figure 13.1 Survival in COPD using long-term domiciliary oxygen (from MRC[4] and NOTT[5] studies), and with nasal ventilation (NIPPV)[25]

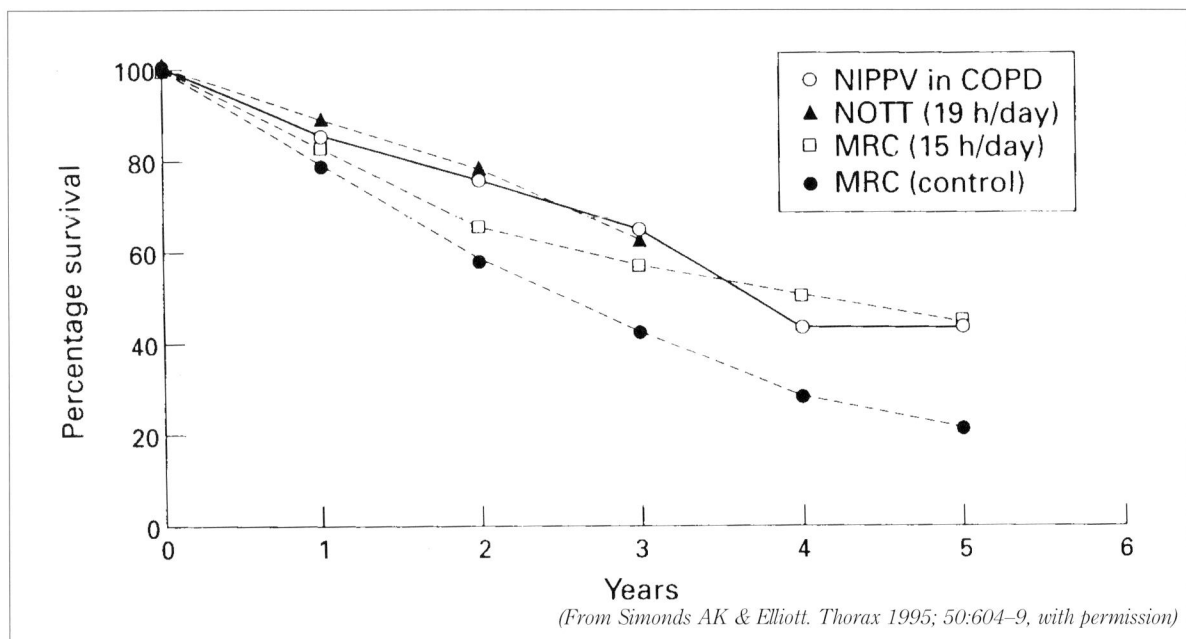

(From Simonds AK & Elliott. Thorax 1995; 50:604–9, with permission)

fire risk, but because of the progressive, deleterious effects of smoking on FEV_1.

Sleep and neuropsychological effects

Many patients with COPD complain of impaired sleep quality. Sleep may be fragmented by hypoxic arousals, bronchospasm, and coughing, or as a result of central stimulant drugs such as theophylline. There is conflicting evidence on the effect of LTOT on sleep.[8,9] The NOTT study showed a high level of neuropsychiatric impairment in hypoxemic patients, with modest improvement seen after six months LTOT. There was no difference in the groups receiving 24 hour versus 12 hour O_2. Despite this evidence of marginal gain, patients did not report any change in emotional status or mood.

Quality of life/hospital admissions

The assessment of health-related quality of life has become an increasingly important part of the evaluation of treatment for chronic disorders over the last decade. There is no convincing evidence that LTOT improves quality of life; indeed, in one recent study comparing LTOT with LTOT plus NIPPV, LTOT produced a deterioration in quality of life measures. The British MRC study[4] showed that LTOT had little effect on the time spent in hospital and on work attendance.

Effects of long-term domiciliary oxygen therapy in COPD

- Benefits proportional to number of hours therapy per day.
- Survival increases.
- Lung function not improved.
- Quality of life unchanged.
- Polycythemia may be reduced.
- Further increases in pulmonary artery pressure may be slowed.

Assessment of patients

As a result of the reduction in mortality attributable to LTOT, guidelines have been issued for the prescription of LTOT in COPD. Oxygen therapy for 15 hours or more each day is recommended in the situations outlined in the 'Indications for domiciliary long-term oxygen therapy' panel (the indications for LTOT are somewhat broader in the USA).

Indications for domiciliary long-term oxygen therapy

Proven benefit (MRC,[4] NOTT[5] trials)

- Patients with chronic obstructive pulmonary disease (COPD) with FEV_1 < 1.5 L, and VC < 2.0 L; PaO_2 < 55 mmHg (7.3 kPa) (SaO_2 < 88%).

Probable benefit (additional USA recommendations)[2]

- PaO_2 < 60 mmHg (8 kPa) (SaO_2 < 90%) in the presence of P pulmonale on the electrocardiogram (EKG), or hematocrit (or PCV) > 56%.
- Nocturnal PaO_2 < 55 mmHg (7.3 kPa) or SaO_2 < 88% with evidence of pulmonary hypertension or cardiac arrhythmias.

Unproven benefit (but often prescribed)

- Patients with other irreversible lung disease (interstitial lung disease, CFA/IPF) with PaO_2 < 55 mmHg (7.3 kPa) or SaO_2 < 88%.
- Palliation of preterminal respiratory failure of any cause.

Non-COPD disorders

There have been no controlled trials of domiciliary oxygen therapy in conditions resulting in end-stage pulmonary fibrosis such as cryptogenic fibrosing alveolitis (idiopathic pulmonary fibrosis) and asbestosis. However, in end-stage interstitial lung disease and lung cancer, oxygen therapy may have a useful palliative role. Oxygen therapy at night in young cystic fibrosis patients does not appear to reduce mortality or morbidity.

Laboratory assessment for domiciliary LTOT

- Measure FEV_1, FVC, D_{LCO}, K_{CO}.
- Check SaO_2 in semi-recumbent position on one (preferably two) occasions when patient is in a stable state (at least three weeks after hospital discharge).
- SaO_2 should be < 88% (< 90% if pulmonary hypertension and polycythemia).
- A walk test may be done: SaO_2 > 90% at rest, but which falls to < 88% at end of exercise, or significant improvement in walking distance or dyspnea on supplementary oxygen may be an indication for ambulatory oxygen.
- Administer 100% oxygen (by nasal cannulae or by route proposed for home use) at 2 L.min^{-1} for 10 minutes, taking average SaO_2 over last 4 minutes. If SaO_2 does not exceed 90%, try flow rate of 3 L.min^{-1} or 4 L.min^{-1}. Flow rates may be increased by 1 L.min^{-1} at night.
- Oxygen concentrators deliver 95% ± 3% O_2 at flow rates up to 4 L.min^{-1}; O_2 percentage is lower at higher flow rates (rarely used).
- Patients, generally with end-stage lung fibrosis, who require > 4 L.min^{-1} O_2 to keep SaO_2 > 90%, will need two concentrator machines (each running at 3–4 L.min^{-1}) for adequate oxygenation.
- Humidification may help at flow rates above 2 L.min^{-1}.
- Patients with known hypercapnia can safely be given LTOT. If in doubt (previous episode of ventilation with $PaCO_2$ > 70 mmHg [9.3 kPa]), use 24% Venturi mask; check $PaCO_2$ in the morning after overnight oxygen breathing, or monitor overnight transcutaneous CO_2.

Oxygen therapy solely at night

Alveolar and arterial PO_2 normally decrease during sleep. Minute ventilation falls because of the reduction in ventilatory drive, increase in upper airway resistance, and decrease in intercostal muscle tone which accompany sleep. If PaO_2 is normal during the day the decrease in oxygenation during sleep is not sufficient to reduce SaO_2 because of the shape of the oxygen dissociation curve. However, significant desaturation may occur during sleep in patients in whom awake PaO_2 is on the 'knee' of the oxygen dissociation curve.

It is arguable whether nocturnal desaturation is an independent prognostic factor. However, a randomised study of oxygen versus air (both given via cylinders) during sleep in COPD patients with a daytime $PaO_2 > 60$ mmHg (8 kPa) but nocturnal desaturation showed some lowering of pulmonary artery pressure in the oxygen therapy group compared to nocturnal desaturators breathing air.[10] Mortality was higher in the COPD patients who desaturated during sleep, but was not reduced by nocturnal oxygen therapy. Further work is needed to clarify the role of oxygen during sleep in the COPD subgroup with daytime $PaO_2 > 60$ mmHg (8 kPa), but who experience nocturnal desaturation.

DELIVERY OF HOME OXYGEN

Whereas there is little evidence to support the use of oxygen therapy for resting breathlessness, patients with exercise-induced dyspnea due to obstructive and interstitial lung disease may derive benefit.[11] Positive responses to oxygen administered during exercise cannot be predicted on the basis of spirometry alone. Many units carry out a baseline 6 minute walk or shuttle walk with oximetry and scoring of breathlessness (e.g. Borg scale – Chapter 8). Oxygen or air from portable cylinders is then given in random order. Portable O_2 is prescribed for individuals in whom correction of hypoxemia occurs, accompanied by a reduction in breathlessness and/or improvement in walk distance.

It is important for patients who are receiving LTOT at home from an oxygen concentrator to realize that portable oxygen systems will enable them to get out and about, and that this will lessen their feelings of isolation.

Oxygen supply

Oxygen concentrators

The concentrator contains a molecular sieve which works using gas chromatography to extract nitrogen from air, producing a gaseous output of approximately 95% O_2, 5% argon at flow rates up to 4 $L.min^{-1}$. In the UK, concentrators may be prescribed on a National Health Service prescription and installed by commercial contractors. The flow rate and intended daily duration of use of the concentrator (usually 15 or more hours) should always be specified. Flow rates (commonly 1–2 $L.min^{-1}$) should be based on laboratory testing (see earlier). For patients needing oxygen therapy for more than 3 months, concentrators are a more economical option than oxygen cylinders. A recent field study in Upper Egypt[12] has shown that concentrators are also a reliable and cost effective mode of supplying oxygen in rural areas in the developing world. Oxygen concentrators are serviced once a year by the suppliers.

Portable oxygen cylinders

In the home, though rarely in hospitals nowadays, oxygen may still be supplied in stand-alone cylinders. Oxygen can also be given to patients, when they move around, in small 'portable' cylinders, carried in a backpack or over the shoulder, or wheeled on a trolley. Portable cylinders provide patients with more mobility, both within the home and outside. Standard flow meters provide 2 $L.min^{-1}$ at medium setting and 4 $L.min^{-1}$ at high setting. If patients need lower flow rates, a separate flow meter needs to be supplied.

The problem with portable cylinders has been their weight and the short period of oxygen supply from them. Conservation devices have been developed to deliver O_2 more economically from cylinders. These devices allow patients to spend longer periods away from home before a refill is required. They take the form either of reservoirs incorporated into the delivery system, which are simple but rather obtrusive, or the more efficient demand devices which allow O_2 flow only during inspiration. The Oxylite™ demand system (Life Support, Europe Ltd.) (Figure 13.2) is a portable electronic conserver which pulses 35 ml of oxygen during inspiration. At a setting of 4 on the Oxylite™ a pulse is delivered with each breath approximately equivalent to 4 $L.min^{-1}$ continuous flow of oxygen. At a setting of 2, a pulse is delivered with alternate breaths equivalent to a continuous flow rate of 2 $L.min^{-1}$. Hence an Oxylite™ 240 (containing 240 L O_2 and weighing 5 lb [2.3 kg]) will last approximately 9 hours on a setting of 2, and 4.5 hours on a setting of 4. Overall oxygen saving ratios vary from 4:1 to 11:1 (average 7:1). However, it cannot

Figure 13.2 The Oxylite™ PS-240 portable oxygen conservation system

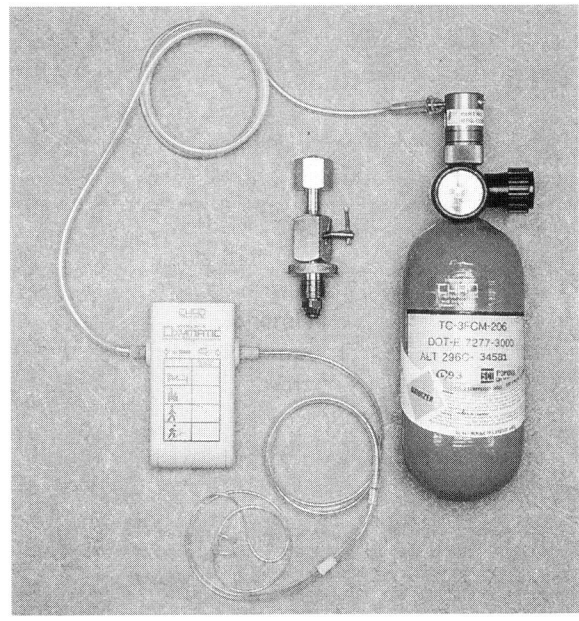

be assumed that exact equivalence with continuous flow rates will be achieved during exercise in patients with severe desaturation.[13] The Oxylite™ costs around $1250 [£800].

The effective 'life' of any cylinder will be reduced by (a) increased respiratory rate and (b) how full the filling cylinder is when topping up the portable device. A half full mother cylinder will result in a half full daughter cylinder.

Liquid oxygen

This is not currently available in the UK, but is used by patients elsewhere in Europe and in the USA. A reservoir is kept by the patient and is regularly filled by the supplier. Small, portable containers of liquid oxygen last for around 8 hours making this a convenient system for ambulant patients[14] although home delivery may be expensive.

Oxygen delivery

Face masks

Depending on their design, masks can deliver either high but uncontrolled oxygen concentrations (up to 60%) or low, but controlled, concentrations in the

Portable (ambulatory) oxygen

- Assess patients with a walk test, breathing air and oxygen, in random order.
- Not usually indicated for attacks of breathlessness at rest.
- Weight of the cylinder is a disadvantage.
- Inspiratory demand valve or reservoir system will extend cylinder life.

range 24–35%. Controlled oxygen concentrations are given through Venturi masks. Oxygen (100%) enters the mask through a constriction and entrains air downstream (the Venturi principle) in a controlled way. By varying the size of the orifice and the design of the entry port, the entrainment ratio (air:oxygen) can be modified to give a range of inspired oxygen concentrations, i.e. 24:1 for 24%, 10:1 for 28%, 4.6:1 for 35%. In normal subjects, the actual concentrations delivered are close to expected.[15] Factors which help to 'stabilize' the inspired O_2 concentration are (a) a large mask volume (c. 300 ml) which acts as a reservoir, and (b) a high *total* inflow (45–50 L.min^{-1}). Factors which reduce the nominal FiO_2 are (a) hyperventilation (the peak inspiratory flow rate of the patient may exceed the flow rate into the mask) and (b) reinspiration of dead space from the mask at the onset of inspiration. For tachypneic patients (fR > 30 min^{-1}) the recommended oxygen inflow rate should be increased (from 2 to 3 L.min^{-1} for FiO_2 24%, and from 4 to 6 L.min^{-1} for FiO_2 28%).[15] Venturi masks delivering 40 and 60% inspired oxygen are available. The 60% oxygen mask has an entrainment ratio of 1:1; 15 L.min^{-1} oxygen delivery still only gives a total flow rate of 30 L.min^{-1}. Actual inspired oxygen concentrations delivered by this mask are about 50%.[15]

To give high inspired oxygen concentrations (50–60%), high oxygen flow rates are required to overcome mask dead space and leaks. Masks of a non-Venturi type are usually used, and inspired oxygen concentrations are uncontrolled and unknown. They may vary – depending on the oxygen flow rate, the design and fit of the mask, and the patients ventilation (either higher or lower than normal) – from 30% to 90%.

Nasal prongs

Many individuals find nasal cannulae more convenient for home overnight use. At a flow rate of 2

> **Oxygen by facemask**
>
> ■ Venturi masks give controlled and steady FIO_2 at 24%, 28%, and 35% levels because of high flow rates into the mask (45–50 L min^{-1}).
>
> ■ Non-Venturi masks give uncontrolled and unknown FIO_2 depending on the conditions.
>
> ■ FIO_2s of 50–60% are the maximum achievable with facemasks unless the patient is hypoventilating.

L.min^{-1} via cannulae, FIO_2s of 24–35% were achieved in COPD patients.[16] Higher concentrations of oxygen may be obtained in patients who hypoventilate, particularly during sleep or after sedating drugs. This variability means that a venturi mask is therefore a safer choice if controlled low concentration oxygen therapy is essential (e.g. in a hypercapnic patient with depressed hypercapnic ventilatory drive who is reliant on hypoxemia to stimulate ventilation).

Transtracheal O_2

Delivery of oxygen directly to the trachea by a surgically implanted microcatheter may reduce delivered oxygen requirements by up to 50%, by decreasing dead space and leakage. Transtracheal O_2 is suitable for individuals who need continuous long-term oxygen. Complications such as infection, sputum impaction, and dislodgment limit the applicability of the system.

Problems and limitations of domiciliary oxygen therapy

Although oxygen therapy improves survival, some patients find that LTOT is tedious and restricts their lifestyle. The provision of ambulatory oxygen systems could improve their quality of life. In Scotland, over 40% of patients prescribed LTOT use it for less than 15 hours per day, and around 14–20% continue to smoke,[17] despite advice to the contrary. In addition, audits have shown that oxygen is still inappropriately prescribed in cylinders in many cases, and that treatment is started too late or not attempted in individuals who might benefit.[11,17] Further education of patients and medical and paramedical staff is needed to address these problems. Respiratory Teams are best placed to assess patients for LTOT and carry out follow-up. Compliance is likely to be improved by the greater availability of portable oxygen therapy.

Air travel

Commercial aircraft fly at altitudes of up to 41 000 feet (12 500 meters), with cabin pressure maintained at a level equivalent to 5–8000 feet above sea level. In a normal individual PaO_2 will fall to around 68 mmHg (9.0 kPa), but as this value lies on the near-horizontal section of the dissociation curve arterial oxygen saturation will only decrease to 92%. However, marked hypoxemia may develop in a patient who has a baseline PaO_2 on the steep part of the dissociation curve. Some pulmonary function laboratories are able to carry out 'fitness to fly' tests in which arterial blood gas tensions are measured with patients breathing from Douglas bags containing 15% O_2 which mimics FIO_2 at cabin pressure. Nomograms (see Smeets, Table 13.1) can predict PaO_2 in normocapnic COPD at altitude. The extent of arterial hypoxemia may be surprisingly severe; a rough guide is given in Table 13.1.

Table 13.1 Likely levels of hypoxemia in COPD patients at altitude [Smeets F. Thorax 1994; 49: 77–81]

	Moderate hypoxemia		Severe hypoxemia	
	PaO_2 mmHg [kPa]	SaO_2 %	PaO_2 mmHg [kPa]	SaO_2 %
Sea level	75 [10]	93.5	60 [8]	90
6000 ft (1830 m) 'jet airliners'	54 [7.2]	86	47 [6.3]	82
10 000 ft (3048 m) 'high alpine pass'	46 [6.1]	81	36 [4.8]	69

As a rule of thumb, individuals with a SaO_2 of < 94% at rest at sea level are likely to need oxygen therapy at altitude. Airline carriers need advance warning of oxygen requirements with specification of flow rates. Patients are not allowed to carry portable cylinders as cabin luggage. For most patients flow rates of 2–4 L.min^{-1} should suffice. It should also be remembered that desaturation during air flights will worsen further during sleep, so that daytime and short haul flights, where possible, are advisable. It is helpful for patients to take nasal cannulae with them if they prefer this delivery method.

> **Home oxygen: conclusions**
>
> ■ Appropriate in chronic lung disease with daytime PaO$_2$ < 55 mmHg (7.3 kPa).
>
> ■ For chronic lung disease oxygen concentrators should replace home use of oxygen cylinders.
>
> ■ Domiciliary oxygen is underprescribed and underutilized.
>
> ■ Ambulatory oxygen is used even less, but O$_2$ conserving systems and lighter cylinders now make it more acceptable.

ASSISTED VENTILATION

Ventilatory pump failure occurs if the capacity of the ventilatory system is compromised by weak/inefficient respiratory muscles, a reduction in central drive, *and/or* the load on the system is excessively increased. In view of the overall reduction in central drive and altered ability to adapt to fluctuations in load during sleep, chronic ventilatory insufficiency first develops during sleep. Then as hypoxemia, hypercapnia, arousals, and sleep deprivation further depress ventilatory drive, hypoventilation becomes manifest during the day resulting in hypercapnia and cor pulmonale if the vicious cycle is not broken.

Modes of assisted ventilation for domiciliary use

Ventilation can be delivered either invasively or non-invasively:

Non-invasive:	*Invasive:*
Nasal ventilation	Tracheostomy ventilation
Negative pressure ventilation	Diaphragm pacing
Mouthpiece ventilation	

The choice of ventilatory technique is based on a number of considerations:

- the underlying pathophysiological process
- degree of ventilator dependency
- bulbar function (particularly effectiveness of swallow and cough)
- social circumstances
- patient preference.

Non-invasive ventilatory support is suitable for individuals who require assisted ventilation during sleep and/or for part of the day. For those with bulbar insufficiency and near 24 hour ventilatory dependence (e.g. cervical spine trauma) ventilation via a tracheostomy is usually required.[19]

Nasal intermittent positive pressure ventilation (NIPPV)

This technique was introduced in the early 1980s and is now the most widely used form of home ventilatory support. Approximately 2000 people in the UK receive domiciliary NIPPV, with most needing nocturnal support alone. NIPPV is also used in hospital to treat acute exacerbations of chronic respiratory failure.[20–22] Oxygen can be entrained into the circuit for patients with severe arterial hypoxemia (see Appendix 13.I). Ventilators delivering NIPPV can be categorized as volume preset or pressure preset.

There is no evidence that any one type of ventilator is superior. In theory, volume preset equipment may compensate for changes in ventilatory load more effectively than pressure preset models, but the latter may better compensate for leaks.[23(pp 16–37)] The BiPAP (Respironics Inc.), VPAP (Rescare), and DP90 (Taema) ventilators differ from volume preset equipment and other pressure preset systems (e.g. NIPPY ventilator) in providing pressure support ventilation with the availability of positive pressure during expiration (EPAP). EPAP may be helpful in reducing atelectasis and offsetting the increased inspiratory threshold load in patients with intrinsic PEEP due to severe airflow obstruction. Most nasal ventilators are used in assist/control mode, i.e. inspiration is triggered by the patient, but back-up ventilatory cycling will occur if the patient becomes apneic. Triggered mode (spontaneous setting S on the BiPAP) may be sufficient if ventilatory drive is intact.

The interface of the ventilator with the patient is central to the success of NIPPV. Close fitting silicone nasal or full face masks are available from a variety of manufacturers and it is possible to customize individual masks. Nasal plugs or seals are an alternative which may be helpful in claustrophobic individuals or those who develop pressure sores from the mask.[23(pp 16–37)]

Mouthpiece ventilation

This is a variant of mask ventilation. Ventilation is delivered via a mouthpiece, which is usually constructed by orthodontic techniques to ensure a good fit. Disadvantages include dislodgment of the mouthpiece during sleep and deformity of the teeth. However mouthpiece ventilation has been successfully employed in many patients with respiratory muscle weakness due to previous poliomyelitis.

Negative pressure ventilation (nPV)

The iron lung or tank ventilator is the most mechanically efficient negative pressure system. Here ventilation is accomplished by enclosing patient from the neck down in a chamber which is evacuated by negative pressure pump to generate inspiration. Expiration occurs passively. The cuirass, pneumosuit, and Hayek oscillator (in which high frequency oscillation is superimposed on intermittent negative pressure) are smaller nPV systems. They are rarely used to support ventilation in the home. nPV may, however, be particularly helpful in infants, and the iron lung is still used in some centers to treat acute hypercapnic exacerbations of chronic lung disease.

Tracheostomy-intermittent positive pressure ventilation (T-IPPV)

A minority of ventilator dependent individuals in the UK receive T-IPPV, and usually have cervical spine lesions or end-stage neuromuscular disease. There are considerable practical problems associated with discharging a patient on T-IPPV, including the provision of suction, humidification, homecare assistance, and back-up ventilatory support in the event of a power cut etc.; these problems are dealt with elsewhere.[18]

Diaphragm pacing

Implantation of a pacemaker to stimulate the phrenic nerve can produce effective ventilation in individuals with central alveolar hypoventilation or high spinal cord lesions. Progressive neuromuscular disease or chest wall/lung pathology should be seen as contraindications to diaphragm pacing. These limitations coupled with technical problems mean that diaphragm pacing is only carried out in a small number of patients.

Assessment of patients for assisted ventilation

Acute NIPPV

There is now evidence from three randomised controlled studies[19–21] that NIPPV may be of value in patients with severe acute exacerbations of COPD. NIPPV reduces the need for endotracheal intubation, the duration of ventilatory support, and length of hospital stay compared with a group receiving conventional therapy. Mortality and complication rates were found to be largely related to intubation. Brochard et al[20] have shown an absolute reduction in mortality rate of 20% (9% mortality in NIPPV group, 29% mortality in group treated conventionally, without NIPPV). Adults and children with acute ventilatory failure due to other causes such as chest wall and neuromuscular problems are also likely to benefit from NIPPV. The selection of patients remains crucial, however. A suggested guide for the initiation of NIPPV in acute ventilatory failure is given in Appendix 13.I. Further practical details are provided elsewhere.[23(pp 45–49)]

Domiciliary ventilation

Candidates for home ventilatory support have chronic symptomatic hypercapnic respiratory failure which is unresponsive to standard measures. In restrictive chest wall or neuromuscular disorders patients with a vital capacity or respiratory muscle strength of less than 30% predicted are at risk of developing ventilatory insufficiency. In COPD patients with respiratory failure LTOT remains first line treatment, but the addition of NIPPV may improve arterial blood gas tensions and quality of life in a subgroup with marked hypercapnia and sleep fragmentation.[24] The role of NIPPV in COPD is currently being investigated in a multicenter European study. Table 13.2 shows

Table 13.2 Selection of patients for domiciliary non-invasive ventilation

Established indications		
Chest wall/pulmonary	*Neural/muscular*	*Central/obstructive*
Scoliosis	Old poliomyelitis	Primary alveolar hypoventilation
Thoracoplasty (old TB)	Myopathies e.g.	Overlap syndrome
Fibrothorax	*Nemaline, central core*	(OSA with hypercapnia)
Rigid spine syndrome	*Acid maltase deficiency*	
	Spinal muscle atrophy	
	Muscular dystrophies	
	Polyneuropathies	
Selected subgroups		
COPD	Cervical cord trauma	Brain stem CVA
Bronchiectasis	Motor neurone disease	Cerebrovascular disease

the conditions in which home ventilatory support has been demonstrated to be of benefit.

Individuals with chronic respiratory failure usually present with features of nocturnal hypoventilation which include morning headaches, poor sleep quality, breathlessness, and fatigue. In children, failure to thrive, anorexia, and concentration problems at school predominate. Patients with these symptoms should undergo overnight monitoring of ventilation which includes measurement of SaO_2 and CO_2 tensions, and diurnal arterial blood gas measurement. Most authorities would consider that ventilatory support is indicated if nocturnal $PaCO_2$ exceeds 53 mmHg (7kPa) in extrapulmonary restrictive disorders.

Outcome of domiciliary ventilation

Both domiciliary positive and negative pressure devices improve survival in patients with chronic ventilatory failure due to chest wall and stable neuromuscular disease. Five year survival figures for patients receiving domiciliary NIPPV at night are shown in Figure 13.3.[25] Similar results were obtained in a recent multicenter French study.[26] Long-term improvements in arterial blood gas tensions and quality of life are seen. The results in COPD patients who fail LTOT are encouraging, but confirmation of this impression is awaited from a randomised controlled study of LTOT versus NIPPV plus LTOT. It is likely that only a subgroup of patients with COPD will be suitable, as discussed above. While it was previously felt inappropriate to provide ventilatory assistance to individuals with respiratory muscle weakness due to progressive neuromuscular disease (Duchenne muscular dystrophy, motor neurone disease) it is now clear that useful palliation of breathlessness and nocturnal hypoventilation may be achieved in some patients with these conditions.[23(pp 96–101)]

Mechanism of action of nocturnal non-invasive ventilatory support

At first sight it may appear strange that ventilatory support provided during sleep improves function dur-

Figure 13.3 Survival using NIPPV at night in COPD and restrictive lung diseases

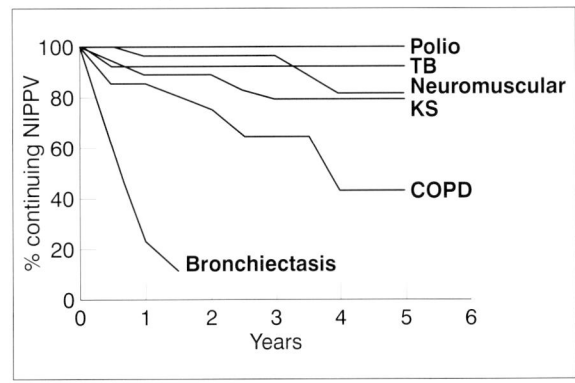

TB = post-tuberculous fibrosis; KS = kyphoscoliosis
(From Simonds AR and Elliott M, *Thorax* 1995; 50:604–9, with permission[25])

ing the day. Possible mechanisms responsible for improvement include:

- increase in ventilatory drive
- improvement in respiratory muscle strength
- reduction in ventilatory load.

Although respiratory muscle fatigue is widely postulated to exist in chronic ventilatory failure, the assessment of fatigue is difficult and many measures of respiratory muscle strength are dependent on the cooperation of the patient (see Chapter 4). In one long-term study of COPD patients receiving domiciliary NIPPV, a significant improvement in arterial blood gas tensions was not accompanied by any increase in respiratory muscle strength. However, nocturnal hypoventilation was controlled and, as a result, chemosensitivity increased.[27] Withdrawal of ventilatory support in patients with restrictive chest wall disease provoked an early return in symptoms of nocturnal hypoventilation in the absence of any lung function changes.[28] The predominant mechanism of action therefore appears to be via control of hypoventilation, although independent effects on chest wall characteristics in some subgroups cannot be excluded.

Maintenance of ventilatory support equipment

Most ventilators require a once or twice yearly service and electrical safety check. All ventilator-dependent patients should have ready access to technical and medical advice to deal with equipment and respiratory problems.

ASSISTED VENTILATION CONCLUSIONS

- Nasal intermittent positive pressure ventilation (NIPPV) in acute ventilatory failure may reduce the need for endotracheal intubation and improve survival.

- Domiciliary ventilation should be considered in adults and children with symptomatic chronic hypercapnic respiratory failure.

- Non-invasive respiratory support, particularly NIPPV, is suitable in most patients with nocturnal hypoventilation.

References

1. Bardsley PA & Howard P. Respiratory failure in COPD. In: Brewis RAL, Gibson GJ & Geddes DM (eds) *Respiratory Medicine*. London: Bailliere Tindall 1990: 534–44.
2. Tarpy SP & Celli BR. Current concepts. Long term oxygen therapy. *N Engl J Med* 1995; **333**: 710–14.
3. Jeffrey AA, Warren PM & Flenley DC. Acute hypercapnic respiratory failure in patients with chronic obstructive lung disease: risk factors and use of guidelines for management. *Thorax* 1992; **47**: 34–40.
4. Medical Research Council Working Party Report. Long term domiciliary oxygen therapy in chronic hypoxic cor pulmonale complicating chronic bronchitis and emphysema. *Lancet* 1981; **i**: 681–5.
5. Nocturnal Oxygen Therapy Trial Group. Continuous or nocturnal oxygen therapy in hypoxaemic chronic obstructive lung disease. *Ann Intern Med* 1980; **93**: 391–8.
6. Strom K. Survival of patients with chronic obstructive pulmonary disease receiving long-term domiciliary oxygen therapy. *Am Rev Respir Dis* 1993; **147**: 585–91.
7. Gorecka D, Gorzelak K, Sliwinski P, Tobiasz M, Zielinski J. Effect of long term oxygen therapy on survival in patients with chronic obstructive pulmonary disease with moderate hypoxemia. *Thorax* 1997; **52**: 674–9.
8. Calverley PMA, Brezinova V, Douglas NJ, Catterall JR, Flenley DC. The effect of oxygenation on sleep quality in chronic bronchitis and emphysema. *Am Rev Respir Dis* 1982; **126**: 206–10.
9. Fleetham JA, West P, Mezon B, Conway W, Roth T, Kryger M. Sleep, arousals, and oxygen desaturation in COPD. *Am Rev Respir Dis* 1982; **126**: 429–33.
10. Fletcher EG, Luckett SGW, Miller CG, Qian W, Costarangos-Galarza C. A doubleblind trial of nocturnal supplemental oxygen for sleep desaturation in patients with chronic obstructive pulmonary disease and a daytime PaO2 above 60 mmHg. *Am Rev Respir Dis* 1992; **145**: 1070–6.
11. Walters MI, Edwards PR, Waterhouse JC, Howard P. Long term domiciliary oxygen therapy in chronic obstructive pulmonary disease. *Thorax* 1993; **48**:1170–7.
12. Dobson M, Peel D & Khallaf N. Field trial of oxygen concentrators in upper Egypt. *Lancet* 1996; **347**: 1597–9.
13. Roberts CM, Bell J & Wedzicha JA. Comparison of the efficacy of a demand flow delivery system with continuous low flow oxygen in subjects with stable COPD and severe oxygen desaturation on walking. *Thorax* 1996; **51**: 831–4.
14. Lock SH, Blower G, Prynne M, Wedzicha JA. Comparison of liquid and gaseous oxygen for domiciliary portable use. *Thorax* 1992; **47**: 98–100.
15. Jones HA, Turner SL & Hughes JMB. Performance of the large reservoir oxygen mask (Ventimask). *Lancet* 1984; **i**: 1427–31.
16. Bazuaye EA, Stone TN, Corris PA, Gibson GJ. Variability of inspired oxygen concentration with nasal cannulas. *Thorax* 1992; **47**: 609–11.
17. Morrison D, Skwarski K & Macnee W. Review of the prescription of domiciliary long term oxygen therapy in Scotland. *Thorax* 1995; **50**: 1103–5.
18. Simonds AK. Discharging the ventilator-dependent patient. *Brit J Int Care Med* 1998; **8**: 47–51.

19. Muir JF. Home mechanical ventilation. *Thorax* 1993; **48**: 1264–73.
20. Brochard L, Mancebo J, Wysocki M *et al.* Noninvasive ventilation for acute exacerbations of chronic pulmonary disease. *N Engl J Med* 1995; **333**: 817–22.
21. Bott J, Carroll MP, Conway JH *et al.* Randomised controlled trial of nasal ventilation in acute ventilatory failure due to chronic obstructive airways disease. *Lancet* 1993; **341**: 1555–7.
22. Kramer N, Meyer TJ, Meharg J, Cece RD, Hill NS. Randomized prospective trial of non-invasive positive pressure ventilation in acute respiratory failure. *Am J Respir Crit Care Med* 1995; **151**: 1799–806.
23. Simonds A K (ed). *Non-invasive Respiratory Support.* London: Chapman & Hall Medical 1996.
24. Meecham Jones DJ, Paul EA, Jones PW, Wedzicha JA. Nasal pressure support ventilation plus oxygen compared to oxygen therapy alone in hypercapnic COPD. *Am J Respir Crit Care Med* 1995; **152**: 538–44.
25. Simonds AK & Elliott MW. Outcome of domiciliary nasal intermittent positive pressure ventilation in restrictive and obstructive disorders. *Thorax* 1995; **50**: 604–9.
26. Leger P, Bedicam JM, Cornette A *et al.* Nasal intermittent positive pressure ventilation. Long term follow-up in patients with severe chronic respiratory insufficiency. *Chest* 1994; **105**: 100–5.
27. Elliott MW, Mulvey DA, Moxham J *et al.* Domiciliary nocturnal intermittent positive pressure ventilation in COPD: mechanisms underlying changes in arterial blood gas tensions. *Eur Respir J* 1991; **4**: 1044–52.
28. Hill NS, Eveloff SE, Carlisle CC, Goff SG. Efficacy of nocturnal nasal ventilation in patients with restrictive thoracic disease. *Am Rev Respir Dis* 1992; **145**: 365–71.

APPENDIX 13.1

Guidelines for institution of NIPPV for acute exacerbations[23]

Suitability of patient

1. ↑$PaCO_2$, pH < 7.3, RR > 30 min^{-1}, PaO_2 < 45 mm/Hg [6kPa] on air with no response to standard therapy.

2. Able to cooperate with therapy (mild confusion not a contraindication).

3. No severe bulbar weakness or hemodynamic instability.

Considerations

Results are less good in patients with severe bronchospasm and pneumonia. Age is no bar. Before you start NIPPV, decide whether it is appropriate to proceed to intubation and conventional ventilation if NIPPV fails.

Equipment

Probably no advantage to any particular type of ventilator. Familiarity with performance and good fitting mask probably more important. Pressure preset ventilation may be preferable in the presence of bullous lung disease or pneumothorax.

Technique

1. Explain to the patient what you are going to do. Check that the ventilator is functioning and circuitry is complete before taking it to the bedside.

2. Ensure a good mask fit. A full face mask may be better in confused patients. Allow the patient to hold in place at first to reduce any sensation of claustrophobia. The mask can then be secured with the headgear.

3. Ventilator settings. For pressure preset ventilator it is usual to start with an inspiratory positive airway pressure of around 12–15 cmH_2O in adults. If expiratory pressure is available a usual setting is 2–5 cmH_2O. If baseline PaO_2 < 7.0 kPa, entrain oxygen into the circuit at a flow rate of 1–3 L.min^{-1} to achieve a SaO_2 of > 90%. For volume ventilator either a flow rate, e.g. 0.7–1.0 L.s^{-1}, or tidal volume, e.g. 500–800 ml, needs to be set. These volumes seem large as NIPPV is inevitably inefficient with air leaks occurring from around the mask and/or the mouth.

4. Take into account feedback from the patient and increase pressure or flow rate if he/she feels that he/she is not getting 'big enough' breaths. The most commonly used mode enables patients to trigger their own respiratory rate. A back-up rate of 12–15 per minute is usually sufficient in adults.

5. Aim to use NIPPV for periods of several hours at a time and particularly during sleep. At least 6–8 hours NIPPV a day, preferably 10–16 hours, is likely to produce the best results. Treatment is usually continued for several days to 1 week to allow correction of daytime blood gas tensions.

Monitoring

Monitor SaO_2 during initiation of NIPPV (and transcutaneous PCO_2 if available), and check arterial blood gas tensions after 40–60 minutes of NIPPV. Do not expect a complete correction of $PaCO_2$ – you are aiming to reduce acidosis, by achieving improved oxygenation, and a gradual decrease in $PaCO_2$. A failure of pH and $PaCO_2$ to improve after 1 hour of NIPPV is a poor prognostic sign. In this situation an increase in inspiratory positive pressure or flow rate may improve $PaCO_2$. However, if the situation continues to deteriorate with the development of progressive acidosis, conventional ventilation should be considered, if appropriate.

Problems with NIPPV

Problem	Management
Nasal bridge sore	Better fitting mask Can try bubble mask or nasal plugs
Mouth leaks	Improve mask fit, try full face mask Keep any dentures in situ
Rhinitis, nasal congestion	Try humidification Short term: ephedrine nose drops Longer term: nasal steroids Deal with mouth leaks
Gastric distension	Adjust position in bed Lower inspiratory positive pressure or flow rate
Expectoration of secretions	Ensure humidification adequate Consider bronchodilators plus steroids Carry out physiotherapy during NIPPV

Section IV
APPLICATIONS WITHIN THE ROUTINE LABORATORY

14 Assessment of Airway Responses and the Cough Reflex

P W Ind and N B Pride

Measurement of the airway response
Site and nature of the airway response

■ **BRONCHOCONSTRICTOR RESPONSES**
Terminology
Mechanisms of hyper-responsiveness
Choice of provocative stimulus
  Method of administration of inhaled pharmacological stimuli
  Other routes of administration of drugs
  Responses to physical agents
Pharmacological blockade
Conduct of provocation tests
  Safety
  Patient preparation
Dose-response curves to constrictor stimuli
Interpretation and clinical usefulness

■ **BRONCHODILATOR RESPONSES**
Dose and choice of bronchodilator
Timing of measurements
Expressing the response
  FEV_1
  Other tests of airway function
Interpretation and clinical usefulness

■ **SENSITIVITY OF THE COUGH REFLEX**
Cough reflex
Laboratory evaluation
  Increased frequency of cough
  Assessing the sensitivity of the cough reflex
  Capsaicin cough responsiveness
  Monitoring frequency of cough
  Cough in asthma
Decreased cough effectiveness

Measurement of the airway response

Assessing whether airway function improves after bronchodilator drugs is one of the most important clinical services provided by the pulmonary function laboratory. Bronchoconstrictor responses are examined less frequently and do not contribute so directly to treatment but can be particularly useful for excluding or confirming the diagnosis of asthma. Most commonly the airway response is assessed by spirometry, particularly in UK and North America, but in some countries body plethysmography is popular. A variety of other tests of airway function can be used (Table 14.1). More details of these tests are given in Chapters 1 and 2.

The most important practical distinction is between tests that require a deep inflation (DI) to total lung capacity (TLC) and those that are made either during tidal breathing or at volumes close to those used during tidal breathing. A DI can considerably modify airway responses; indeed the difference in response before and after a DI has been used to localize the site of a response. In some circumstances where cooperation is difficult, an indirect assessment can be made. The basic lung function techniques used to measure response are discussed in other chapters: this chapter concentrates on the use of pharmacological and other agents to stimulate responses, the analysis of the responses, and the differences that may occur between the response in different tests of airway function.

Site and nature of the airway response

Responses that acutely improve or decrease airway function are usually assumed to be due to relaxation or contraction of airway smooth muscle. Changes in mucosal edema or airway secretions could also conceivably occur, but these are likely to be more important in the inflammatory response and fall in FEV_1 that occurs late (i.e. several hours) after the inhalation of allergen in a sensitized individual.

The site of narrowing or dilatation within the airway is usually not known. For acute responses it is probably in the conducting airways but some investigations have shown that the glottis and trachea may be involved in acute constrictor responses, while peripheral airway narrowing may be prominent in the late constrictor response to antigen. Indeed, recent work in animals has suggested that constrictor agents may increase lung tissue resistance; whether this occurs in humans is unknown. The constrictor response does not affect all parallel airways equally. When a constrictor response in extrathoracic airways is suspected, measuring reduction in maximum inspiratory flow may be particularly useful.

BRONCHOCONSTRICTOR RESPONSES

Terminology

'Bronchial (or airway) hyper-responsiveness' is used to describe an enhanced tendency to narrowing. This may be specific – that is responses to allergens, occupational agents, and occasionally drugs, which are confined to individuals who have become sensitized – or non-specific, such as the enhanced constrictor responses shown to low doses of agents such as histamine and methacholine. In vitro, such direct acting agents invariably constrict airway smooth muscle; in vivo, it is not possible to induce constriction in all subjects but non-specific hyper-responsiveness is usually regarded as the sensitive end of a unimodal distribution in the population.

The airway response may not be confined to the bronchi, and so some prefer to use the term 'airway hyper-responsiveness' but in the remainder of this section *bronchial* provocation, *broncho*dilatation and *broncho*constrictor will be used, as remains the most common practice. Hyper-responsiveness can be described more precisely in terms of the different features of a dose-response curve to a specific provocative agent (see later).

Mechanisms of hyper-responsiveness

Acute constrictor responses involve contraction of airway smooth muscle; even in the late response to antigen the narrowing can be reduced by inhaled β_2-adrenergic agonist drugs such as salbutamol* or terbutaline.

The precise reasons for enhanced constrictor responses in asthma (and to a lesser extent in other diseases of the intrapulmonary airways) are surprisingly uncertain and probably vary between different individuals.[1] The conventional view is that in asthma

---

* Known as albuterol in USA

Table 14.1 Measuring the airway response

Test	Advantages	Disadvantages	Indication
TESTS OF AIRWAY FUNCTION			
(a) Requiring a deep inflation			
FEV_1	Simple, highly repeatable	Relatively insensitive; particularly for studies of normal pharmacology	Most clinical studies of dilator and constrictor responses
PEF	Simplest	Less reliable than FEV_1	Field studies, exercise-induced responses. Young children
FVC	Indicates extent of airway closure/ opening	Repeated forced expiration tiring, may enhance constrictor response	Examining airway closure
Inspiratory capacity	Indicates level of hyperinflation	Not obtainable on all spirometers	Useful supplement to forced expiration tests
Maximum expiratory and inspiratory flow-volume curves	Widely available; good quality control of repeatability	Tiring, requires repeated forced expiration and may not add to FEV_1, FVC	Most useful in combination with partial forced expirations
(b) Not requiring a deep inflation			
Body plethysmography	Indicates tidal airway dimensions, usually combined with FRC	Complex equipment, repeatability poorer than tests of forced expiration	Best method for normal pharmacology; best alternative to spirometry for clinical responses
Forced oscillation	Indicates tidal airway dimensions during natural breathing.	Not widely available, FRC not obtained	Alternative to body plethysmography
Partial forced expiration	More sensitive to constrictor or dilator response than tests requiring a forced expiration from TLC	More variability, requires more subject cooperation	Research studies may indicate site of response. Alternative for normal pharmacology
Functional residual capacity	Indicates changes in hyperinflation but requires multi-breath equilibration	Slow; and requires direct test of airway function also	Limited place in assessing dilator response
INDIRECT ASSESSMENT			
Exercise tests, including 6 minute walk distance or shuttle walk	Simple	Tests motivation as well as lung function	Supplements bronchodilator assessment
Onset of wheeze	Simple	Sensitivity may be improved by acoustic method	Assess constrictor responses in young children or other poorly cooperative subjects
Transcutaneous PO_2	Simple	More sensitive than oximetry	Assess constrictor response in children < 5 years

the airway smooth muscle is unduly 'twitchy' and primed to contract in response to enhanced neural stimulation or the release of inflammatory mediators. But structural factors may amplify the response – there is an increased amount of airway smooth muscle, increased thickening of the airway wall, and possibly less restraint on airway narrowing by the surrounding attachments to the lung alveoli in asthma. (It has been proposed that lung-airway coupling may be impaired by an increase in outer diameter of the airway and peri-airway inflammation.) Proportionate changes in resistance to airflow are also greater when the initial caliber is reduced.

In contrast, in normal subjects the surrounding lung attachments greatly restrict the narrowing of airways induced by histamine or methacholine, resulting in a plateau of maximum narrowing. In addition, a deep inflation is much more effective in reducing induced airway narrowing in normal subjects than in asthmatic subjects.

Choice of provocative stimulus

A wide range of pharmacological and physical stimuli have been used (Table 14.2). Direct-acting agents themselves cause contraction of airway smooth muscle; indirect stimuli provoke mediator release or activate neural stimuli that in turn lead to contraction of airway smooth muscle. Indirect stimuli are often used to investigate the protective actions of drugs.

Histamine and methacholine are the most commonly used direct-acting agents. Although responses to similar concentrations of the two drugs are approximately equivalent, methacholine can be increased to a higher dose than histamine, whose maximum dose is limited by systemic side effects (flushing, headache). Thus, methacholine is particularly useful for population surveys.

Exercise is the most commonly used physical stimulus, particularly in school children. It has the advantage of being a natural stimulus and provokes airway narrowing by changes in temperature and osmotic conditions of the airway epithelium.

Inhalation of sulfur dioxide (SO_2) or sodium metabisulfite, which causes release of SO_2, stimulates a vagal reflex.

- Non-specific bronchial hyper-responsiveness to histamine or methacholine is due to a direct action contracting airway smooth muscle: it is short-lived and rapidly reversed by β_2-adrenergic drugs.

- Indirect acting stimuli such as exercise, adenosine monophosphate, or sodium metabisulfite involve interactions with cells or nerve endings in the airway mucosa and probably are closer to the pathophysiology of a spontaneous asthmatic reaction.

- The response sites within the bronchial tree are not known, but airway narrowing is not uniform.

Table 14.2 Pharmacological and physical agents used for inhaled provocation tests

DIRECT	INDIRECT	
Pharmacological	**Pharmacological**	**Physical**
Histamine*	Metabisulfite/SO_2	Exercise*
Methacholine* and other cholinergic analogues (carbachol, acetyl choline)	Potassium chloride	Hyperventilation
	Propranolol†	Cold air/airway drying
	Neuropeptides (neurokinin A)	Osmotic: hypertonic saline
Prostaglandins (PGF$_{2\alpha}$, PGD$_2$)	Adenosine monophosphate	hypotonic saline
Leukotrienes (LTC$_4$, LTD$_4$, LTE$_4$)		distilled water
Bradykinin		mannitol powder

* Those challenges most used in clinical practice.
† Causes prolonged airway constriction.

Method of administration of inhaled pharmacological constrictors

Three delivery systems for administering successively increasing doses of inhaled pharmacological agents are in general use:

- continuous tidal breathing of nebulized agent[2]
- breath-actuated dosimeter[3]
- 'Yan method' – investigator-activated dosimeters.[4]

The method chosen will be influenced by a number of factors including the need for portability, the subject population (adult or child), and the purpose of the challenge (clinical or research; epidemiological or pharmacological). Whichever delivery system is selected, a pre-filled nebulizer of an appropriate bronchodilator solution (usually a β_2-agonist such as salbutamol or terbutaline) should be prepared before administration of the first dose of challenge agent.

Tidal breathing methods require the subject to breathe with a normal pattern through a mouthpiece or face mask while the challenge agent is nebulized. Delivery is dependent upon the rate and depth of breathing and an attempt is often made to regulate this by asking the subject to breathe in time with a metronome or at a specified rate. This method can be time consuming because each concentration is administered for two minutes, and successive concentrations are given at five minute intervals.

A breath-actuated dosimeter is a device designed to accurately deliver small volumes of nebulized solution. Delivery of a brief (1 s) burst of mist is triggered either manually or automatically by air flow over a heat sensitive sensor (thermistor) at the onset of inspiration. An appropriate delay ensures optimal timing of delivery to maximize the inhaled dose. Doses may be increased by repeated doses of the same concentration or by increasing concentration. This method is accurate but requires relatively expensive and delicate equipment.

The method of Yan et al[4] uses simple, cheap and portable equipment while retaining satisfactory reproducibility. At the start of a full, slow inspiration from functional residual capacity (FRC) to total lung capacity (TLC) the investigator administers a single puff of agent from a hand-held glass bulb nebulizer (e.g. De Vilbiss no. 40) placed between the subject's teeth. The subject then breath-holds for 3 seconds at TLC. For histamine, 2 or 4 doses are given on consecutive full inhalations for each concentration. Doubling doses are delivered by using stronger concentrations or more puffs of the same concentration. FEV_1 is measured one minute after the last puff of histamine and the next dose is delivered within three minutes to maintain a cumulative effect.

Other routes of administration

In the past, drugs such as histamine were given in small doses intravenously; although this has the advantage of providing a uniform dose to all parts of the peripheral lung it is rarely used now. Provocation tests using drugs such as aspirin* may be given orally but are only performed in laboratories with specialized experience. The same applies to attempts to reproduce responses to inhaled occupational agents – solder, flour etc. – in the laboratory since it is difficult to control the exposure at safe and predictable levels.

Responses to physical agents

During exercise there is mild bronchodilatation. However, some asthmatics bronchoconstrict *after* exercise; this can therefore be used as a physiological challenge, particularly in children. Free running in open air with peak flow measurements before and after is effective; however a standardized regime using a treadmill or cycle ergometer and measuring ventilation, air temperature, and humidity is preferable. Airway narrowing characteristically is greatest 5–15 minutes after exercise. Specificity is excellent, a greater than 15% fall in FEV_1 being diagnostic of asthma. Sensitivity is relatively poor and reproducibility is less than that of pharmacological challenges. Near-maximal exercise usually has to be undertaken and it is not easy to obtain a graded response to different intensities of exercise. Provocation of post-exercise airway narrowing is followed by a prolonged refractory period to repeated exercise.

Of the other physical stimuli, hyperosmolar concentrations of saline or distilled water generated by an ultrasonic nebulizer are the most used. Stimulation is graded by gradually building up the period of exposure and reporting the cumulative volume of fluid to which the subject is exposed. A simpler

---

* Inhaled lysine-aspirin is a safer alternative

method to deliver an osmotic challenge may be to use successive doses of mannitol powder.[5] The response to cold air requires specialized equipment which restricts its use.

Pharmacological blockade

β_2-adrenergic agonists are very effective in blocking the response to all direct and indirect acting agents, again demonstrating the central role of contraction of airway smooth muscle. Other direct acting agents (such as histamine, methacholine and leukotrienes) can be blocked by specific antagonists. Indirect acting agents are often antagonized by inhaled anticholinergic drugs, furosemide (frusemide), and cromones (cromoglycate, nedocromil). Corticosteroids have little acute effect but continued treatment – usually for 2 weeks or more – attenuates responsiveness in asthma even to direct acting drugs such as methacholine and histamine.

Table 14.3 Drugs to be withdrawn before provocation tests

Drug	Period of abstinence
β_2-agonists	
Short-acting inhaled	6 hours
Long-acting inhaled	36 hours
Oral	24 hours
Methylxanthines	
Short-acting	12 hours
Sustained release	48 hours
Anticholinergics	
Short-acting (e.g. ipratropium)	6 hours
Cromones (before indirect challenges)	24 hours
Antihistamines (before histamine challenges)	72 hours

The normal practice is for relevant drugs to be withdrawn before assessing airway constrictor responses (Table 14.3). Oral or inhaled corticosteroids are continued unchanged. Sometimes it may be difficult for subjects to avoid taking relieving β_2-agonists, so the recent history of bronchodilator use should be checked before proceeding to the test.

Conduct of provocation tests

Safety

Over the last 20 years, vast numbers of provocation tests have been conducted with very few ill-effects when standard agents such as histamine or methacholine or, in young people, exercise provocation, are used. Important precautions are shown in Table 14.4.

Most tests are conducted in subjects with no or mild air flow obstruction; they are rarely valuable in established obstruction except for specialized research. Most constrictor responses are rapidly reversed by inhaling nebulized β_2-agonists and are inherently short lived.

The following provocation tests, however, require special care and specialized experience:

- Allergens in sensitized individuals: the effective dose varies widely and the acute response is followed some hours later by a late deterioration in airway function. A single allergen provocation test may increase non-specific responsiveness to histamine or methacholine for the following 7–14 days.

- Drugs in sensitized individuals: the most common example is aspirin and other non-steroidal anti-inflammatory drugs. These can give extremely severe reactions at low dose.

- Propranolol and other β-adrenergic blocking agents. These can result in prolonged constrictor responses, which may only respond to large doses of anticholinergic and β_2-adrenergic drugs.

- Occupational asthma (antigens or irritants) in sensitized individuals: usually the diagnosis is suspected from the history and peak flow measurements during and remote from exposure to the putative agent. Attempts to mimic occupational exposure in the laboratory should only be made in specialized laboratories where the 'dose' can be tightly controlled.

Patient preparation

Patients should be rested in the laboratory for at least 15 minutes. Recent bronchodilator use and clinical history should be checked, particularly for recent

Table 14.4 Safe conduct of provocation tests

- Adequate facilities for treatment of acute severe asthma. (Prepare nebulizer with solution of salbutamol 2.5–5 mg or terbutaline 5–10 mg; oxygen should be available.)
- The subject must be physically and mentally capable of cooperating.

Absolute contraindications
- Severe airway narrowing (baseline $FEV_1 < 1.2$ L in adults) or recent severe acute asthma
- Myocardial infarction or cerebrovascular accident within the last 3 months
- Arterial aneurysm

Relative contraindications
- Moderate airway narrowing (tests rarely indicated)
- Spirometry induced airway obstruction
- Recent upper respiratory tract infection
- During an exacerbation of asthma
- Hypertension
- Pregnancy
- Epilepsy

Study termination
- Pre-calculate the airway function at which the study will be terminated (e.g. the absolute value of FEV_1 which allows the dose causing a 20% fall to be obtained)
- Stop if excessive breathlessness, wheeze or cough develops
- Stop if uncomfortable side effects develop (e.g. flushing or headache with histamine)
- If excess loss of airway function or symptoms are induced give nebulized salbutamol or terbutaline
- Supervision should continue until the FEV_1 has returned to at least 90% of baseline

instability of asthma or other medical problems. Time of day and caffeine use should also ideally be standardized, particularly for sequential studies which usually require similar baseline conditions for correct interpretation.

Dose-response curves to constrictor stimuli

Pharmacological agents can be assessed using successive doubling doses. The starting dose should be sufficiently small that no constrictor response is expected. This ensures safety and also familiarizes the subject with the technique.

The *threshold* dose at which constriction is first seen indicates the *sensitivity*; it may not become obvious that the change is greater than the signal-noise ratio until the subsequent dose induces a bigger change. Above the threshold dose, the response increases progressively and the slope represents the *reactivity* of the subject. In most, but not all, normal subjects and in mild asthma, there is a *plateau of maximum response* (typically in normal subjects after $< 30\%$ fall in FEV_1 and in mild asthma after $< 50\%$ fall in FEV_1). The occurrence of a limited maximum response indicates that asthma is mild or well controlled. In more severe asthma and in COPD there is no maximum response, or at least not in the range of fall (maximum 40–50% below baseline) that it is safe to induce. In routine clinical use only the initial part of the curve is studied. This represents a compromise between inducing a constriction large enough to be definitely outside the signal-noise ratio, without causing symptoms that are too severe.

Responses are conventionally expressed as % of baseline function. The dose is calculated as the *provocative concentration* (PC) for tidal breathing methods (using the final concentrations) and as the *provocation dose* (PD) for dosimeter methods (where usually the total cumulative dose is used). For FEV_1, a PC_{20} or PD_{20} is usually measured; although the value is influenced by the *reactivity* (slope between 0 and 20% fall in FEV_1) it is chiefly an indication of *sensitivity*. For airway resistance PD and PC are usually calculated for a 35 or 40% rise. The actual PD or PC is obtained by linear interpolation on a plot of log-

Figure 14.1 Dose-response curve to inhaled methacholine

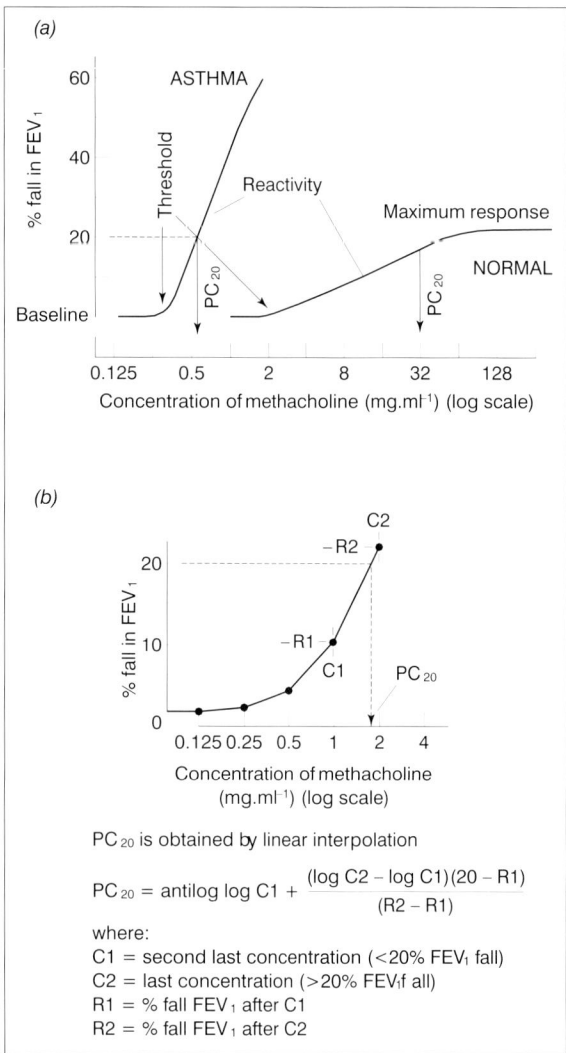

PC$_{20}$ is obtained by linear interpolation

$$PC_{20} = \text{antilog} \log C1 + \frac{(\log C2 - \log C1)(20 - R1)}{(R2 - R1)}$$

where:
C1 = second last concentration (<20% FEV$_1$ fall)
C2 = last concentration (>20% FEV$_1$ fall)
R1 = % fall FEV$_1$ after C1
R2 = % fall FEV$_1$ after C2

dose versus response. Repeatability of PD or PC should be within one doubling concentration, but can be difficult to establish rigorously as tachyphylaxis – particularly to histamine and some indirect stimuli – can be present for several hours after first testing. When responses are small, a 15% or even a 10% fall in FEV$_1$ may be used; another way to obtain confirmation of a small response is to study the curve of the response versus time and measure the area under the curve instead of relying on only one early time point.

In asthma there are changes in all three features of the dose-response curve (loss of plateau of maximum response, steeper slope – i.e. increased reactivity, and reduced threshold dose – i.e. increased sensitivity), but probably the most striking change is leftward shift of the whole curve to lower threshold doses.

Interpretation and clinical usefulness

Bronchial hyper-responsiveness is a key pathophysiological feature of bronchial asthma and is included in its definition. Histamine and methacholine (and, in children, exercise) are the constrictor stimuli that have been studied most on a population basis; those patients with clinical asthma probably represent the most sensitive segment of a normally distributed population. Subjects with a family history of asthma or with atopic features show some enhanced responsiveness even when they have no respiratory symptoms. Although non-specific bronchial hyper-responsiveness is usual in active asthma a very small proportion of subjects are not hyper-responsive, most frequently in the context of occupational asthma. Non-specific hyper-responsiveness in asthma is usually reduced by treatment with inhaled corticosteroids but it may take 6 months or more of treatment to reach maximum attenuation. There are loose correlations between the severity of asthma and of hyper-responsiveness.

Non-specific hyper-responsiveness, albeit less severe, is also found in other diseases associated with airflow obstruction, such as COPD, cystic fibrosis, and bronchiectasis. The presence and intensity of hyper-responsiveness in COPD predicts the future rate of decline in airway function. There may be a different type of responsiveness in smokers and patients with COPD from that associated with asthma and atopy; certainly non-specific responsiveness is not attenuated by inhaled corticosteroids in COPD, in contrast to their beneficial effect in asthma. Structural changes may be more important than active airway inflammation; these include loss of alveolar attachments to the airway perimeter in emphysema.

There are some studies showing non-specific hyper-responsiveness in left ventricular failure and in association with severe viral respiratory tract infections, but these changes appear less consistent. In general women show more hyper-responsiveness than men. Young children are more hyper-responsive than older children; this may relate to smaller baseline caliber of the airways.

> - Non-specific bronchial hyper-responsiveness (BHR) is characteristic of, but not exclusive to, asthma.
> - Failure to demonstrate BHR does not totally exclude asthma.
> - Specific responses to inhaled allergens, occupational agents and drugs are only present in sensitized subjects, are often associated with late responses, and should only be tested in specialized laboratories.

BRONCHODILATOR RESPONSES

The response to bronchodilator drugs is assessed to confirm the diagnosis of asthma and often to decide on the need for bronchodilator treatment.

As with bronchoconstrictor tests, spirometry is the most commonly used test for clinical studies, but body plethysmography or partial expiratory flow-volume curves are necessary to conduct pharmacological studies in normal subjects. With small responses, particularly in patients with COPD in whom there is a large, irreversible component to the airflow obstruction, additional tests may be required (Table 14.1).

Dose and choice of bronchodilator

Ideally the initial bronchodilator assessment in the laboratory should be conducted with a large dose of a nebulized β_2-agonist (2.5–5 mg salbutamol, 5–10 mg terbutaline) at a time when the effects of pre-existing bronchodilator treatment are zero or small. This entails appropriate withdrawal of bronchodilators such as theophyllines or long-acting β_2-agonists (salmeterol or formoterol – Table 14.3) and an interval of about 6 hours after the last dose of short-acting inhaled bronchodilators. This is not always achieved, and so differences in percentage or absolute response to different drugs may be influenced by initial values (including diurnal variation), but the most important measurement is the post-bronchodilator value.

Although most patients (except a few on home nebulizers) will be subsequently treated with much smaller doses of bronchodilators, patients with severe airflow obstruction tend to need larger doses to obtain a maximum response and it is important not to miss a potentially useful response by using too low a dose. Large doses of inhaled β_2-agonists result in significant systemic absorption so reduced doses (1 mg of salbutamol) may be indicated when cardiac stimulation or tachycardia should be avoided. Most laboratories assess only β_2-agonist response on a routine basis, but some consider that a combination of a β_2-agonist and a cholinergic antagonist (such as ipratropium), or even the latter alone, should be used to assess the response in older patients, especially those with COPD. When giving nebulized ipratropium care should be taken to avoid spray reaching the eyes, where it can cause dilatation of the pupil and an increase in intraocular pressure.

Of course, subsequent to the initial 'large-dose' assessment it may be more relevant to measure the bronchodilator response with the usual doses given by the device used by the patient, and so assess whether changes in dose, drug or a combination of drugs, or device are required. Formal dose-response curves to bronchodilators, using doubling or more widely separated dose increments, can be performed in a manner analogous to dose-response curves to constrictor drugs. These can be used to establish whether a plateau of maximal effect is achieved, to establish the dose to obtain 50% of maximum dilatation, or to study the displacement of the curve by antagonist or synergist drugs. While useful for research, they are not commonly done in clinical practice.

Timing of measurements

Basal lung function is at its lowest in the early hours of the morning and is lower at 8.00–9.00 h than at 15.00–18.00 h. This is related to greater vagal tonic activity in the morning; because this is readily removed by bronchodilators, the bronchodilator response may be greater in a morning than an afternoon test.

The time taken to develop a full bronchodilator response varies with the drug used. Some β_2-agonists develop a full action within 5 minutes, but it is preferable to leave an interval of 15 minutes after a dose before testing. The full response to ipratropium may take 30–60 minutes to develop.

Expressing the response

FEV_1

FEV_1 is the most repeatable test of airway function but, even with excellent technique, intra-session variability in an individual may be up to 140 ml; the absolute size of this variation is similar in those subjects with near-normal and with greatly reduced FEV_1.

Bronchodilator response used to be most commonly expressed as a percent improvement over baseline.[6] This results in a given absolute improvement being a higher percentage of a low than a high baseline (Table 14.5). Although it can be argued that a small improvement on a low baseline can be very useful in terms of improvement in symptoms, the between-test variability of a low FEV_1 is large (i.e. about 20% of a FEV_1 of 0.7 L).[7] Certainly, reports should show the absolute as well as any percent change. Since normal lung function varies with age, height, and gender – broadly correlating with ventilatory demands during activity – probably the best way of expressing bronchodilator response is as a percent of *predicted* FEV_1.

Other tests of airway function

Changes are invariably expressed as percent change from baseline, analogous to the normalization that is used for assessing constrictor responses. This is because predicted normal values are much less precise than for FEV_1. Percentage change after bronchodilators and baseline variability are often much larger for these other tests, but care has to be taken before equating a larger percentage increase to a more useful clinical effect.

Interpretation and clinical usefulness

Because bronchodilator responses are inevitably measured after baseline measurements there is always a possibility that improvement in the values after bronchodilator is due to an improvement in technique. Generally, good repeatability at baseline indicates good technique.

A large acute improvement (> 15% predicted value) in FEV_1 is important in the diagnosis of asthma and usually results in treatment with inhaled corticosteroids and bronchodilators as appropriate. Such large FEV_1 changes are usually accompanied by consider-

Table 14.5 Expressing bronchodilator response

1.	Absolute change	FEV_1 post-bd – FEV_1 pre-bd	The absolute change must be ≥ 0.2 L to be significant
2.	Percent initial value	$\dfrac{FEV_1\ \text{post-bd} - FEV_1\ \text{pre-bd}}{FEV_1\ \text{pre-bd}}$	The best of several attempts should be recorded pre and post bronchodilator.
3.	Percent predicted value	$\dfrac{FEV_1\ \text{post-bd} - FEV_1\ \text{pre-bd}}{FEV_1\ \text{predicted}}$	
4.	Percent 'possible' improvement	$\dfrac{FEV_1\ \text{post-bd} - FEV_1\ \text{pre-bd}}{FEV_1\ \text{predicted} - FEV_1\ \text{pre-bd}}$	

Examples:	Values of FEV_1 (L)			Improvement after bronchodilator			
	pre-bd	post-bd	predicted	Absolute ΔFEV_1 (L)	% initial value	% predicted value	% possible
(a)	0.4	0.6	3.1	0.2	50	6.5	7.4
(b)	2.1	2.3	3.1	0.2	9.5	6.5	20

- Percent initial value is highly sensitive to absolute initial level, and is the least reproducible.
- Percent possible value assumes a 'best' level of 100%, whereas the normal range covers 80–120% predicted.
- Percent predicted value is probably the best index, allowing for different age, height and gender.

able improvements in all other tests of airway function and a reduction in functional residual capacity (FRC).

Problems arise with smaller improvements in airway function. At the extreme, patients with COPD may claim considerable symptomatic benefit when there is no change in FEV_1. The problem then is to decide whether this is a placebo effect or an effect on airway function which reduces symptoms (such as dyspnea on effort) which is not picked up by FEV_1. There is no difficulty in imagining possible ways in which this could happen: there could be improvements in airway dimensions during tidal breathing or a reduction in FRC (reducing the work that has to be done by the inspiratory muscles) which were not reflected in the FEV_1. Both changes could be picked up by body plethysmography measuring inspiratory and expiratory resistance and FRC (see Table 14.1). Sometimes, small improvements in 6 minute walking distance after a bronchodilator appear to relate better to improvement in forced vital capacity (FVC) than in FEV_1; the most likely explanation is that an increase in FVC is associated with a fall in FRC at rest, and perhaps in the extent of dynamic hyperinflation that takes place on exercise. In addition, changes in FVC can be useful to assess changes in airway closure.

Maximum effort flow-volume curves may also be useful. After bronchodilation complete expiratory and inspiratory curves (started from TLC and RV respectively) usually show improvement throughout in maximum flows (i.e. no striking differential effects between inspiration and expiration or between large and small lung volumes) and an improvement in FVC (Figure 14.2), but when the changes are small some may reach statistical significance and others may not. An advantage of using maximum effort flow-volume curves to detect small change is that the reproducibility of the curves throughout the FVC can be visualized. A more informative, but less often applied, technique is to

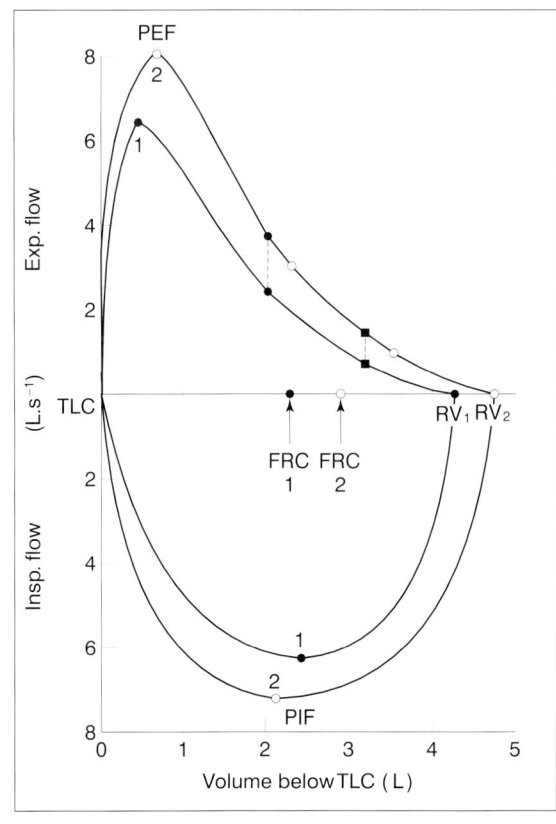

Figure 14.2 Maximum expiratory and inspiratory flow-volume curves before (1) and after (2) bronchodilation

Comment: In this subject there is expansion of the whole maximum flow-volume envelope on both volume and flow axes after bronchodilation (open circles). Peak expiratory flow (PEF) and peak inspiratory flow (PIF) are produced at slightly different lung volumes before and after bronchodilation. Because forced vital capacity (FVC) has increased (note RV_2), maximum expiratory flows at 50% and 25% of FVC are measured at smaller absolute lung volumes after bronchodilation (see open circles), reducing the difference compared to the change in flow at the same absolute volume below total lung capacity (TLC), indicated by the vertical dashed lines between curves 1 and 2. Fall in functional residual capacity (FRC) was detected by recording the tidal flow-volume curve and inspiratory capacity immediately before recording the maximum expiratory flow-volume curve.

measure flows during a partial forced expiration starting from the end-inspired tidal volume (see Chapter 1 p18 and Figure 1.14). In this technique tidal flow-volume curves are first measured, to establish how far FRC is below TLC (inspiratory capacity); in the subsequent partial forced expiration, maximal flow at about 30–40% of FVC remaining to be expired is measured ($\dot{V}p$) and compared to the subsequent flow at the same volume below TLC on the standard full forced expiration from TLC ($\dot{V}m$). These measurements are all repeated after a bronchodilator. Increases in $\dot{V}p$ are characteristically greater than in $\dot{V}m$; changes in FRC can also be detected. The problem with having so many ways of detecting a response to bronchodilators lies in assessing their relative importance when some tests are positive and others are not. Fortunately, because bronchodilators in moderate dose have few adverse effects, the clinician usually prescribes them in COPD even if the results of tests of airway function are divergent or marginal!

Differences between responses in tests of forced expiratory flow and of airway resistance in the tidal range are not solely due to differences in sensitivity and accuracy but represent true physiological differences. Thus in normal subjects bronchodilators reduce airway resistance considerably, while producing only a small increase in maximum expiratory flow on full forced expiration from TLC. These differences are discussed more fully in Chapter 1.

- Initial laboratory bronchodilator tests usually should be made using large doses of β_2-adrenergic agonists (and possibly anticholinergic drugs in older subjects).

- Increases in FEV_1 are best expressed as absolute change (L) or % predicted.

- Small bronchodilator changes in normal subjects or COPD are often assessed better by measuring resistance or $\dot{V}p$ than by tests of maximum expiration from TLC.

SENSITIVITY OF THE COUGH REFLEX

Cough reflex

A cough is an explosive burst of high velocity expiratory airflow which clears airway secretions. The reflex is initiated by stimulation of sensory nerve endings in the larynx, trachea, and lower airways. Afferent impulses are carried via the vagus nerve to the medulla (brain stem), where they are influenced by the cortex which may inhibit (as when attending a concert) or indeed initiate voluntary cough. The efferent limb involves contraction of abdominal and intercostal muscles to raise abdominal and intrathoracic pressure and activation of pharyngeal and laryngeal muscles first to close and then rapidly open the glottis. There is often associated vagal efferent activation resulting in brief contraction of airway smooth muscle (and a rise in airflow resistance) and mucus secretion.

Cough is an important protective mechanism for removing increased airway secretions, as in acute and chronic infections, bronchiectasis, cystic fibrosis, and the chronic bronchitis of smokers. Non-productive cough may also have a 'protective' effect in detecting inhalation of a foreign body or exposure to fumes or gases and, in a more chronic sense, by indicating development of lung diseases such as tuberculosis or cancer.

Laboratory evaluation of cough

Increased frequency of cough

Most of the common causes of cough mentioned above are identified by the initial clinical investigation and chest X-ray; in these patients the cough is performing its protective function and the sensitivity of the cough reflex is normal. But some patients develop a persistent 'dry' (non-productive) cough which has no obvious protective function and whose cause may not be obvious. The laboratory can help investigate these patients by:

- testing the sensitivity of the cough reflex (this is analogous to testing bronchoconstrictor responsiveness in asthma)
- monitoring cough over periods up to 24 hours
- exclusion of a variant form of asthma in which cough is prominent but symptoms due to airway narrowing (wheezing and breathlessness) are less obvious.

Assessing the sensitivity of the cough reflex

The cough reflex can be assessed by recording the number of coughs that occur after controlled doses of substances which provoke cough ('tussigens'). Several different pharmacological tussigens have been used, including some also used as bronchoconstrictor stimuli (SO_2, bradykinin, prostaglandins, neuropeptides, hypertonic saline, low chloride solutions etc.). Most experience has been gained however with citric acid and capsaicin* (extract of hot pepper) which are thought to stimulate slightly different airway receptors. A problem with citric acid challenge is that tolerance develops rapidly to its effects; this is less of a problem with capsaicin. For both agents, tidal breathing and breath-activated dosimeter techniques have been used. In recent years most experience has been gained with capsaicin using a breath-activated dosimeter:[8]

Capsaicin cough-responsiveness[8]

Method A breath-activated dosimeter which nebulizes 5 μL of a range (0.5–500 μMol) of doubling concentrations of capsaicin is used. The number of coughs in the first 60 s after each dose is counted. Increasing concentrations of capsaicin are interspersed with normal saline to minimize cortical influences.

Analysis The number of coughs after each dose is plotted against log capsaicin concentration (Figure 14.3).

Figure 14.3 Cough response to inhaled capsaicin

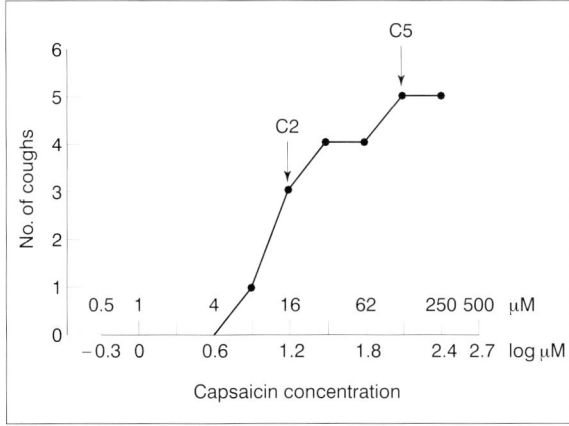

The threshold is measured as the minimum concentration causing at least two coughs (C2). The minimum concentration causing at least five coughs is also recorded (C5); it is not useful to try to produce more coughs as this causes discomfort. Some normal subjects do not cough with the highest dose (500 μMol). Repeatability should be one doubling concentration or less. To avoid tolerance, tests should be at least one hour apart. Cortical influences may act in either direction; C_2 and C_5 are usually somewhat higher with the initial test in an individual. Instructions should emphasize the transient nature of the response and that the subject should not attempt to actively suppress cough.

Interpretation – clinical usefulness Capsaicin cough-responsiveness (CCR) is usually normal when excessive cough is productive, but is enhanced in most patients with chronic non-productive cough. In most patients with asthma CCR is normal, but it is enhanced in a subgroup of variant asthma with predominant cough. Compared with the wide variations in response to bronchoconstrictor challenge, variations in CCR show a much narrower range, making it more difficult to show change with disease or treatment. Nevertheless, CCR is robust enough to provide useful results in clinical investigation and to show effects of cough suppressants in normal subjects. CCR may be greater in women than in men. A tidal breathing technique has been used in children.[9]

Inhaled capsaicin (and other tussigens) provoke small and short-lived (< 2 min) increases in airflow resistance; usually hypersensitivity of the cough reflex is not associated with bronchial hyper-responsiveness.

Clinical conditions in which CCR is *enhanced* include the development of troublesome cough with gastro-esophageal reflux, following viral respiratory tract infections, variant asthma, during treatment for hypertension or chronic heart failure with angiotensin converting enzyme (ACE) inhibitor drugs, and, occasionally, nasal disease. If these conditions can be treated effectively CCR returns to the normal range. There have been few investigations of conditions such as strokes which might be associated with *diminished* CCR.

Monitoring frequency of cough

Until recently the severity of cough was only monitored by diary cards and visual analogue scores, and

---

* Capsaicin is not licensed for inhalation use in some countries. It is extremely irritant in strong concentrations and higher doses should not be used; great care has to be taken in preparing solutions for laboratory use.

responses to systematic questions provided by the subjects. Ambulatory recorders are now available which use microphones and upper abdominal surface electromyograms but analysis of 24 hour records at present remains time consuming, comparable to the early days of heart rate monitoring. 24 hour records are useful because there is often a large difference in cough frequency when the patient is asleep and awake. A particular application is in investigating the relation of cough to acid regurgitation from the stomach into the esophagus (gastro-esophageal reflux) when cough recording is combined with monitoring esophageal pH with an intra-esophageal electrode.

Cough in asthma

Cough in asthma usually responds to anti-asthma treatment. Sometimes asthma presents as troublesome, non-productive cough with little wheezing or breathlessness, so the correct diagnosis is not made. Such patients have increased bronchoconstrictor responsiveness to methacholine and often an enhanced CCR. For this reason it is useful to check bronchoconstrictor responsiveness (and sometimes measure peak expiratory flow variability and examine induced sputum) as well as CCR in the investigation of unexplained cough.

Decreased cough effectiveness

The efferent limb of the cough reflex can be ineffective when there is inability to generate high abdominal and intrathoracic pressures as happens in some muscle diseases, with traumatic lesions of the spinal cord, or when abdominal muscle contraction is inhibited by pain as after abdominal surgery.

The expiratory pressures generated during a cough can be directly measured by esophageal and gastric balloons or indirectly from the mouth pressure measured against an occluded mouthpiece during a maximum expiratory effort or simulated cough ($P_{E}max$). The expiratory flow pattern may also be measured with a pneumotachograph; on glottal opening there should be transient peaks of flow considerably above the level on the standard MEFV curve. (see Figure 1.17) Although airway disease is associated with reductions in maximum expiratory flow, there is no loss of expiratory pressure and there is enhanced dynamic compression of central intrathoracic airways, so that the effectiveness of cough is preserved.

■ Sensitivity of the cough reflex may be increased in patients with chronic non-productive cough.

■ Common causes of chronic non-productive cough include gastro-esophageal reflux, following viral respiratory infections, some types of asthma, and ACE inhibitor drugs.

■ The cough reflex can be assessed by counting coughs after increasing concentrations of citric acid, capsaicin, or other tussigens.

■ Tussigens provoke mild and transient bronchoconstriction, but usually hypersensitivity of the cough reflex is not associated with bronchial hyper-responsiveness.

References

1 Moreno RH, Hogg JC & Paré PD. Mechanics of airway narrowing. *Am Rev Respir Dis* 1986; **133**: 1171–80.
2 Cockcroft DW, Killian DN, Mellon JJ, Hargreave FF. Bronchial reactivity to inhaled histamine: a method and clinical survey. *Clin Allergy* 1977; **7**: 235–43.
3 Sterk PJ, Fabbri LM, Quanjer Ph.H et al. Airway responsiveness. *Eur Respir J* 1993; **6**(suppl 16): 53–83.
4 Yan K, Salome C, Woolcock AJ. Rapid method for measurement of bronchial responsiveness. *Thorax* 1983; **38**: 760–5.
5 Anderson SD, Brannan J, Spring J et al. A new method for bronchial-provocation testing in asthmatic subjects using a dry powder of mannitol. *Am J Respir Crit Care Med* 1997; **156**: 758–65.
6 Quanjer Ph.H, Tammeling GJ, Cotes JE, Pedersen OF, Peslin R, Yernault, JC. Lung volumes and forced ventilatory flows. *Eur Respir J* 1993; **6**(suppl 16): 24–5.
7 Tweeddale PM, Alexander F, McHardy GJR. Short term variability in FEV_1 and bronchodilator responsiveness in patients with obstructive ventilatory defects. *Thorax* 1987; **42**: 487–90.
8 Choudry, NB, Fuller RW. Sensitivity of the cough reflex in patients with chronic cough. *Eur Respir J* 1992; **5**: 296–300.
9 Chang AB, Phelan PD, Robertson CF. Cough receptor sensitivity in children with acute and non-acute asthma. *Thorax* 1997; **52**: 770–4.

15 Pre-Operative Evaluation for Thoracic Surgery

P A Corris

- **INTRODUCTION**
- **SURGERY FOR LUNG CANCER**
  Curative surgery
  Estimation of postoperative lung function using spirometry and perfusion scanning
  Direct assessment of lobar ventilation
  Exercise testing
  Arterial PO_2 and PCO_2
  Coexistent risk factors
  Conclusions
  Palliative surgery
- **SURGERY FOR LUNG BULLAE**
  Assessment for surgery
  Results of surgery
- **LUNG VOLUME REDUCTION SURGERY**
  Theoretical basis
  Selection of patients
  Results of surgery
- **LUNG TRANSPLANTATION**
  Introduction: types of operation
  Selection of patients
  Lung function after transplantation
  Spirometry and static lung volumes
  Other tests
  Physiology of the denervated lung
  Monitoring after transplantation
  Acute rejection
  Chronic rejection
- **CONCLUSIONS**

INTRODUCTION

Two contrasting types of thoracic surgery are performed. Surgery for lung cancer involves removing functioning lung tissue, so pulmonary function is inevitably impaired postoperatively. Other procedures such as bullectomy, lung volume reduction surgery, and lung transplantation aim to improve, and certainly not to worsen, lung function.

The decision to operate on a patient who requires thoracic surgery is dependent upon a satisfactory preoperative evaluation based on the answer to two questions:

1. Is the patient's condition suitable for surgical treatment?
2. Is the proposed surgery safe for the patient?

Preoperative pulmonary function testing may predict the likelihood of postoperative complications and postoperative disability. Poor pulmonary function may itself be a contraindication to surgery. On the other hand, pulmonary function must be sufficiently impaired in non-malignant conditions for the patient to gain worthwhile benefit from an operation with its own risks and morbidity (very small if the patient is reasonably fit and well). Examples include surgery for lung bullae and lung volume reduction surgery (LVRS) in patients with emphysema. The level of abnormality in pulmonary function is an important factor in deciding when to undertake heart and heart-lung transplantation in patients with end-stage pulmonary and pulmonary vascular disease. In general, the more complex the surgical procedure and the greater the risk of postoperative morbidity and mortality, the more disabled the patient has to be before such major surgery is undertaken. In the case of organ transplantation, the shortage of donor hearts and lungs in relation to the need also means that careful functional assessment becomes an important part of the preoperative selection process. The correct application of new surgical techniques such as video-assisted thoracoscopy, lung volume reduction surgery, and transplantation depends heavily on an accurate functional assessment, indicating the continued clinical usefulness of physiological science.

In addition to the more conventional methods of testing lung function, measurement of regional lung function using radioisotopes plays an important part in preoperative assessment.

> **Role of the pulmonary function laboratory in preoperative evaluation**
>
> ■ Prediction of postoperative function and, thus, postoperative disability.
>
> ■ Postoperative predictions may be so poor that surgery is postponed – temporarily or permanently.
>
> ■ Assessment of timing for transplantation surgery, based on a threshold level of disordered function.
>
> ■ Objective evaluation (combined with measurements postoperatively) of surgical procedures for non-malignant conditions, especially lung volume reduction surgery and transplantation.

SURGERY FOR LUNG CANCER*

Curative surgery

Curative surgery for lung cancer involves removal of the tumor and usually the removal of adjoining functional lung tissue. The amount of functioning tissue removed depends upon the extent of the surgical resection, being least for wedge resection, intermediate for lobectomy, and greatest for pneumonectomy. The preoperative assessment comprises two aspects:

1. defining the functional capacity preoperatively
2. estimating the loss of functional capacity consequent upon surgery.

One might have predicted a strictly anatomic reduction in preoperative values of TLC, VC, and FEV_1 as a consequence of pneumonectomy (Figure 15.1). The left lung has nine segments, the right lung ten segments; as a consequence, in the normal situation, the left lung contributes 45% and the right lung 55% to overall function. So, left or right pneumonectomy might be expected to result in a 45% or 55% fall in lung volumes respectively. In practice, the reductions

---

* Thoracotomy alone leads to a temporary decrease in vital capacity which usually resolves by the sixth post operative week but may persist for up to three months[1]. Median sternotomy results in smaller but identifiable fall in VC which lasts for a similar period. This section deals with predicting lung function when it has stabilized after these early post-operative changes.

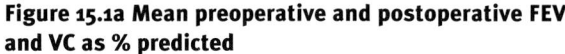

Figure 15.1a Mean preoperative and postoperative FEV$_1$ and VC as % predicted

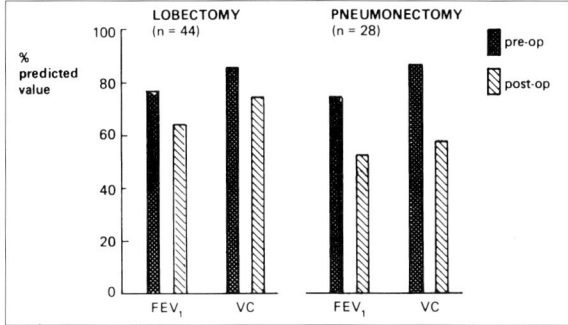

Figure 15.1b Individual postoperative changes in FEV$_1$ as % predicted

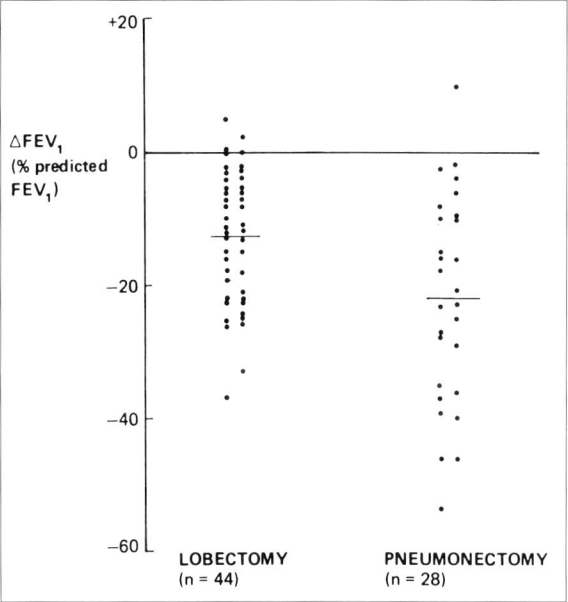

Note wide variation depending on contribution of lobe or lung to preoperative function.

in both VC and TLC tend to be less than expected after pneumonectomy.[2,3] Figures 1a and 1b show the loss in FEV$_1$ and VC in a series of patients undergoing lung resection at Freeman Hospital; there is a large range of loss of functioning lung volumes which is explained by marked differences in the preoperative functional contribution of the lobe or lung that was resected. In some patients, the functional consequences of surgery may be less than anticipated. Accordingly it is wise not to consider an absolute level of preoperative lung function to determine operability, but to estimate the functional consequences of resection and predict the postoperative function. Miller et al[4] applied a set of minimum pulmonary function criteria to 500 patients undergoing pulmonary resection and suggested that a predicted postoperative FEV$_1$ of more than 0.8 L yielded an acceptable rate of morbidity and mortality. This figure has received widespread acceptance although it should be appreciated that a tall 40-year-old man is likely to be more disabled with this FEV$_1$ than a shorter 65-year-old woman. Preoperatively, patients are usually assessed in terms of their likelihood to survive pneumonectomy because this is the most extensive procedure they may undergo. The single-breath D$_{LCO}$, assuming a normal value preoperatively, falls to between 60 and 80% of the predicted value after pneumonectomy, and the K$_{CO}$ is often greater than normal.[5]

Estimation of postoperative lung function using spirometry and perfusion scans

Pneumonectomy Fortunately the prediction of post-pneumonectomy FEV$_1$ can be made easily by the use of preoperative perfusion lung scanning using 99m-technetium (^{99m}Tc) labeled macro-aggregates.[6,7] The relative percentage of perfusion to the affected lung is proportional to its contribution to overall function, so that postoperative FEV$_1$ can be estimated as:

$$\text{Postop FEV}_1 = \text{preop FEV}_1 \times \%\dot{Q} \text{ to lung which remains}$$

It may seem illogical to use a perfusion rather than ventilation scan to predict FEV$_1$. But whereas ^{99m}Tc perfusion scans give both posterior and anterior images and an accurate assessment of unilateral function, 81m-krypton ventilation scans are not available at all centers, and an alternative (133-xenon) generally only provides a posterior image. However, studies comparing 81m-krypton ventilation scans with ^{99m}Tc perfusion scans show that both are usually well matched and equally effective in assessing function. The relative ease of access to ^{99m}Tc perfusion scans rather than ventilation scans has led to the more widespread and successful use of perfusion scanning (Figure 15.2).

Example: Tumor in right main bronchus requiring right pneumonectomy for clearance

Preop FEV_1	3.0 L
Perfusion scan	60% perfusion to left lung
	40% perfusion to right lung
Estimated postop FEV_1	= 60% of 3.0 L = 1.8 L

Some patients will have much larger perfusion defects than predicted from their preoperative chest radiograph (Figure 15.3). Although such patients will lose very little function should pneumonectomy be possible, in practice most will have disease in the mediastinum and be unsuitable for radical surgical treatment.

Lobectomy Attempts have been made to calculate postoperative lung function following lobectomy by the use of a standard perfusion scan and knowledge of the number of anatomical segments to be removed.

It is apparent, however, that this method can easily under- or overestimate the functional contribution of the affected lobe, if ventilation distribution is not matched to that of perfusion. This may be critical in an individual patient with borderline function so a ventilation scan, if available, should always be done as well as the perfusion scan.

Figure 15.2 Estimated post-pneumonectomy FEV_1 versus observed FEV_1

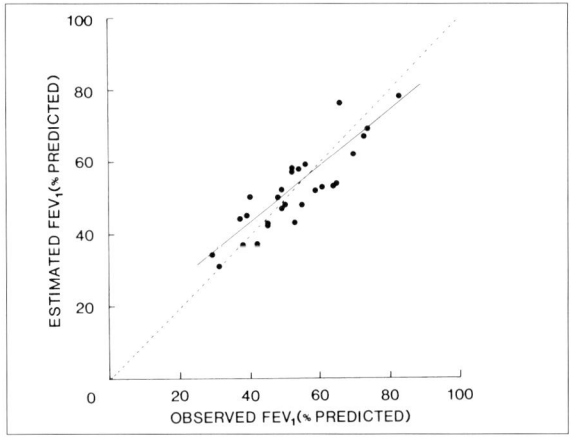

The solid line represents the line of regression, and the dotted line the line of identity.

Figure 15.3 Absent blood flow to right lung on perfusion scan

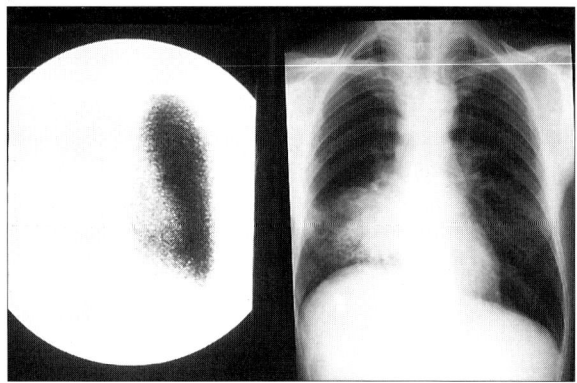

Anterior perfusion scan and corresponding chest radiograph showing absent perfusion to right lung which has a central tumor. Note the right lung remains expanded on chest radiograph.

Although lobectomy and pneumonectomy are usually performed to remove lung cancer, similar assessments should be made when resection is required for localized bronchiectasis, aspergilloma, benign tumors, etc.

Example: Tumor in right upper lobe requiring right upper lobectomy for clearance

Preop FEV_1	= 3.0 L
Perfusion scan	= 60% perfusion to left lung
	40% perfusion to right lung
Total number of lung segments on right	= 9
Number of segments to be removed	= 3
Therefore: estimated *loss* of FEV_1	$= \dfrac{3}{9} \times \dfrac{40}{100} \times 3.0 \text{ L}$ = 0.4 L
Therefore: postop FEV_1	= 2.6 L

Direct assessment of lobar ventilation

In the 1950s there was much interest in bronchospirometry using a Carlens double lumen catheter as an endotracheobronchial tube during bronchoscopy to predict the effects of pneumonectomy. This technique lost favor, but regional tests of lung function using the single breath argon-freon test and occlusion of lobar bronchi by a balloon catheter applied via a fiberoptic bronchoscope have been used prospectively to estimate the loss in lung function consequent upon lobectomy. They have, however, remained a tool for research.[8]

Exercise testing

Many authors have explored the value of exercise testing and measuring pulmonary hemodynamics in the prediction of postoperative morbidity and mortality. Corris et al[9] have shown that the changes in maximum ventilation and maximum oxygen consumption are proportional to changes in FEV_1 in such patients and hence formal exercise testing is not necessary for the majority of patients. Olsen[10] has demonstrated that there is a high risk of complications and a poor outcome when mean pulmonary artery pressure is greater than 35 mmHg at rest and maximum oxygen consumption on exercise is less than 15 ml.kg^{-1} min^{-1}. Postoperative complications are more frequent if the preoperative D_{LCO} is less than 50% predicted.

Measurements of pulmonary hemodynamics and exercise tests should be reserved for patients who appear more disabled than one would predict from simple spirometry and those with coexistent interstitial lung disease such as idiopathic pulmonary fibrosis (fibrosing alveolitis).

Arterial PO_2 and PCO_2

Arterial blood gases should be performed on patients with an FEV_1 < 50% predicted and those falling into the categories outlined above. Patients with an arterial PCO_2 > 45 mmHg (6 kPa) should not be considered suitable for pneumonectomy since it is associated with a high postoperative mortality.[11]

Coexistent risk factors

Major thoracic surgery for lung cancer is most commonly undertaken in patients who have increased risk factors for myocardial ischemia. Symptomatic ischemic heart disease increases the morbidity and mortality associated with thoracic surgery and such patients should be given a wider margin of safety in terms of preoperative lung function and estimate of postoperative FEV_1. There are no hard and fast rules concerning the limits, but the estimated postoperative FEV_1 should preferably be greater than 30% and the preoperative D_{LCO} greater than 50% predicted.

Conclusions

It is difficult to offer hard and fast rules for surgical suitability on the basis of lung function (Figure 15.4). No single test can predict reliably the risks of postoperative complications but the FEV_1 is a simple and robust measure. If the FEV_1 is greater than 2.0 L or

Figure 15.4 Presurgical assessment of patients with lung cancer

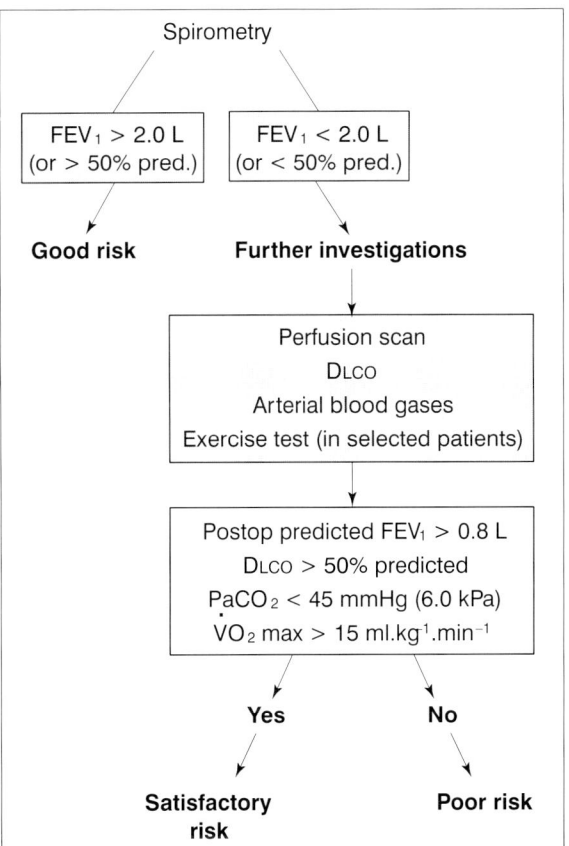

(Adapted from Olsen[10])

50% predicted, patients rarely have major complications (sensitivity 96%, negative predictive value 99%) and thus simple spirometry is a useful screening test.[12]

- The loss in lung function associated with pulmonary resection is directly proportional to the preoperative functional contribution of that lobe or lung.
- For pneumonectomy this can easily be calculated from a quantitative perfusion scan.
- FEV_1 is a simple robust guide of functional adequacy.
- An estimated postoperative $FEV_1 > 0.8$ L is associated with an acceptable outcome in most patients.
- Patients with coexistent interstitial lung disease or unexpected disability require greater investigation, including D_{LCO} (T_{LCO}).
- Patients whose FEV_1 is less than 50% predicted should have blood gases performed preoperatively.
- Resting preoperative arterial $PCO_2 > 45$ mmHg (6 kPa) is a contraindication to pneumonectomy.

Palliative surgery

Obstructing tumors of the trachea or central bronchi are commonly inoperable but suitable for palliative measures. Patients usually present with signs and symptoms of stridor, and maximum inspiratory and expiratory flow-volume curves are very useful to confirm the presence and quantify the severity (see Chapter 1). Flow-volume curves can identify whether the central airflow obstruction is extra- or intrathoracic in its site of obstruction and differentiate between tracheal and main bronchial occlusion. There are many techniques to relieve both intra- and extraluminal components of endotracheal and endobronchial obstruction including diathermy, laser bronchoscopy, brachytherapy, and stenting. Flow-volume curves are useful tests to demonstrate and quantify improvement after these palliative methods.

SURGERY FOR LUNG BULLAE

The majority of bullae are recognized when a standard chest radiograph is taken in a patient presenting with exertional dyspnea and airflow obstruction. They appear as hyperlucent areas with thin curvilinear boundaries, which may displace a fissure and compress surrounding lung. Pulmonary function abnormalities include:

1. Reduced FEV_1 and FEV_1/VC due to coexisting emphysema with loss of elastic recoil.
2. Hyperinflation with a proportionally greater increase of RV and FRC compared with TLC. Since most bullae do not ventilate during tidal breathing, plethysmographic TLC greatly exceeds helium dilution TLC or V_A as measured during a single breath measurement of D_{LCO}.
3. Gas exchange is usually impaired and manifested with a low PaO_2 on air and a reduced D_{LCO}. The K_{CO} is a useful measure in patients with non-ventilated bullae; reductions in K_{CO} are proportional to the degree of emphysema affecting the surrounding lungs.

Assessment for surgery

The identification of patients who are suitable for resection of lung bullae is difficult. The use of X-ray CT scanning and radionuclide imaging has helped define the anatomy, but the functional criteria for selecting those patients who may benefit remain difficult to identify. Paradoxically, it is patients with large bullae (greater than 1.0 L volume) with few symptoms and well preserved lung function who show the best functional improvement!

Patients with bullae less than 1.0 L in volume and poor overall function due to widespread emphysema in general show insufficient improvement to justify the operation.[13] The following tests of pulmonary function have value in selecting those patients who may benefit most.

> **Criteria for surgical resection of bullae**
>
> ■ Large bullae (> 1.0 L) from a CT scan estimate of volume of the bulla.
>
> ■ Preservation of K_{CO} (D_L/V_A).
>
> ■ Relative preservation of FEV_1 percent predicted and a shallow slope in phase III of the single breath nitrogen washout curve.[14]
>
> ■ Evidence of well ventilated, poorly perfused bullae by high V_D/V_T on exercise and appropriate radionuclide ventilation and perfusion scans. This is rare.

Bullae occupying greater than 50% of a hemithorax or greater than 1 liter in volume with evidence of crowded vessels and airways in adjacent lung are associated with a good outcome after surgical excision or plication (collapse and oversewing). Preoperative functional abnormalities relate more to the degree of emphysema in the surrounding or non-bullous lung and not to the bulla itself. This allows the physician or surgeon to make judgments on the potential benefit of bulla surgery using preoperative functional indices as listed above.

Results of surgery

Most series suggest that successful bullectomy increases FEV_1 by about 0.5 L, with a mortality of 1–10% in well selected patients. Postoperatively, exercise performance improves with an increase in maximum oxygen consumption and a reduced ventilation for a given oxygen consumption. The persistence of improvement after surgery is variable. Once removed, giant bullae usually do not recur and the immediate postoperative functional improvement is well maintained. In most patients, the subsequent rate of deterioration is related to the condition of the remaining lung and varies from stability to an annual decline in FEV_1 which is similar to that of other patients with COPD.

LUNG VOLUME REDUCTION SURGERY

The introduction of lung volume reduction surgery (LVRS) in selected patients with emphysema represents one of the most exciting recent developments in thoracic surgery. LVRS employs a different concept offering pulmonary resection to patients with diffuse emphysema without evidence of a large bulla. Both bullectomy and LVRS aim to reduce thoracic gas volume. The bulla is clearly the target for the former, and bullectomy is usually a unilateral procedure. LVRS involves identification of target areas of the lungs which are most affected with emphysema and then removing them using a bilateral approach, aiming to reduce up to 30% of the lung volume in this way.

Theoretical basis

The procedure is based on pioneering work carried out by Dr Otto Brantigan over 35 years ago. He suggested that, in patients with over-expanded lungs, there was loss of elastic traction on bronchioles leading to expiratory collapse. Brantigan's theory was that lung elastic recoil could be increased and the circumferential pull on the airways restored by reducing the size of the lung. Moreover the characteristic hyperinflation in patients with emphysema results in shortening of the inspiratory muscles, particularly the diaphragm, leading to mechanical inefficiency and requiring a greater motor input to produce a given tension. This partly explains the extreme breathlessness associated with emphysema. A reduction in the end-expiratory volume of the lung should lead to an improvement in diaphragmatic function and potentially a reduction in breathlessness. Interestingly, it was the observation that the configuration of the chest wall and diaphragm improved significantly after lung transplantation for emphysema, when normal sized lungs were placed in the hyperexpanded thorax, which provided the spur and confidence for Cooper in St Louis to review Brantigan's approach. In 1995 Cooper et al[15] reported preliminary results of bilateral pneumectomy (usually termed lung volume reduction surgery) for patients with diffuse emphysema which have vindicated Brantigan's theories.

The surgical technique of Cooper et al[15] involves exposure of both lungs through a median sternotomy, allowing one lung to deflate while ventilating the contralateral lung. The healthy parts of the deflated lung undergo absorption atelectasis (being previously ventilated with a high FIO_2) leaving the avascular and emphysematous parts fully inflated. These parts are excised and the lung edges are stapled with bovine pericardium to reduce air leaks. The lung is reinflated, and the procedure repeated on the other lung. Other groups have excised lung tissue with an Nd:YAG laser, or have scarified the whole lung surface (to produce scarring which would inhibit expansion of underlying tissue) after surgical excision of lung tissue has been completed.

Selection of patients[15]

Pulmonary function testing plays a vital role in selection of patients for LVRS. Current criteria, which are evolving as experience accrues, include:

1. FEV_1 < 35% predicted
2. Heterogeneity of emphysema identified on radionuclide perfusion scanning and computed tomography of the lungs, ideally with the worst disease in the upper zones
3. RV and FRC > 220% predicted
4. TLC > 125% predicted
5. $PaCO_2$ < 55 mmHg (7.5 kPa)
6. Age < 75 years

These criteria, together with evidence of marked disability, should be present after patients have completed a six week (minimum) pulmonary rehabilitation program.

Absolute contraindications are severe kyphoscoliosis, previous thoracotomy or pleurodesis, significant coronary artery disease, severe airway disease (bronchiectasis, chronic bronchitis, asthma), pulmonary hypertension, and *current smoking*.

Results of surgery[15]

Significant improvements have been seen in FEV_1, forced vital capacity (FVC), TLC, RV, PaO_2 and the MRC dyspnea scale (see Chapter 8), as listed in Table 15.1. There was no change in $PaCO_2$. The six minute walking distance improved significantly (see Figure 15.5). Quality of life indices, using validated questionnaires, showed that nearly all patients rated their health as 'much better'. There was also a reduction in the requirements for supplemental oxygen in 70% of those requiring oxygen on exercise, and yet the PaO_2 improvement at rest breathing air was very modest (Table 15.1). Some of these changes are nec-

Table 15.1 Pulmonary function and dyspnea assessment in 20 patients before and up to six months after lung volume reduction surgery for diffuse emphysema.[15] Mean values with, for lung volumes, percent predicted [ ].

	No of patients	Pre-operative	Post-operative	P value
FEV_1 (L)	20	0.77 [25]	1.4 [44]	< 0.001
FVC (L)	20	2.2 [56]	2.8 [73]	< 0.05
TLC (L)	20	8.5 [140]	6.6 [110]	< 0.001
RV (L)	20	5.9 [228]	3.6 [171]	< 0.001
PaO_2 air (mmHg) [kPa]	18	64 [8.5]	70 [9.3]	< 0.05
MRC dyspnea scale (0–5)	11	2.9	0.8	

essarily rather subjective, and have not been tested against controls or placebo therapy. Nevertheless, the functional changes documented in Table 15.1 and Figure 15.5 are more than could have occurred spontaneously.

Using a combined excision and Nd:YAG laser scarifying technique, Sciurba et al[16] found P_Lmax increased from 9.5 ± 3.2 to 12.1 ± 3.2 cm H_2O (p < 0.001) and the coefficient of retraction (P_Lmax/TLC) increased from 1.3 to 1.8 cm $H_2O.L^{-1}$. The shift to the right in the pressure-volume curve was related to improvements in walking distance.

- Selected patients with heterogenous emphysema but without giant bullae may benefit from LVRS.
- Suitable patients should have airflow obstruction with an FEV_1 < 35% predicted and marked hyperinflation.
- Targeted areas with minimal perfusion and severe parenchymal destruction to be removed, up to 30% of the lung volume.
- Postoperatively, patients have an increase in lung function, improved exercise performance, and better quality of life.
- Improvement has been sustained for at least one year (Figure 15.5), but longer term follow-up studies are awaited.

LUNG TRANSPLANTATION

Introduction: types of operation

The modern era for lung transplantation began in 1981 when Bruce Reitz and colleagues in Stanford University introduced heart-lung transplantation for patients with pulmonary vascular disease. Indications for combined heart and lung transplantation (HLT) were subsequently widened to include various pulmonary conditions. In 1986 the Toronto group reported success with single lung transplantation (SLT) in patients with fibrosing lung disease, and in 1988 a double lung transplantation using an en bloc transplantation of both lungs with a tracheal anastomosis was introduced by Paxton and colleagues. By 1989 this procedure had been largely abandoned owing to problems with airway healing to be replaced by a bilateral sequential lung transplantation (BLT) with separate hilar anastomoses of each main bronchus from a pulmonary artery and left apical cuff.

Selection of patients

Table 15.2 provides broad guidelines of when patients should be considered for transplantation on simple functional criteria.

Pulmonary function testing plays a pivotal role in the selection of patients for transplant assessment. The pattern of impairment of pulmonary function depends on the underlying lung disease. Four main groups of patients are referred for transplantation.

Idiopathic pulmonary fibrosis (IPF); cryptogenic fibrosing alveolitis (CFA) The two year survival of patients with IPF is only 20%[17] in those whose initial vital capacity is ≤ 60% predicted and who do not show a response to oral prednisolone (rise in vital capacity > 10%). This survival falls to 10% in those with PaO_2 < 60 mmHg (8 kPa) breathing air. Other studies showed similar results with only 50% surviving two years when the vital capacity is less than 70% predicted.

Accordingly patients with IPF should be referred for lung transplantation when the VC is less than 60–70% of predicted and there has been no response to immunosuppressive medication. The majority of patients will be hypoxemic breathing air at rest by this stage. Hypercapnia is usually associated with a prognosis of a few months, and death occurs before transplantation can be carried out.

Cystic fibrosis (CF) The risk of death within 2 years has been reported to be 50% when the FEV_1 is less than 30% predicted, vital capacity is < 40% predicted, PaO_2 is < 53 mmHg (7.3 kPa) and $PaCO_2$ is > 53 mmHg (7.3 kPa).[18] Most CF centers now refer patients for consideration for transplantation when the FEV_1 falls to 30% of predicted or if there is a sudden acceleration in decline of FEV_1.

Emphysema The mean two year survival of patients whose post-bronchodilator FEV_1 (the best predictor of outcome[19]) was less than 30% predicted is 60–70%.[20] For an individual, however, the estimate of prognosis has wide confidence limits. Moreover, the treatment of hypoxemic patients with emphysema with long term home oxygen (LTOT, see chapter 13) has improved prognosis. Most patients with emphysema will be referred on account of severe dyspnea and in general the FEV_1 will have fallen to 20–25% predicted. The six minute walking distance should be

Table 15.2 Guidelines for appropriate transplant operation

Condition	When to refer for transplantation	Operation
IPF (CFA)	VC < 60% predicted and no response to immunosuppressive treatment	SLT
Cystic fibrosis	FEV_1 < 30% predicted or accelerating loss of FEV_1 toward 30%	BLT
Emphysema	FEV_1 < 25% predicted 6 minute walk test < 300 meters	SLT/BLT
Pulmonary hypertension	Right atrial pressure > 10 mmHg (1.3 kPa) Cardiac index < 3.0 L min^{-1}m^{-2} Mixed venous oxygen saturation ($S\bar{v}O_2$) < 63% at rest No response to vasodilators	HLT

less than 300 meters, and many will show oxygen desaturation (using pulse oximetry) on exercise.

Pulmonary hypertension All patients who present with unexplained pulmonary hypertension should undergo catheterization with an acute vasodilator trial in order to assess prognosis. Patients who fail to show significant response to vasodilators should be considered for transplantation. Indicators of a poor prognosis are a mean right atrial pressure of greater than 10 mmHg, a cardiac index of less than 3.0 L.min^{-1} m^{-2}, and a mixed venous oxygen saturation of less than 63%.[21] These form an appropriate baseline for transplant assessment, however all symptomatic patients with primary pulmonary hypertension should be referred to a transplant center.

Lung function after transplantation

The lung function of the transplant recipient is affected by: (a) factors relating to the operation itself, (b) post-transplant complications, and (c) pre-transplant factors relating to native lung disease in recipients of single lungs. Mechanical factors such as surgical incision, pleural complications, and phrenic nerve injury all affect lung function independently of lung allograft function.

Spirometry and static lung volumes

Heart-lung recipients Initially patients have mild to moderate restriction of lung volume which may take 12–18 months to improve to their best although some patients reach their maximum by six months. The volumes obtained ultimately are close to those predicted by the age, sex, and size of the recipient. There is adaptation of the chest wall in recipients with preoperative hyperinflation toward the predicted normal TLC of the recipient, although elevation of RV and FRC may persist.

Bilateral lung transplantation Mild reduction of lung volumes may persist 12–18 months post transplantation, but one large series reported a maximum vital capacity of 90% predicted in fit patients.

Single lung transplantation The lung volumes in single lung recipients reflect the lung mechanics of the transplant lung and the function of the remaining native lung. There is generally little further improvement in spirometry after the first six months following single lung transplantation.

Chronic obstructive pulmonary disease A persisting obstructive defect is seen with an FEV_1 of 50% predicted reported by most authors at 3–6 months. Figure 15.5 presents a comparison of SLT, BLT, and lung volume reduction surgery (LVRS) as treatment for severe and diffuse emphysema.[22] The striking fact is that the very large gain in FEV_1 after BLT (compared to SLT and LVRS) is accompanied by much less improvement in the six minute walking distance for BLT versus the other two operations.

Restrictive lung disease A persistent restrictive defect is seen, with authors reporting an FEV_1 of about 80% predicted for medium term recipients after SLT.

Other tests

Flow-volume curves Flow-volume curves after HLT and BLT generally show mild restriction. An obstructive curve may be caused by the development of an airway anastomotic complication such as malacia or stricture. The early development of obliterative bronchiolitis may be indicated by a reduced FEV_1 or MMEF (see below, Chronic Rejection).

The shape of the flow-volume curve in SLT depends upon the pathology of the native lung. Biphasic flow-volume curves following single lung transplantation carried out for obstructive lung disease are in part reflecting different time constants for each lung (see Chapter 1, Figure 1.9).

Diffusing capacity When corrected for hemoglobin, D_{LCO} (T_{LCO}) remains lower than predicted values in stable HLT and BLT recipients. There are proportional reductions in both capillary volume and membrane diffusing capacity.

Provocation testing A high prevalence of airway hyper-responsiveness to methacholine has been reported, possibly as a consequence of airway denervation. Transplant recipients demonstrate only sporadic and inconsistent results to other agents such as distilled water or histamine.

Figure 15.5 Functional status pre/post thoracic surgery

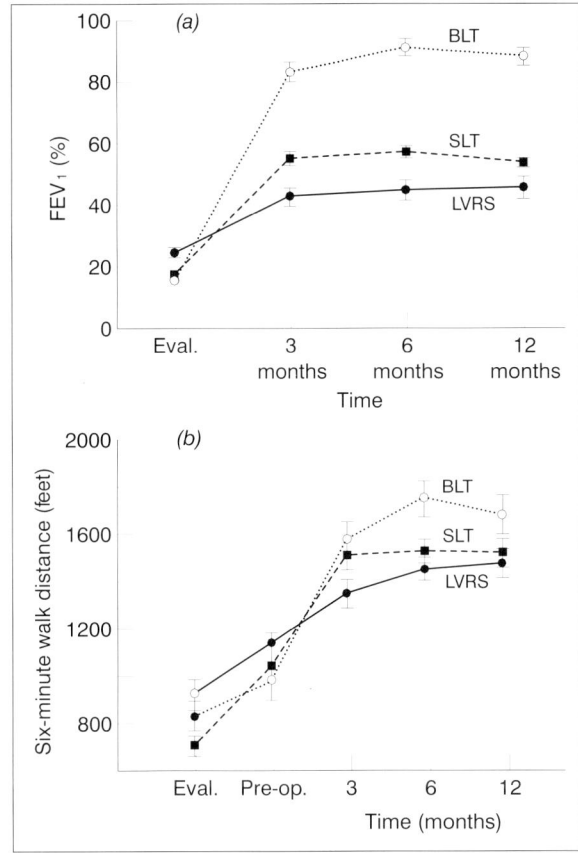

[a] FEV_1 (% predicted) and [b] 6 min Walking Distance at Evaluation (Eval), Pre-op and after Single (SLT) [n=39], or Bilateral (BLT) [n=25] Lung Transplantation or Lung Volume Reduction Surgery (LVRS) [n=33], all for COPD

(From Gaissert HA, Trulock EP, Cooper JD, Sundaresen RS, Patterson GA. Comparison of early results after volume reduction or lung transplantation for COPD. J Thorac Cardiovasc Surg 1996; 111:296–307, with permission)

Exercise testing A significant degree of exercise limitation has been reported 12 months following HLT, BLT, or SLT. Recipients maximum oxygen consumption ranges from 45–52% predicted. Leg fatigue is the most common reason for terminating the exercise test and an early anaerobic threshold has been noted. There is no evidence of ventilation limitation in HLT or BLT recipients.

Physiology of the denervated lung

The lungs remain denervated post transplantation, but the pattern of breathing at rest is normal. Increase in ventilation on exercise is achieved with a smaller tidal volume and an increased frequency compared to normal. This probably reflects a mild restrictive defect in the subjects studied.

Monitoring after transplantation

Acute rejection

Over the first few postoperative days graft function may be monitored physiologically by pulse oximetry and arterial blood gas analysis. Thereafter, lung function, in particular spirometry and diffusing capacity, should be monitored. The daily use of a hand-held spirometer to detect falls in FEV_1 has been advocated by many groups as a useful and simple monitoring device. A sustained fall in FEV_1 of greater than 10% is associated with a high chance of finding rejection or infection in the pulmonary allograft and indicates the need to proceed to transbronchial lung biopsy and lavage. Acute rejection is associated, in general, with falls in vital capacity of the same magnitude as FEV_1. Occasionally falls in the D_{LCO} are the earliest indication of rejection or infection of the allograft.

Chronic rejection

Approximately 40% of intermediate survivors of lung transplantation develop obliterative bronchiolitis, which is a manifestation of chronic rejection. The severity of this complication is assessed by the % fall in the best post-transplant value of the FEV_1.[23]

Measurements of MMEF have been proposed as a more sensitive indicator of development of obliterative bronchiolitis, but the innate variability of this measurement within an individual compared to the FEV_1 remains a problem and in practice the FEV_1 is still used to define and classify obliterative bronchiolitis functionally.

CONCLUSIONS

- Prediction of post-operative lung function is the aim when lobectomy or pneumonectomy is contemplated, usually for lung cancer.
- The demand for lung transplantation (single or bilateral lung) is high in relation to the number of available donor lungs. Young patients with cystic fibrosis and pulmonary hypertension have priority. Post transplantation, serial pulmonary function tests are essential for monitoring acute or chronic rejection.
- Patients with severe emphysema will probably gain little more in terms of quantity and quality of life from lung transplantation than from more palliative procedures such as bullectomy or lung volume reduction surgery. There is a need for careful monitoring of pulmonary function in assessing the benefit of these operations in these patients.

References

1. Locke TJ, Griffiths TL, Mould H, Gibson GJ. Rib cage mechanics after median sternotomy. *Thorax* 1990; **45**: 465–8.
2. McIlroy MB & Bates DV. Respiratory function after pneumonectomy. *Thorax* 1956; **11**: 303–11.
3. Miller RD, Bridge EV, Fowler WS *et al*. Pulmonary function before and after pulmonary resection in tuberculosis patients. *J Thorac Surg* 1958; **35**: 651–61.
4. Miller JI, Crossman GD & Hatcher CR. Pulmonary function criteria for operability and pulmonary resection. *Surg Gynaecol Obstet* 1981; **52**: 813–17.
5. Ogilvie C, Harris LH, Meecham J, Ryder G. Ten years after pneumonectomy for carcinoma. *Br Med J* 1963; **1**: 1111–15.
6. Boysen PG, Block AJ, Olsen GN *et al*. Prospective evaluation for pneumonectomy using the technetium quantitative perfusion lung scan. *Chest* 1977; **72**: 422–5.
7. Olsen GN, Block AJ & Tobias JA. Prediction of post pneumonectomy pulmonary function using quantitative macroaggregate lung scanning. *Chest* 1974; **66**: 13–16.
8. Williams SJ, Pierce RJ, Davies NJH, Denison DM. Methods of studying lobar and segmental function of the lung. *Br J Dis Chest* 1979; **73**: 97–112.
9. Corris PA, Ellis DA, Hawkins T, Gibson GJ. Use of radionuclide scanning in the assessment of resectability of bronchial carcinoma. *Thorax* 1987; **42**: 285–90.
10. Olsen GN. The evolving role of exercise testing prior to lung resection. *Chest* 1989; **95**: 218–25.
11. Tisi GM. Preoperative identification and evaluation of the patient with lung disease. *Med Clin North Am* 1987; **71**: 399–412.
12. Boushey SF, Billing DM, Norton LB, Helgasan AH. Clinical course related to preoperative and postoperative pulmonary function in patients with bronchogenic carcinoma. *Chest* 1971; **59**: 383–91.
13. Gaensler EA, Cugell DW, Davidson RJ *et al*. Surgical management of emphysema. *Clin Chest Med* 1983; **4**: 443–63.
14. Ohta M, Nakahara K, Yasumitsu T *et al*. Prediction of postoperative performance status in patients with giant bullae. *Chest* 1992; **101**: 668–73.
15. Cooper JD, Trulock EP, Triantafillou AN *et al*. Bilateral pneumectomy (volume reduction) for chronic obstructive pulmonary disease. *J Thorac Cardiovasc Surg* 1995;**109**: 106–19.
16. Sciurba FC, Rogers RM, Kennan RJ *et al*. Improvement in pulmonary function and elastic recoil after lung reduction surgery for diffuse emphysema. *N Engl J Med* 1996; **334**: 1095–9.
17. Carrington CB, Gaensler EA, Contu RE, Fitzgerald MX, Gupta RT. Natural history and treated course of usual and desquamative interstitial pneumonia. *N Engl J Med* 1978; **298**: 801–809.
18. Kerem E, Reisman J, Copry M, Canny GJ, Levison H. Prediction of mortality in patients with cystic fibrosis. *N Engl J Med* 1992; **326**: 1187–91.
19. Postma DS, Sluiter HJ. Prognosis of chronic obstructive pulmonary disease. The Dutch experience. *Am Rev Respir Dis* 1989; **140**: 5100–105.
20. Anthonisen NR, Wright EC, Hodgkin JE *et al*. Prognosis in chronic obstructive pulmonary disease. *Am Rev Respir Dis* 1986; **13**: 14–20.
21. Fuster V, Steele PM, Edwards ED, Gersh BJ, McGoon MD, Frye RL. Primary pulmonary hypertension, natural history and the importance of thrombosis. *Circulation* 1984; **70**: 580–7.
22. Gaissert HA, Trulock EP, Cooper JD, Sundaresen RS, Patterson GA. Comparison of early results after volume reduction or lung transplantation for COPD. *J Thorac Cardiovasc Surg* 1996; **111**: 296–307.
23. Cooper JD, Billingham M, Egan T *et al*. A working formulation for the standardization of nomenclature and for clinical staging of chronic dysfunction in lung allografts. *J Heart Lung Transplant* 1993; **12**: 713–6.

16 Pulmonary Vascular Disease
J M B Hughes

- **INTRODUCTION**
- **PULMONARY HYPERTENSION**
  Pulmonary venous hypertension
  Pulmonary embolic disease
  Sickle-cell disease
  Primary pulmonary hypertension
  Pulmonary vasculitis
  > *Wegener's granulomatosis*
  > *Churg-Strauss syndrome*
  > *Behçet's disease*
  > *Connective tissue diseases*
  > *Systemic lupus erythematosus*
- **MICROVASCULAR INJURY**
  Alveolar hemorrhage
- **PULMONARY HYPOTENSION**
  Intrapulmonary shunting
  > *Hereditary hemorrhagic telangiectasia (HHT)*
  > *Idiopathic pulmonary arteriovenous malformations (non-HHT)*
  > *Hepatopulmonary syndrome*
- **CONCLUSIONS**

INTRODUCTION

In lung disease confined to the pulmonary vasculature, the expected pattern of pulmonary function is:

- normal lung volumes
- no airflow obstruction
- low diffusion (transfer factor), both D_{LCO} (T_{LCO}) and D_L/V_A (K_{CO}).

Lung volumes may be reduced in severe or longstanding disease, for reasons that are not really understood. There may be active alveolar hemorrhage, which will raise D_{LCO} and K_{CO}. If there is a right to left shunt (intrapulmonary or intracardiac), PaO_2 and SaO_2 will be reduced. Most cases of pulmonary vascular disease are associated with pulmonary hypertension (a raised pulmonary artery pressure) caused by pulmonary arterial obstruction with thrombus or inflammation of the arterial wall. The small pulmonary vessels, which accompany the small bronchi and bronchioles, may become involved in bronchiolar inflammation, e.g. obliterative bronchiolitis. Occasionally, asthma and vasculitis come together as in the Churg-Strauss syndrome.

PULMONARY HYPERTENSION

Pulmonary venous hypertension

A raised pulmonary venous pressure most commonly results from mitral valve disease or left ventricular dysfunction of any cause. Pulmonary venous hypertension leads to pulmonary vascular congestion and pulmonary edema. The high capillary pressure causes endothelial and epithelial cell rupture with scarring (but only minimal fibrosis) and loss of vessels in the microvascular bed. Pulmonary arterial hypertension of moderate degree (mean pulmonary arterial pressure up to 50 mmHg) ensues with medial hypertrophy and intimal thickening of arterial vessels.

Pulmonary function has been studied extensively,[1] particularly in cases of longstanding mitral stenosis in the days before mitral valve surgery became routine. With increasing severity of disease, first vital capacity (up to 40% decrease), and then TLC (up to 30% decrease) decline. FRC does not change, but residual volume increases by 40%. In chronic mitral stenosis, there is a progressive fall in D_{LCO} with increasing severity of disease, mostly due to a reduction in the membrane diffusing capacity (D_M) component of the D_{LCO} (see Chapter 6 for partitioning of D_{LCO}) rather than capillary volume (Q_c). The changes in chronic heart failure due to left ventricular muscle dysfunction are broadly similar[2] as shown in Table 16.1.

In mitral stenosis, static lung compliance is reduced, mostly because of the loss of lung volume. $P_{L}max$ is not increased, unlike diffuse lung fibrosis (see Chapter 3). Below FRC, P_L is increased for a given lung volume (either as % predicted or as % actual TLC); this shift to the left in the pressure-volume curve is thought to be caused by vascular engorgement, since it can be reproduced in normal subjects with elevations of central venous pressure.

Wheezing is common in patients with pulmonary vascular congestion, but the rise in airway resistance (in non-smokers) is mild and FEV_1/VC ratios are fairly normal. Airway hyper-responsiveness to methacholine has been reported in some patients with congestive heart failure, but the incidence is no more than 20% and the predisposing and precipitating factors are not yet known. There is probably overall skeletal muscle weakness in chronic heart failure, and tests of respiratory muscle strength ($P_I max$ and $P_E max$) and endurance show mild to moderate abnormalities.

Arterial PO_2 is reduced in congestive heart failure, especially if pulmonary edema is present. SaO_2, in well controlled heart failure, is generally $\geq 93\%$ and it does not fall significantly further on exercise. Exercise capacity is reduced out of proportion to most of the respiratory abnormalities, because of an inability to increase cardiac output in relation to the increased metabolic demand, and excessive ventilation.

In the supine posture, patients with pulmonary vascular congestion behave in a unique way in that FRC does not fall on lying supine compared to sitting or standing erect (normal ΔV = c.0.7 L), and yet airway resistance rises in the supine position *more* than in normal subjects. Possible explanations are that the central blood volume is more 'fixed' than in normal subjects and that the enlarged heart in the supine posture compresses the larger bronchi.

If the pulmonary venous pressure which has been elevated for many years is suddenly made normal (as a result of mitral valve surgery) the abnormal pulmonary function does not improve because the structural damage to the lung is irreversible. Exercise capacity, however, improves considerably because of a better cardiac output.

Pulmonary embolic disease

Thrombi which form in the veins of the calf, often following surgical operations or in those who have inherited a 'thrombotic tendency' propagate into the femoral and iliac veins; pieces of thrombus may become

Table 16.1 Pulmonary function in left ventricular muscle dysfunction

NYHA class	Age/ No	FEV_1/VC ratio	VC % pred	D_{LCO} % pred	K_{CO} % pred	V_A % pred	D_M % pred	Q_c % pred
II	61/40	0.72	82	80	95	85	63	111
III	62/10	0.71	76	72	85	75	33	137

Comment: One patient in each group was female. NYHA Classification II is symptomatic breathlessness walking up an incline, and Class III is breathlessness when walking on the level. Note Class III group results worse than Class II, except for Qc. Volume loss (VC and V_A: TLC loss would have been similar) with minimal airflow obstruction (normal FEV_1/VC at age 61 = 0.75). Reduction of K_{CO} in relation to lowered V_A implies alveolar-capillary damage. Membrane diffusing capacity (D_M) is most severely affected, especially in Class III.

detached from the vessel wall and lodge eventually in the pulmonary circulation. These emboli obstruct one or more medium-sized vessels, generally at the level of segmental arteries. The diagnosis of pulmonary embolism (PE) is usually confirmed following a radioisotope ventilation and perfusion scan, which classically shows a mismatched pattern (wedge-shaped defects in the periphery of the lung on the perfusion scan accompanied by a normal ventilation scan). Alternatively, the diagnosis may be made from a helical (spiral) CT scan, or from pulmonary angiography.

Patients frequently have a moderate degree of arterial hypoxemia due to $\dot{V}_A/\dot{Q}$ mismatching, amplified by a low mixed venous PO_2 if cardiac output is reduced. There is hyperventilation leading to a low $PaCO_2$. In mild to moderate PE, PaO_2 may be within the normal range because of hyperventilation, but the alveolar-arterial oxygen gradient (A-a)PO_2 will be increased (see Chapter 5). On the other hand, a normal (A-a)PO_2 and $PaCO_2$ (breathing air) virtually excludes *severe* pulmonary embolic disease.

The dead space-tidal volume ratio (V_D/V_T) is often high because unperfused lung is being ventilated. Interestingly, V_D/V_T may be normal because the lung distal to the vascular obstruction is perfused by the bronchial circulation (there are anastomoses between the bronchial and pulmonary circulations) and CO_2 excretion continues to take place even though the increase in arterial oxygen content is necessarily small. This is also the reason why the D_{LCO} is usually well preserved in pulmonary embolic disease. Bronchial-pulmonary artery anastomoses are the reason why pulmonary infarction (necrosis of lung tissue) is uncommon following pulmonary vascular obstruction from any cause.

Pulmonary function tests are rarely performed in the acute stage of pulmonary embolic disease; they have no diagnostic role. Two studies[3,4] have measured D_{LCO} within one week of an acute embolic episode, in 34 patients overall; D_{LCO} was 60–70% predicted normal, increasing to 68–78% predicted 3–6 months later. Lung volumes were reduced by about 10%, but recovered at 3 months. K_{CO} was 104% predicted in one study[3] and 81% in the other.[4]

Acute pulmonary vascular obstruction from emboli usually resolves satisfactorily with anticoagulant treatment. A proportion of patients experience repeated episodes of pulmonary emboli which are not recognized or which do not resolve on treatment. They may have a genetic predisposition to venous thrombosis or one or more risk factors such as immobility, smoking, or multiple operations. Their pulmonary function profile is similar to that described in acute embolic disease, though the fall in lung volume may be greater if pulmonary infarction has occurred.[5]

Sickle-cell disease

Sickle-cell disease is an inherited hemoglobinopathy in which both copies of normal Hb A are replaced by the variant hemoglobin S. The heterozygous state (Hb A.S), when only 50% of total hemoglobin is HbS (sickle-cell 'trait'), is not associated with any morbidity. Hb S can associate with other abnormal hemoglobins (Hb S.C or Hb S.βThalassemia) but the disease is less severe than with the SS form. Oxygenated Hb S behaves like Hb A but it tends to polymerize and crystallize in the deoxygenated form. The red cells become 'stiff' and take on 'sickle' and 'holly leaf' shapes, becoming trapped in capillaries.[6] Microvascular occlusion and infarction ensue, especially in the spleen. The lung is frequently involved and microvascular occlusions cause alveolar wall necrosis and scarring. The end result is loss of lung units. In a population study, the loss of lung volume in Hb SS disease averaged 20%. When corrected for anemia (average Hb 8.0 g.dL^{-1}) the reduction in D_{LCO} was only 8%.[7] The pulmonary function laboratory is, of course, likely to see those most severely affected with larger volume and D_{LCO} loss than observed in population surveys.

Table 16.2 Sickle cell disease

Age/sex	FEV_1/VC ratio	VC % pred	D_{LCO} % pred	K_{CO} % pred	V_A % pred
46/F	0.74	71	70	133	63

Comment: Severe disease with 'loss of units' pattern (low volumes and D_{LCO} with compensatory increase of K_{CO}). D_{LCO} and K_{CO} corrected for her low Hb of 9.4 g dL^{-1}.

Primary pulmonary hypertension (PPH)

PPH is a condition of unknown cause in which the pulmonary artery pressure is often at systemic level, associated with obliteration of medium and small pulmonary arteries by smooth muscle hypertrophy and intimal cellular proliferation with or without fibrosis. Lung volumes are often moderately reduced, but less so than the D_{LCO} and K_{CO}. The arterial hypoxemia can be severe if there is a patent foramen ovale (between the right and left atrium) through which blood can shunt from right to left because of the high pressure in the right atrium and ventricle. In most patients, the hypoxemia can be explained by intrapulmonary 'shunts' ($\dot{V}_A/\dot{Q}$ ratios < 0.1), the effects of which are aggravated by low mixed venous oxygen levels because of a low cardiac output.[8]

Table 16.3 Primary pulmonary hypertension

Age/sex	FEV$_1$/VC ratio	VC % pred	D$_{LCO}$ % pred	K$_{CO}$ % pred	V$_A$ % pred
18/F	0.95	91	58	58	107

Comment: Normal volumes and FEV$_1$/VC ratio (0.95 within normal range for her age) but reduced diffusing capacity and K$_{CO}$ typical of pulmonary vascular involvement.

Pulmonary vasculitis

Some causes of pulmonary vasculitis are listed in Table 16.4. The specific causes for these conditions have not yet been identified. Vascular inflammation and obliteration is only part of the disease process.

Wegeners granulomatosis

The upper respiratory tract (nose and sinuses) is frequently involved with ulcerating lesions. Necrotizing granulomas and cavitation occur in the lung and pursue a chronic course. A serious complication is microvascular inflammation (capillaritis) which can lead to severe lung hemorrhage (see Alveolar Hemorrhage). In our local experience of 28 cases, and in the absence of lung hemorrhage, the D$_{LCO}$ was < 80% predicted in 18 (64%) but K$_{CO}$ was low in only 5 (18%). If the lung volume reduction is minor, the D$_{LCO}$ and K$_{CO}$ abnormalities could be attributed to 'vasculitis. With lung volume reduction and normal or high K$_{CO}$, the predominant pathology is 'loss of units'.

Airflow obstruction occurred in 46% and was associated with a low D$_{LCO}$ in 25% of the patients. Low FEV$_1$/VC ratios occur also in non-smokers. Bronchial disease with granulomas and inflammation

Table 16.5 Wegener's granulomatosis

Age/sex	FEV$_1$/VC ratio	VC % pred	D$_{LCO}$ % pred	K$_{CO}$ % pred	V$_A$ % pred
65/M	0.62	71	65	108	65

Comment: The patient was a non-smoker. This pattern of airflow obstruction with 'loss of units' (low D$_{LCO}$ with preserved K$_{CO}$) would also be compatible with bronchiectasis, although the diagnosis of Wegeners was not in doubt.

Table 16.4 Common causes of pulmonary vasculitis

Disease	Other pathological features
Wegener's granulomatosis	Necrotizing granulomas and cavitation
	Upper respiratory tract involved
Microscopic polyarteritis	
Churg-Strauss syndrome	Eosinophilia, asthma, lung consolidation
Behçet's disease	Thrombosis, large vessel aneurysms
Connective tissue disorders	
Rheumatoid arthritis	Pleurisy, fibrosing alveolitis, bronchiolitis, lung nodules
Systemic sclerosis/ CREST* syndrome	Fibrosing alveolitis (common)
Mixed connective tissue disease	Fibrosing alveolitis (rare)
Systemic lupus erythematosus (SLE)	Pneumonitis, pleurisy, atelectasis, diaphragm weakness

* CREST is **c**alcinosis, **R**aynaud's phenomenon, **e**sophageal dysmotility, **s**clerodactyly and **t**elangiectasia.

is seen in < 20% of patients at bronchoscopy, so inflammation of the small bronchi and bronchioles probably contributes to the airflow obstruction.

Churg-Strauss syndrome

Patients with the Churg-Strauss syndrome often have a history of many years of allergic rhinitis.[9] They may present with pulmonary infiltrates and eosinophilia. They also have asthma and evidence of systemic vasculitis, characteristically a mononeuritis multiplex. Pathologically, there is tissue eosinophilia and a necrotizing vasculitis with granuloma formation. Pulmonary function tests may show airflow obstruction (day-to-day variations would be seen on peak flow charts), low D_{LCO} and K_{CO}, and low lung volumes if there are infiltrates on the chest radiograph.

Table 16.6 Churg–Strauss syndrome

Date/ months:	FEV_1/VC ratio	VC % pred	D_{LCO} % pred	K_{CO} % pred	V_A % pred
0	0.9	87	83	101	87
11	0.89	67	34	54	66
11.5	0.9	83	45	57	83
21	0.75	100	93	89	111

Comment: Female, age 30. Initial presentation (0 months) was with mild infiltrates and reduction of D_{LCO} greater than expected just from small VC loss. 11 months later, infiltrates were very extensive, with gross volume loss, and low D_{LCO} and K_{CO} out of proportion to low VC and indicative of pulmonary vascular involvement. SaO_2 at this time was 89%. Treatment with high dose prednisolone and azathioprine led to rapid improvement at 11.5 months; SaO_2 returned to normal (97%). At 21 months, volume loss had completely recovered and vasculitis (in terms of D_{LCO} and K_{CO}) had satisfactorily resolved. Peak flow charts confirmed intermittent and reversible airflow obstruction.

Behçet's disease

Behçet's disease is a multisystem disorder associated with oral and genital aphthous ulceration, venous thrombosis, uveitis, synovitis, and cutaneous vasculitis. There is a generalized vasculitis with thrombosis of the large veins and arteries and arterial aneurysms. When the lungs are involved (most often in young men), there is a necrotizing vasculitis of arteries, capillaries, and veins. Hemoptysis is common, probably

Table 16.7 Behçet's disease

Date/ months:	FEV_1/VC ratio	VC % pred	D_{LCO} % pred	K_{CO} % pred	V_A % pred
65/M	0.69	132	84	67	129

Comment: FEV_1 normal (105%) and low FEV_1/VC ratio (< 0.75) caused by large VC and does not suggest airflow obstruction (flow-volume curve of normal contour). Low D_{LCO} and K_{CO} are compatible with pulmonary vasculitis.

from erosion of bronchi by pulmonary arterial aneurysms. The vital capacity, D_{LCO}, and (usually) K_{CO} are reduced.[10]

Connective tissue diseases

Mixed connective tissue disease (MCTD) is a syndrome with features of SLE, systemic sclerosis (scleroderma), Sjögren's syndrome, and polymyositis. It mostly affects females (8:1 ratio); about 80% of patients with MCTD have pulmonary involvement.

Table 16.8 Mixed connective tissue disease

Date/ months:	FEV_1/VC ratio	VC % pred	D_{LCO} % pred	K_{CO} % pred	V_A % pred
28/F	0.9	100	61	61	105

Comment: Typical example of a referral from the rheumatological service with a pattern suggesting pulmonary vasculitis. Patients with fibrosing alveolitis (CFA/IPF) may have normal lung volumes when there is coexistent emphysema or gross 'honeycomb' lung pathology but D_{LCO} and K_{CO} would be lower.

Systemic lupus erythematosus (SLE)

SLE is a multisystem immunological disorder characterized by arthropathy, skin lesions, and a systemic vasculitis. Antibodies to deoxyribonucleic acid (DNA) are found in the blood. The lung is involved in most cases (72% [n = 117] of patients tested by us had a D_{LCO} < 80% predicted). The lungs show a rather nonspecific 'diffuse alveolar damage' picture, often called lupus pneumonitis, with an interstitial cellular infiltrate, edema, and hyaline membrane formation. This is associated with micro-atelectasis in the lung periphery (often difficult to detect even with a CT scan) which may be apparent as streaks of 'plate atelectasis' on the chest radiograph.

Respiratory abnormalities in SLE

- Interstitial pneumonitis
- Alveolar hemorrhage
- Vasculitis and infarction
- Thromboembolism
- Obliterative bronchiolitis
- Pleurisy and pleural effusion
- Diaphragm weakness

The exuberant fibrosis seen in other connective tissue disorders (so-called 'fibrosing alveolitis') is rarely seen in SLE. Thus, the K_{co} is better preserved than D_{LCO} (40% of patients with $D_{LCO} < 80\%$ had a normal K_{co}), but it was rarely > 100% even when lung volumes were reduced. A reduction in K_{co} (or lack of an appropriate compensation for volume reduction) suggests a vasculitic element.

Alveolar hemorrhage is a serious complication, but fortunately a rare one. Patients are usually too ill for a diffusion measurement which would show a raised D_{LCO} and K_{co}. A pure vasculitic picture without lung volume loss is unusual. Vasculitis may be associated with pulmonary embolism and 'pro-thrombotic' factors in the blood, or with obliterative bronchiolitis.

A vital capacity < 80% predicted occurred in 33% of 117 of our local patients, but a much lower incidence (< 10%) occurs in 'unselected series.[11] (The frequency of TLC reduction will be similar once smokers have been excluded, since airflow obstruction is not a feature of SLE.) A most dramatic, though unusual, presentation is that of shrinking or vanishing lungs.[12] Lung volumes are severely reduced, with the VC < 50%. The diaphragms are elevated on the chest radiograph, and move 'sluggishly' on fluoroscopy. Gibson et al[13] studied six patients with SLE with VC < 72% predicted. Mouth pressures ($P_I$max and $P_E$max) and maximum-transdiaphragmatic pressures (Pdi max) were reduced. Static lung compliance and maximum lung recoil pressures at TLC ($P_L$max) were low. Similar findings were reported by Martens et al[14] in 7 out of 26 consecutive referrals to the pulmonary function service from the rheumatological department. Their seven patients had VCs ranging from 36–63% predicted with low mean values for TLC (67%), D_{LCO} (55%) and K_{co} (89%, which is low for the lung volume). The low $P_L$max argues against pleural thickening or atelectasis as a cause of the volume reduction. A generalized myositis occurs frequently in SLE (often subclinically) and the diaphragm may sometimes be the muscle most severely affected. Nevertheless, the reduction in lung volume is sometimes greater than that expected from diaphragm weakness alone, and atelectasis may be a

Table 16.9 Diagnosis: SLE with 'shrinking lungs' syndrome

Age (years)	$P_I$max cmH$_2$O	$P_E$max cmH$_2$O	FEV$_1$ [L]	VC [L]	D$_{LCO}$* ml.min^{-1} mmHg^{-1}	K$_{co}$‡	V$_A$ [L]	TLC [L]
21	−12	+31	2.2	2.5	14.7	6.0	2.1	3.5
21.5			0.6	0.9				2.0
25	−36	+60	2.1	2.4	15.6	5.7	2.8	3.0
28	−10	+25	0.4	0.4				
42	−75	+78	1.9	2.25	13.7	8.0		
Predicted								
age 21	<−40	>+70	2.9	3.4	27.9	5.7	4.5	5.0
age 42			2.7	3.1	18	4.8	4.3	4.8

*D$_{LCO}$ and ‡K$_{co}$ (ml.min^{-1} mmHg^{-1} L^{-1}) in traditional units. Divide by 3 for SI units.
Comment: Severe case of shrinking lung syndrome in SLE with recurrent episodes (3 in toto) of volume loss and generalized and respiratory muscle weakness (reduced P$_E$max and P$_I$max). Each episode of volume loss was reversed eventually with corticosteroid treatment.

Pulmonary Vascular Disease 251

Figure 16.1 Detection of alveolar hemorrhage using single-breath K_{CO} and external counting of inhaled $C^{15}O$

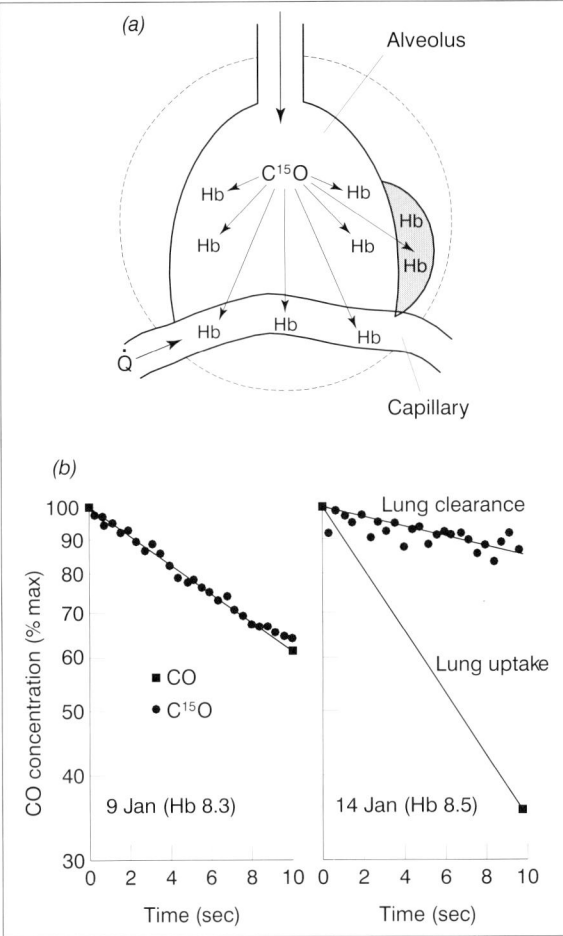

(a) Uptake of radioactive carbon monoxide ($C^{15}O$) by hemoglobin (Hb) in alveolar space, pulmonary interstitium (stippled), and capillary blood. Interrupted circle represents field of view of a detector over the lung. Uptake of $C^{15}O$ will be high in presence of extra (shed) Hb, but removal from counting field will be delayed because of the stagnant pool of Hb.

$\dot{Q}$ represents capillary blood flow.

(b) Carbon monoxide concentration (as percent initial value) plotted against time for inhaled CO (measured in expired air at 10 s) and inhaled $C^{15}O$ (counts recorded by an external counter). Note slopes of CO and $C^{15}O$ uptake are the same (**left panel**) in absence of lung hemorrhage but diverge from each other (**right panel**) when bleeding occurs and a stagnant pool of Hb is present. (From Ewan et al,[16] with permission.)

contributory factor. In fact, Martens et al found that static lung compliance returned to normal in two patients following passive inflation of the lungs to transpulmonary pressures > 30 cmH$_2$O.

Diagnoses associated with transient elevations of D_{LCO} and K_{CO}[17]

	Number
■ Goodpasture syndrome (anti-GBM disease)	21
■ Wegener's granulomatosis	4
■ Microscopic polyangiitis	7
■ Systemic lupus erythematosus	1
■ Idiopathic pulmonary hemosiderosis	1
■ Pulmonary edema	2
■ Thrombocytopenia	3

Laroche et al[15] studied 12 patients (3M/9F) with SLE and volume reduction (VC range 37–72%: mean 54%). Several patients who had borderline values for PLmax, and/or low PImax and low Pdi max, developed a twitch Pdi within the normal range during electrical stimulation of the phrenic nerves. The hypothesis was that the diaphragm weakness in SLE could be 'functional', due to the patients inability to activate the diaphragm fully. Therefore, if a low PImax is found in SLE, in a well-motivated patient, referral to a specialist center for non-volitional tests (phrenic nerve stimulation) might be appropriate (see Chapter 4).

The shrinking lung syndrome, even at its most severe, may be reversible with treatment as shown in Table 16.9 (see facing page).

MICROVASCULAR INJURY

Alveolar hemorrhage

The diagnosis of alveolar hemorrhage on the basis of elevated levels of D_{LCO} and K_{CO} was demonstrated by Ewan et al.[16] They used radioactive $C^{15}O$ to show that transient elevations in D_{LCO} and K_{CO} in 11 patients with Goodpasture syndrome (an immunological disease with anti-glomerular basement membrane [anti-GBM] antibodies directed against the lung and the kidney) were associated with 'trapping' of the inhaled carbon monoxide in the lung itself, as shown in Figure 16.1.

After the initial studies with $C^{15}O$ had established the reason for the high D_{LCO} and K_{CO} values[16] (it is

Table 16.10 Cryoglobulinemia

Date/ days:	FEV$_1$/VC ratio	VC % pred	D$_{LCO}$ % pred	K$_{CO}$ % pred	V$_A$ % pred
0	49	52	56	97	57
22	40	46	100	170	57
29	55	58	79	99	61

Comment: Female, age 62. Mixed cryoglobulinemia is an unusual cause of systemic vasculitis with purpura, arthritis, hepatitis, and glomerulonephritis. Pulmonary capillaritis is uncommon, but alveolar hemorrhage is suggested in this case by the 75% rise in K$_{CO}$ and its subsequent fall over the period of one month. This diagnosis was supported by the simultaneous occurrence of hemoptysis (not severe) and alveolar shadowing on the chest radiograph.

essential to apply a Hb correction because these patients have fluctuating levels of anemia), a diagnosis of alveolar hemorrhage could be made on the basis of a reversible rise of K$_{CO}$ of 50% or more above baseline values. Greening and Hughes[17] reported such a rise on 61 occasions in 39 patients, and 77% of episodes were accompanied by at least two 'traditional indicators of pulmonary hemorrhage, i.e. hemoptysis, an abrupt fall in Hb concentration, or chest X-ray opacities. The changes in D$_{LCO}$ and K$_{CO}$ were not accompanied by any significant changes in vital capacity or alveolar volume except when bleeding was very severe. The elevations of D$_{LCO}$ and K$_{CO}$ represented active bleeding. In some instances the elevated K$_{CO}$ returned to baseline with a t½ of 1.7 days, consistent with abrupt cessation of hemorrhage and macrophage ingestion of the extravascular erythrocytes. In contrast to the elevation of D$_{LCO}$ and K$_{CO}$, the appearances of alveolar hemorrhage on the chest radiograph are non-specific, until infection and edema have been excluded, and may persist for some time after active bleeding has ceased, or may be absent or delayed.[18] See Chapter 17 for an example of serial measurements of diffusing capacity in alveolar hemorrhage.

The initial papers focused on Goodpasture's syndrome, where the likelihood of alveolar hemorrhage is much greater in cigarette smokers. Subsequently, 53 patients with Wegener's granulomatosis and 36 patients with microscopic polyangiitis were reported.[19] 32/89 patients had hemoptysis which was considered to be due to alveolar hemorrhage and 20 had a transient elevation of K$_{CO}$ (a further 5 had only a single raised value). Microvascular capillaritis is a feature of Wegener's. Autopsies have documented extensive alveolar hemorrhage. Unlike anti-GBM disease there is no association of hemorrhage with cigarette smoking.

PULMONARY HYPOTENSION
Intrapulmonary shunting

Intrapulmonary shunting presents a quite different physiological pattern of abnormality when contrasted with pulmonary vasculitis and pulmonary embolic disease. There is no pulmonary hypertension because of the 'run-off' effect of the shunts; in fact, there is *pulmonary hypotension*. Arterial hypoxemia may be severe. Paradoxically, patients with pulmonary shunts complain much less of exertional dyspnea, and their exercise tolerance is surprisingly well preserved. They are well adapted because they have no difficulty in raising cardiac output to compensate for arterial hypoxemia.[20] Patients with *pulmonary hypertension* cannot increase their cardiac output so easily.

Causes of intrapulmonary shunting

- Hereditary hemorrhagic telangiectasia with pulmonary arteriovenous malformations.
- Idiopathic pulmonary arteriovenous malformations.
- Hepatopulmonary syndrome.

Hereditary hemorrhagic telangiectasia (HHT)

HHT is a disorder of vascular development which has an autosomal dominant inheritance. It is characterized by frequent epistaxes, usually beginning in childhood, mucocutaneous telangiectasia, and a clear-cut family history. The telangiectasias are recognizable from about the age of 20 years as pin-point cherry-red spots on the lips, palate, tongue, and buccal mucosa. Bleeding from the gastrointestinal tract occurs in about 30% of those affected with HHT, but generally after the age of 50 years. The other vascular lesions of HHT are arteriovenous malformations (AVMs=), which are similar to superficial telangiectasias but much larger, with direct communication between larger arteries and veins (Figure 16.2). The most common site for these 'macro-telangiectasias' is the lung, with a frequency of 15–30%.[21]

In the majority of patients with HHT, there is a mutation in the gene for endoglin located on chromosome 9. Endoglin has high levels of expression in human vascular endothelium. Endoglin binds TGF-β_1 and associates with other signaling receptors to modify TGF-β_1 signal transduction. TGF-β_1 plays a role in maintaining the integrity of the interstitial matrix which surrounds and supports capillary vessels. Other families have a mutation on chromosome 12, which also results in dysregulation of TGF-β_1.

Large pulmonary arteriovenous malformations (PAVMs) are easily recognized once the diagnosis has been thought of. There are characteristic shadows on the chest radiograph, and the arterial oxygen saturation (SaO_2) is reduced, more so in the erect position than the supine; this is because the majority of the larger PAVMs are in the lower lobes and receive a greater fraction of pulmonary blood flow in the erect position. The arterial hypoxemia is caused by an intrapulmonary anatomic shunt. This can be measured by the classical 100% O_2 breathing method or by an intravenous injection of radiolabeled albumin macroaggregates (^{99m}Tc-MAA) (see Chapter 5). There is a further fall in SaO_2 on exercise caused by the normal fall in the mixed venous oxygen content of the shunted blood. The shunt fraction through the PAVMs may increase or decrease on exercise, exaggerating or minimizing the fall in SaO_2.[22] Cardiac output is increased, by an amount approximately equal to the R-L shunt, both at rest and on exercise.[20] A further adaptive mechanism, but not occurring in all patients, is polycythemia. As already mentioned, exercise capacity is well preserved in spite of the low SaO_2. Maximum workloads exceeding 70% predicted were frequently found.

There is wide variation in the arterial hypoxemia according to the number of PAVMs and their blood flow. Arterial PCO_2 tends to be low. Lung volumes are normal and there is no airflow obstruction. Diffusion for carbon monoxide is reduced, D_{LCO} being 78 ± 3.2 (SEM) % predicted and K_{CO} 85 ± 3.2 % (n = 53).[23] Those with the lowest D_{LCO} and K_{CO} have the most widespread vascular malformations. A vascular steal might contribute to the low diffusion values because of the low vascular resistance of PAVMs. This is unlikely for two reasons: (a) there is usually only a small rise in K_{CO} after macroscopic PAVMs have been eliminated by embolization techniques; (b) pulmonary blood flow to non-shunting lung is normal.

Figure 16.2 Pulmonary arteriovenous malformation (PAVM) before and after embolization

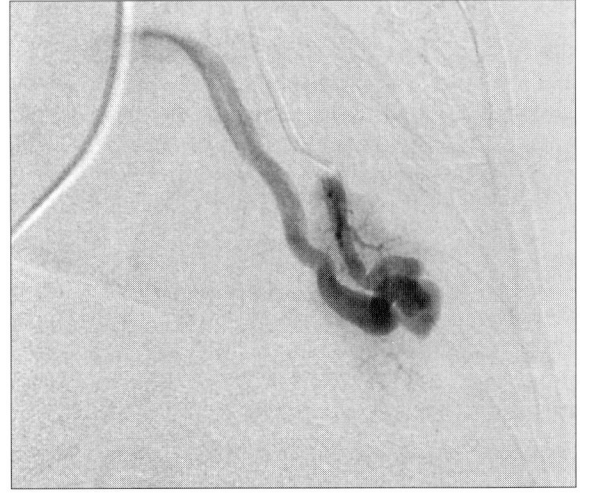

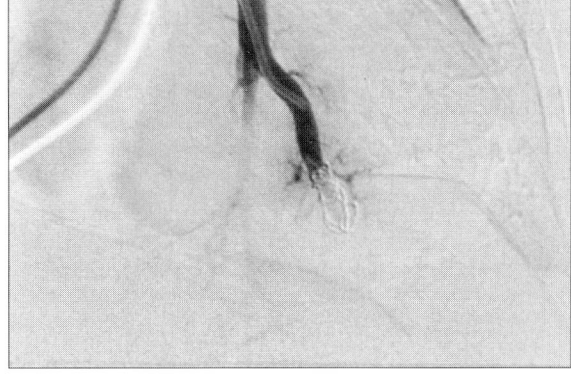

(a) Super selective digital subtraction angiogram of a PAVM showing feeding arterial vessel (containing catheter tip), the sac-like replacement of the normal capillary bed, and the draining vein. Note small normal pulmonary arterial vessels and large size of the draining vein, probably secondary to high blood flow.

(b) Same field after occlusion of feeding artery with five stainless steel coils. No draining vein visible.

(Courtesy of Dr JE Jackson, Hammersmith Hospital.)

The seriousness of PAVMs lies not so much in the hypoxemia (except in the severest cases), but in the frequency of paradoxical embolization, leading to cerebral transient ischemic attacks (TIAs), ischemic stroke, and cerebral abscess. The overall neurological complication rate in patients with PAVMs is about 40%. The incidence of cerebral abscess in different series ranges from 6% to 20%.[20]

In women with extensive and multiple PAVMs, arterial oxygenation improves during pregnancy, only to deteriorate markedly afterwards to a lower level than before pregnancy, associated with enlargement of pre-existing PAVMs.[24] Estrogens and progesterones would seem to be important modifiers of the clinical expression of HHT. PAVMs are more common in females; hemorrhage from the nose or gastrointestinal tract occurs more severely after the menopause, and may be alleviated by hormonal therapy.

The treatment of PAVMs with feeding vessel diameters > 3 mm is by intravascular placement of steel coils which induce a permanent thrombus. The radiologist introduces a catheter into the pulmonary arterial tree (via the femoral vein) and passes it into the artery feeding the PAVM. Up to 30 PAVMs may be occluded in several embolization sessions. Dutton et al[23] found significant improvements in SaO_2 and decreases in R–L shunt in 53 PAVM patients:

	SaO_2% supine	SaO_2% erect	SaO_2% exercise	R–L shunt %	Kco % pred
Pre-emb	89(1)	83(1)	81(2)	23(2)	85(3)
Post-emb	94(1)	92(1)	91(1)	9(1)	90(4)
					(SEM)

Using SaO_2 > 95% and R-L shunt < 5% as criteria of 'normality', supine SaO_2 had returned to normal in 64% of patients, erect SaO_2 in 53% and R-L shunt in 40%. In HHT (most of the cases), there are often multiple small PAVM channels which cannot be embolized, in addition to the larger ones which have been treated. Changes in pulmonary function post embolization were small, only the increase in Kco (from 85% ± 3.2 to 90% ± 4) being significant.[23]

Figure 16.3 Pulse oximetry showing postural fall in SaO_2 in a patient with PAVMs

Supine		
Time	SaO_2	Pulse
1	94	50
2	95	47
3	94	47
4	95	49
5	95	47
6	95	52
7	96	48
8	96	53
9	95	50
10	95	55

Erect		
Time	SaO_2	Pulse
1	93	85
2	93	85
3	93	83
4	94	86
5	93	80
6	93	79
7	93	83
8	93	86
9	92	88
10	92	88

Measurements are continued for 10 minutes to ensure steady state, and would be averaged over minutes 6–10. SaO_2 as %. Pulse as min^{-1}.

Table 16.11a Male, aged 44 years, with diffuse PAVMs

Embolization status	SaO_2 % erect	SaO_2 % supine	SaO_2 % max. ex	R–L shunt % supine	VC % pred	DLCO % pred	Kco % pred
Pre	75	84	69	35	94	62	78
Post	87	94	86	13	96	77	88

Comment: More than 30 PAVMs were embolized over a ten year period, although many small PAVMs, too small for embolization therapy, remain. Nevertheless, oxygenation has improved considerably and R-L shunt has decreased. A remarkable feature is that exercise capacity (progressive cycle ergometer test) has remained normal throughout this period (180 watts; 100% predicted) in spite of profound hypoxemia on exertion.

Table 16.11b Female, 34 years, with PAVMs

Embolization status	SaO$_2$ % erect	SaO$_2$ % supine	SaO$_2$ % max. ex	R-L shunt % supine	VC % pred	D$_{LCO}$ % pred	K$_{CO}$ % pred
Pre	92	95	93	9	97	77	88
Post	96	96	95	3.5	94	96	114

Comment: This patient presented with a right-sided cerebral infarct (with good eventual recovery) within one week of a cholecystectomy operation. HHT and PAVMs were diagnosed. Initially, one PAVM was ligated at thoracotomy, but when further lesions were found she was referred for percutaneous transcatheter embolization. Pre-embolization, note lower SaO$_2$ in erect position compared to supine suggesting a doubling of R-L shunt from its supine value (9%). After embolization of 5 PAVMs, oxygenation improved and R-L shunt decreased. Increase in D$_{LCO}$ and K$_{CO}$ after embolization is greater than is usually seen.

The laboratory measurement in this patient of SaO$_2$, using pulse oximetry, is illustrated in Figure 16.3.

Idiopathic PAVMs (non-HHT)

20% of PAVMs seen on angiography are not associated with HHT, although the angiographic appearances are identical. These patients have no family history, no telangiectasia, and no chronic epistaxes. They are more likely to have polycythemia, because they are not bleeding from the nose or the gastrointestinal tract. They usually have fewer than five abnormal vascular channels, all of which are amenable to embolization. Typically, they are not left with any residual shunt.

Hepatopulmonary syndrome (HPS)

The hepatopulmonary syndrome is a form of intrapulmonary shunting which is quite different anatomically from the PAVMs of HHT, but the physiological effects are very similar. The features of HPS are:

- chronic liver disease
- pulmonary microvascular dilatation
- arterial hypoxemia
- low D$_{LCO}$ and K$_{CO}$.

The liver disease may be mild and unrecognized (as in the case in Figure 16.4), though there is always portal hypertension. Unlike PAVMs (see above) where parts of the capillary bed have never developed, the vascular defect in HPS is acquired and affects individual septal vessels which become dilated up to 20–30 times their normal diameter.[25] The pulmonary angiogram shows dilated 'sacs' between the arteries and veins in PAVMs but it is virtually normal in HPS. Alveolar-capillary equilibration for oxygen is never complete because of the long distance for diffusion between alveolar gas and the central core of flowing blood in the dilated capillaries. This is the cause of the low arterial PO$_2$. Even when 100% oxygen is breathed, a significant alveolar-arterial PO$_2$ gradient remains, indicating an intrapulmonary anatomic shunt. Radiolabeled albumin macroaggregates (^{99m}Tc-MAA)

Figure 16.4 Hepatopulmonary syndrome

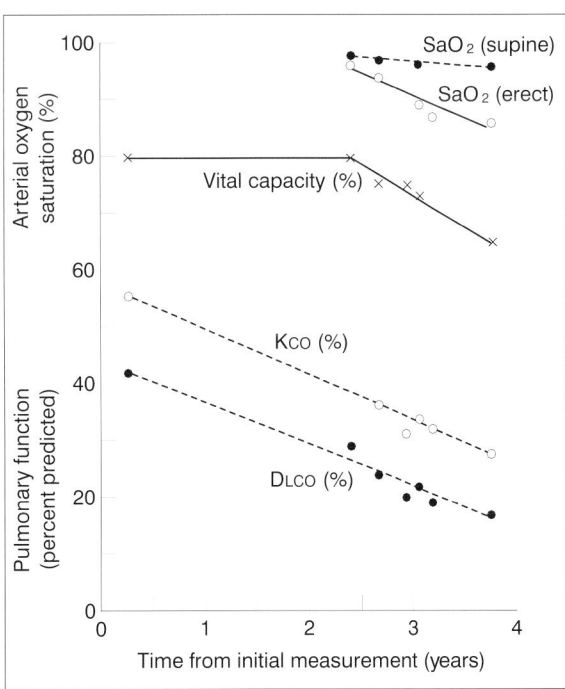

Serial pulmonary function testing in a case of hepatopulmonary syndrome followed for 3.75 years. Arterial oxygen saturation was measured by pulse oximetry. Liver cirrhosis was not diagnosed until 2½ years after initial presentation (liver function tests were normal at that time).

Table 16.12 Male, aged 43 years, with cryptogenic liver cirrhosis, before and after liver transplantation

Transplantation status	SaO$_2$ % erect	SaO$_2$ % supine	SaO$_2$ % max.ex	R-L shunt % 99mTc-MAA	VC % pred	D$_{LCO}$ % pred	K$_{CO}$ % pred
Pre	92	96	72	30	100	50	52
Post	96	96	92	0	98	50	54

Comment: Similar physiological picture to previous patient with diffuse macroscopic PAVMs except for lower D$_{LCO}$ and K$_{CO}$. The R-L shunt (pre-transplant) on 100% oxygen was 12% (not shown), considerably less than the 99mTc-MAA R-L shunt (30%). Following liver transplantation, oxygenation in erect position and on maximum exercise improved, but D$_{LCO}$ and K$_{CO}$ did not. See text for explanation.

injected intravenously pass through these dilated capillaries and an 'anatomic' shunt can be calculated which exceeds the 'quasi-anatomic' shunt measured with 100% O$_2$ where partial equilibration has occurred because of the relatively small size of the shunt vessels and because of their thin walls.[26]

Alveolar-capillary equilibration for carbon monoxide is similarly affected, and D$_{LCO}$ and K$_{CO}$ are always reduced. In very severe cases, lung volumes may be reduced. Figure 16.4 illustrates the progressive decline in pulmonary function, affecting the co diffusing capacity severely for at least two years before gas exchange at rest is significantly compromised (though PaO$_2$ might have been slightly low somewhat earlier). Liver cirrhosis was not detected until 2.5 years from presentation, at a time when D$_{LCO}$ was < 25% predicted.

The circulation is very hyperdynamic and these patients have a high cardiac output. This compounds the problem for oxygen because alveolar-capillary PO$_2$ equilibrium (but not that for CO) will be incomplete if capillary transit times are short. Of great interest is the observation that arterial PO$_2$ improves dramatically following liver transplantation.[27]

The failure of D$_{LCO}$ and K$_{CO}$ to improve after liver transplantation is difficult to explain. The dilated vessels must have become smaller for the 99mTc-MAA R-L shunt to have disappeared. One explanation would be that the dilated pre-capillary vessels have narrowed sufficiently to trap the 20–60 μm albumin particles, but that the septal vessels remain dilated and continue to slow CO uptake. Alveolar-capillary equilibration for oxygen depends on the diffusion:perfusion (D/$\dot{Q}$) ratio; slowing the circulation by reducing the cardiac output ($\dot{Q}$) after liver transplantation may improve the D/$\dot{Q}$ ratio and the PaO$_2$. CO uptake, unlike oxygen, is solely dependent on diffusion and will only increase if the gas exchanging (alveolar septal) vessels decrease in size.

Comparison of two types of intrapulmonary shunting

	PAVMs	HPS
Pathogenesis	Inherited	Acquired
Anatomy	Capillary network replaced	Dilatation of individual capillaries
Angiogram	Sac-like lesions	Normal or 'spongy' appearance
R-L shunt methods	99mTc-MAA = 100% O$_2$	99mTc-MAA > 100% O$_2$
D$_{LCO}$	Normal or reduced	Severely reduced (< 50% pred)
SaO$_2$ erect < supine	Yes	Yes
SaO$_2$ falls on exercise	Yes	Yes
Treatment	Coil embolization	Liver transplantation

CONCLUSIONS

- Pulmonary vascular pathology is characterized by a low D_{LCO} and K_{CO}.
- Lung volumes may be reduced but airflow obstruction is uncommon except in Wegener's granulomatosis and the Churg-Strauss syndrome.
- Transient elevations of D_{LCO} and K_{CO} are compatible with alveolar hemorrhage.
- Low D_{LCO} plus low SaO_2 (erect < supine) suggests intrapulmonary shunting.

References

1. Hughes JMB. The lungs in heart disease. In: Murray JF & Nadel JA (eds) *Textbook of Respiratory Medicine*, 2nd edn. Philadelphia: WB Saunders 1994: 2399–415.
2. Puri S, Baker BL, Dutka DP, Oakley CM, Hughes JMB, Cleland JGF. Reduced alveolar-capillary membrane diffusing capacity in chronic heart failure. *Circulation* 1995; **91**: 2769–74.
3. Fennerty AG, Gunawardena KA & Smith AP. The transfer factor and its subdivisions in patients with pulmonary embolism. *Eur Respir J* 1988; **1**: 98–107.
4. Wimalaratna HSK, Farrel J & Lee HY. Measurement of diffusing capacity in pulmonary embolism. *Respir Med* 1989; **83**: 481–6.
5. Horn M, Ries A, Neven C, Moser KM. Restrictive ventilatory pattern in precapillary pulmonary hypertension. *Am Rev Respir Dis* 1983; **128**: 163–5.
6. Serjeant GR. Sickle-cell disease. *Lancet* 1997; **350**: 926–32.
7. Miller GJ, Serjeant GR, Saunders MJ, Richardson C, Gilson RJC. Interpretation of lung function tests in the sickle cell haemoglobinopathies. *Thorax* 1978; **33**: 85–8.
8. Dantzker DR & Bower JS. Mechanism of gas exchange abnormalities in patients with chronic obliterative pulmonary vascular disease. *J Clin Invest* 1979; **64**: 1050–5.
9. Lanham JG, Elkon KB, Pusey CD, Hughes GRV. Systemic vasculitis with asthma and eosinophilia: a clinical approach to the Churg-Strauss syndrome. *Medicine* 1984; **63**: 65–81.
10. Efthimiou J, Johnston C, Spiro SG, Turner-Warwick M. Pulmonary disease in Behçet's syndrome. *Quart J Med* 1986; **58**: 259–80.
11. Andonopoulos AP, Constantopoulos SH, Galanopoulou V, Drosos AA, Acritidis NC, Montsopoulos HM. Pulmonary function of non-smoking patients with systemic lupus erythematosus. *Chest* 1988; **94**: 312–5.
12. Hoffbrand BI & Beck ER. "Unexplained" dyspnoea and shrinking lungs in systemic lupus erythematosus. *BMJ* 1965; **i**: 1273–7.
13. Gibson GJ, Edmonds JP & Hughes GRV. Diaphragm function and lung involvement in systemic lupus erythematosus. *Am J Med* 1977; **63**: 926–32.
14. Martens J, Demedts M, Vanmeenen MT, Dequeker J. Respiratory muscle dysfunction in systemic lupus erythematosus. *Chest* 1983; **84**: 170–5.
15. Laroche CM, Mulvey DA, Hawkins P *et al*. Diaphragm strength in the shrinking lung syndrome of systemic lupus erythematosus. *Quart J Med* 1989; **71**: 429–39.
16. Ewan PW, Jones HA, Rhodes CG, Hughes JMB. Detection of intrapulmonary hemorrhage with carbon monoxide. Application in Goodpasture's syndrome. *N Engl J Med* 1976; **295**: 1391–6.
17. Greening AP & Hughes JMB. Serial measurements of carbon monoxide diffusing capacity in intrapulmonary haemorrhage. *Clin Sci* 1981; **60**: 507–12.
18. Bowley NB, Hughes JMB & Steiner RE. The chest x-ray in pulmonary capillary haemorrhage: correlation with carbon monoxide uptake. *Clin Radiol* 1979; **30**: 413–7.
19. Haworth SJ, Savage COS, Carr D, Hughes JMB, Rees AJ. Pulmonary haemorrhage complicating Wegener's granulomatosis and microscopic polyarteritis. *BMJ* 1985; **290**: 1775–8.
20. Whyte MKB, Hughes JMB, Jackson JE, Peters AM, Hempleman SC, Jones HA. Cardiopulmonary response to exercise in patients with intrapulmonary shunts. *J Appl Physiol* 1993; **75**: 321–8.
21. Hughes JMB. Pulmonary arteriovenous malformations in hereditary hemorrhagic telangiectasia. In: duBois RM (ed) *Pulmonary Vasculitis. Seminars in Respiratory and Critical Care Medicine* 1997; **19**: 79–89.
22. Whyte MKB, Peters AM, Hughes JMB, Henderson BL, Bellingan GJ, Jackson JE, Chilvers ER. Quantification of right-to-left shunting at rest and during exercise in patients with pulmonary arteriovenous malformations. *Thorax* 1992; **47**: 914–21.
23. Dutton J, Jackson JE, Peters AM, Ueki J, Ussov W, Hughes JMB. Pulmonary arteriovenous malformations: pathophysiology and treatment with coil embolization. *Am J Roentgenol* 1995; **165**: 1119–25.
24. Shovlin CL, Winstock AR, Jackson JE, Peters AM, Hughes JMB. Medical complications of pregnancy in hereditary haemorrhagic telangiectasia. *Quart J Med* 1995; **88**: 879–87.
25. Davis HA, Schwartz DJ, Lefrak SS, Susman N, Schainker BA. Alveolar-capillary oxygen disequilibrium in hepatic cirrhosis. *Chest* 1978; **73**: 507–11.
26. Genovesi MG, Tierney DF, Taplin GV, Eisenberg H. An intravenous radionuclide method to evaluate hypoxemia caused by abnormal alveolar vessels. *Am Rev Respir Dis* 1976; **114**: 59–65.
27. Rodriguez-Roisin R & Krowka MJ. Is severe arterial hypoxaemia due to hepatic disease an indication for liver transplantation? A new therapeutic approach. *Eur Respir J* 1994; **7**: 839–42.

17 Interpretation of the Diffusing Capacity (transfer factor) with special reference to Interstitial Lung Disease

J M B Hughes

- **INTRODUCTION**
- **CLINICAL ANALYSIS OF D_{LCO} (T_{LCO})**
  Alveolar volume and kCO (~ K_{CO}) as the components of D_{LCO}
  Causes of a low alveolar volume (V_A) in the single-breath D_{LCO}
   Loss of alveolar units
   Spectrum of discrete versus diffuse loss of units
   Incomplete alveolar expansion
   Airflow obstruction
  Causes of a low K_{CO}
  Causes of a high K_{CO}
  Interpretation of D_{LCO} and K_{CO} in the presence of a low V_A
   Response of K_{CO} to gain or loss of units
  Intermittent high K_{CO}
- **INTERSTITIAL LUNG DISEASE**
  Sarcoidosis
  Cryptogenic fibrosing alveolitis/idiopathic pulmonary fibrosis
- **CLINICAL ANALYSIS AND TEACHING**
- **CONCLUSIONS**
- **APPENDIX 17.1: CLINICAL EXAMPLES**

INTRODUCTION

This chapter looks at the meaning of a low or high value for the diffusing capacity (D_{LCO}) [transfer factor, T_{LCO}] in physiological and clinical terms. The analysis focuses on the two components (V_A and K_{CO}) from which the D_{LCO} is derived. The problem of how to interpret a low D_{LCO} (T_{LCO}) in the presence of a reduced alveolar volume (V_A) is presented in a new way. The value of studying all three parameters (D_{LCO}, K_{CO} [D_L/V_A] and V_A) is emphasized.

Interstitial lung disease has been chosen as an example to illustrate this analysis.

CLINICAL ANALYSIS OF D_{LCO} (T_{LCO})

Alveolar volume and kco (~Kco) as the components of D_{LCO}

The fundamental relationship (see Chapter 6) is:

alveolar volume (V_A) × kCO = D_{LCO}
number of × *efficiency* = *gas exchange*
contributing units *per unit* *capacity**

Therefore, the cause of a *low* D_{LCO} (T_{LCO}) must be either a low V_A or a low kCO or both. Remember that kCO (the rate of CO uptake from alveolar gas as time^{-1}) is equivalent, except in its units, to K_{CO} (D_{LCO}/V_A). The ratio of kCO (min^{-1}) to K_{CO} (ml.min^{-1} mmHg^{-1} L^{-1}) is 0.8 (or 2.4 if K_{CO} is in SI units [mmol.min^{-1} kPa^{-1} L^{-1}]).

The prediction for V_A is equal to predicted TLC minus predicted V_D (anatomic). A value of 150 ml (± a correction for body weight) is usually taken for V_{Danat}. (V_A + V_{Danat})/TLC, where TLC was measured by plethysmography, was 93.7% ± 6.65,[1] the absolute difference being 390 ml ± 45 (SD). We take predicted V_A as (TLC predicted − V_{Danat} [150 ml] − 350 ml) where the latter is an arbitrary value for 'mixing inefficiency' due to the short (10 second) time interval over which V_A is measured. Because of size differences, V_A in a normal lung could range from 250 to 600 ml less than TLC.

Causes of a low alveolar volume (V_A) in the single-breath D_{LCO}

Loss of alveolar units

Table 17.1 lists some of the pathological processes associated with low V_A. The most common cause is *loss of alveolar units* (Table 17.1 A1 and A2). There are a variety of causes for this, ranging from removal of lung, to lung destruction by disease, to filling of alveolar air spaces with inflammatory or edematous fluid.

The causes of loss of alveolar units can be subdivided into *discrete* loss of lung (either a whole lung or lobe/s or part of a lobe, or units scattered discretely within several lobes or sublobar units) or more *diffuse/generalized* loss with no recognizable anatomic location. **Discrete loss of units** implies that the lung remaining (and contributing to the VC, TLC, V_A, etc.) is essentially normal. In **diffuse loss of units**, on the other hand, the remaining lung in terms of its volume (VC, etc.) is considered to be involved in the primary pathology. Pneumonectomy or collapse or consolidation of the right lower lobe would be an example of *discrete* loss of units. Lung fibrosis affecting more than one lobe is generally part of a *diffuse* disease process. Chronic heart failure, controlled on therapy and in the absence of pulmonary edema, is associated with small lung volumes and diffuse vascular injury induced by high left atrial and microvascular pressures. The volume loss is regained after cardiac transplantation (mean VC and TLC 76% and 79% predicted *before* and 94% and 98% *after* transplantation [n = 47]).[2] This volume gain is thought to be inversely related to the reduction in heart size and central blood vessels (veins).[3]

Spectrum of discrete versus diffuse loss of units

The concept of loss of units is a fundamental one. *Discrete* and *diffuse* refer to the functional status of the lung that remains (or is ventilated), which is normal in the former and diseased in the latter, but all combinations may occur – such as 25% or 75% of the remaining units being normal (or diseased), etc.

For example, the PV curve of the lung and the value of lung compliance (but not specific compliance, necessarily) will be influenced by the number of contributing lung units. If the ventilated lung volume is reduced to 50% of normal, the PV curve will be truncated on its volume axis and the 'chord' compliance will be halved, but the shape factor 'k' (see Chapter 3) will be normal, provided the contributing units retain normal function. The 'apparent stiffness' of the lung in fibrosing alveolitis can sometimes be explained entirely by volume loss[4] ('k' would be normal), but to the extent that some of the remaining units are diseased, the shape ('k' factor) of the PV curve will be affected as well as its position on the volume axis. The same concepts can be applied to the diffusing capacity where K_{CO} is the gas exchange analogue of the shape factor 'k'. But the important difference for D_{LCO} and K_{CO} is that blood volume can be diverted from dis-

---

* Since D_{LCO} is often interpreted alongside spirometric results, note that there is an equivalent mechanical analogy:

vital capacity (VC) × FEV_1/VC = FEV_1
no of × *emptying* = *ventilatory capacity*
contributing units *efficiency*

Table 17.1 Causes of a low alveolar volume (V_A) *(single-breath D_{LCO})*

A1 Loss of alveolar units Discrete	A2 Loss of alveolar units Diffuse	B Incomplete expansion	C Airflow obstruction
1. Pneumonectomy lobectomy	**1. Diffuse fibrosis** Asbestosis Pneumoconiosis Connective tissue diseases IPF/CFA Honeycomb lung	**1. Pleural disease** Thickening, plaques Mesothelioma	**1. Asthma** Churg-Strauss
2. Local destruction Post-pneumonic Post-TB Bronchiectasis	**2. Alveolar infiltrates** Inflammatory EAA Neoplastic Rejection/GVHD PCP	**2. Neuromuscular** Myopathy Neuropathy Myasthenia Spinal cord and cerebral lesions	**2. Emphysema ± bullae**
3. Consolidation or collapse Infective Neoplastic Space occupying lesions	**3. Pulmonary edema**	**3. Chest wall** Kyphoscoliosis Thoracoplasty Trauma or fracture Chest pain Obesity	**3. Chronic bronchitis**
4. Localized alveolar infiltrate Sarcoidosis IPF/CFA (cellular phase)	**4. Vascular** PHT, PE CHF, vasculitis Wegener's, SLE Sickle-cell disease	**4. Space occupying lesion** Pleural effusion Pneumothorax Large tumors	**4. Bronchiolitis** Viral, drugs BPA, GVHD Connective tissue diseases
		5. Poor technique Lack of comprehension Lack of cooperation Facial weakness	**5. Bronchiectasis**

Abbreviations: SLE – systemic lupus erythematosus; EAA – extrinsic allergic alveolitis (hypersensitivity pneumonitis); IPF – idiopathic pulmonary fibrosis; PCP – *Pneumocystis carinii* pneumonia; GVHD – graft versus host disease; PHT – pulmonary hypertension; CFA – cryptogenic fibrosing alveolitis; CHF – congestive heart failure; PE – pulmonary embolic disease; BPA – bronchopulmonary aspergillosis.

eased (or absent) lung to the units which are contributing to the measurement, i.e. 'seeing' the inhaled CO, and this raises their Kco. This is a form of compensation which is not available in lung mechanics.

Fibrosing alveolitis (CFA) or idiopathic pulmonary fibrosis (IPF), often called 'honeycomb' lung, involves the lung diffusely in its end stage but in its early stages the predominant pathology is a localized alveolar infiltrate consisting of protein-rich edema and inflammatory cells. Thus, a disease process may have *discrete loss of units* in the early inflammatory stage and *diffuse loss of units* in the later fibrotic stage. The difference between *discrete* and *diffuse* loss of alveolar units influences the value of Kco (see Figure 17.1), which is normal or increased in the former and reduced in the latter. It is not an absolute distinction, however – the remaining lung may be *partially* involved in the primary disease process, and the level of the Kco will reflect this.

Incomplete alveolar expansion

A second, quite different, cause of a low alveolar volume (V_A) is incomplete expansion of 'normal' lung units (B in Table 17.1), generally due to problems in the chest wall or respiratory muscle weakness. An inadequate inspiration to TLC, as a result of poor comprehension or lack of cooperation, is another cause of lack of alveolar expansion. Space occupying lesions also cause incomplete expansion, but there is often secondary collapse of lung units in regions adjacent to a mass or fluid collection. Thus the low V_A may reflect a combination of incomplete expansion and loss of units. In a similar fashion, collapse of peripheral lung units may contribute to the low V_A seen in respiratory muscle weakness.

Airflow obstruction

The third cause of a low V_A is incomplete mixing within the breath-holding time, between the inspired He/CO gas mixture and the residual gas volume (RV) in the lungs. Thus any cause of airflow obstruction can lead to a low V_A (Table 17.1C). The reason is uneven distribution of inspired He/CO gas mixture with the most 'obstructed' regions receiving little or none of the inspirate. There will also be a *volume gap* between the low V_A and the usually *normal* or even increased TLC (measured by body plethysmography or multibreath inert gas wash-in).

Causes of a low K_{CO}

The most common causes of a low K_{CO} are emphysema, pulmonary vascular disease, and the diffuse lung fibrosis which is generally associated with connective tissue or autoimmune disease. Table 17.2 also lists some of the less common causes. A low K_{CO} is primarily caused by destruction of the microvasculature, and this implies poor local blood flow. Thus units with a low K_{CO} are likely to have high $\dot{V}_A/\dot{Q}$ ratios. In emphysema and fibrosing alveolitis (idiopathic lung fibrosis) a large number of units have high $\dot{V}_A/\dot{Q}$ ratios.

Causes of a high K_{CO}

The causes of a high K_{CO} are listed in Table 17.3. Incomplete alveolar expansion (Table 17.3B) is a reflection of the exponential rise of K_{CO} as the breath-holding lung volume falls (Figure 17.1). Pulmonary hemorrhage is associated with an intermittently high K_{CO} (see page 265). A high K_{CO} with the *discrete loss of*

Table 17.2 Causes of a low K_{CO}

A With airflow obstruction	B Without airflow obstruction
1. Emphysema ± Chronic bronchitis	**1. Diffuse fibrosis** IPF/CFA Sarcoidosis Connective tissue/ autoimmune diseases Asbestosis, etc.
2. Bronchiolitis Viral BPA Drugs Connective tissue diseases GVHD	**2. Pulmonary hypertension** Primary pulmonary hypertension Pulmonary embolism Vasculitis Sickle-cell disease
3. Churg-Strauss syndrome	**3. Intrapulmonary shunting** Pulmonary arteriovenous malformations Hepatopulmonary syndrome
	4. Cardiac Congestive heart failure Eisenmenger syndrome
	5. Pulmonary edema

units type of pathology (Table 17.3A and Figure 17.1) is probably related to a high local pulmonary blood flow per ventilated lung unit. Perfusion is high in the remaining lung units because blood flow has been diverted from unventilated units, either because they are diseased (fibrotic) or hypoxic and therefore vasoconstricted (distal to a bronchial obstruction) or because they are 'absent' (pneumonectomy or lung destruction). Therefore, the remaining units, *provided they are structurally intact*, will have an increased K_{CO} as shown for the lung as a whole when the cardiac output is increased by exercise. In other words, loss of 50% of lung units effectively doubles pulmonary blood flow *per unit volume* in the rest of the lung, and K_{CO} will increase twofold *as if* total cardiac output had increased from 5 L.min^{-1} to 10 L.min^{-1} (see Chapter 6, Fig 7, panel B, which applies equally to D_{LCO} and K_{CO}). Loss of 66% of lung units increases per cardiac output per unit volume threefold. Thus a plot of K_{CO} versus V_A (loss of units) has been constructed (Figure 17.1, panel B) from the previously shown relationship for normal lungs between D_{LCO} and K_{CO} and cardiac output. D_{LCO} (discrete loss of units) is derived from D_{LCO} at the appropriate blood flow per unit lung volume multiplied by the V_A (number of units) as a fraction of the V_A at total lung capacity (TLC).

Note that excess blood flow per alveolus throughout the whole lung in high cardiac output states also increases the microvascular volume and therefore the K_{CO} (Table 17.3D). For example, in left to right intracardiac shunts, D_{LCO} was increased (123% of predicted normal in ventricular septal defect, and 142% in atrial septal defect).[5] Patients with stable asthma often have a slightly raised D_{LCO} and K_{CO} (116% and 117% respectively) which seems to be related to recruitment of blood flow to the lung apices in the erect posture.[6]

Interpretation of D_{LCO} and K_{CO} in the presence of a low V_A

A common pattern associated with a low D_{LCO} is a low V_A and a compensatory high K_{CO}. Some authorities[7] have argued that it should be possible to calculate a [V_A-corrected] D_{LCO}. Unfortunately, this is not possible unless one knows the reason for the low V_A.[8] Figure 17.1 (adapted from Figure 7 in Chapter 6) shows that the relationship between D_{LCO} and K_{CO} and a low V_A caused by *incomplete alveolar expansion* is quite different from that caused by *discrete loss of alveolar units*.

Incomplete alveolar expansion   The reduction in V_A (in the absence of airflow obstruction, $V_A \sim$ TLC) caused by failure, or inability, to inspire maximally (to TLC) is offset in large part by increase in the surface to volume ratio for diffusion per alveolus ($\sim K_{CO}$) which increases exponentially as the alveoli get smaller (Figure 17.1B). Therefore, D_{LCO} (as the multiple of K_{CO} and V_A) is well preserved as a function of V_A, falling by only 3% per 10% fall in V_A (Figure 17.1B).

Discrete loss of alveolar units   Blood flow to units which have been 'lost' is diverted to the remaining units. Discrete loss of units in its 'pure' form probably only exists for lobectomy/pneumonectomy, the assumption being that the remaining units are completely 'normal'. When blood flow to the remaining units increases twofold, the K_{CO} (see Figure 17.1B for V_A/V_A at TLC of 50%) increases by 20%, i.e. to 120%. But if the initial K_{CO} of the remaining units had been only 50% of the predicted value because of pre-existing disease, the K_{CO} (following pneumonecto-

Figure 17.1 Response of D_{LCO} and K_{CO} to fall in alveolar volume (V_A)

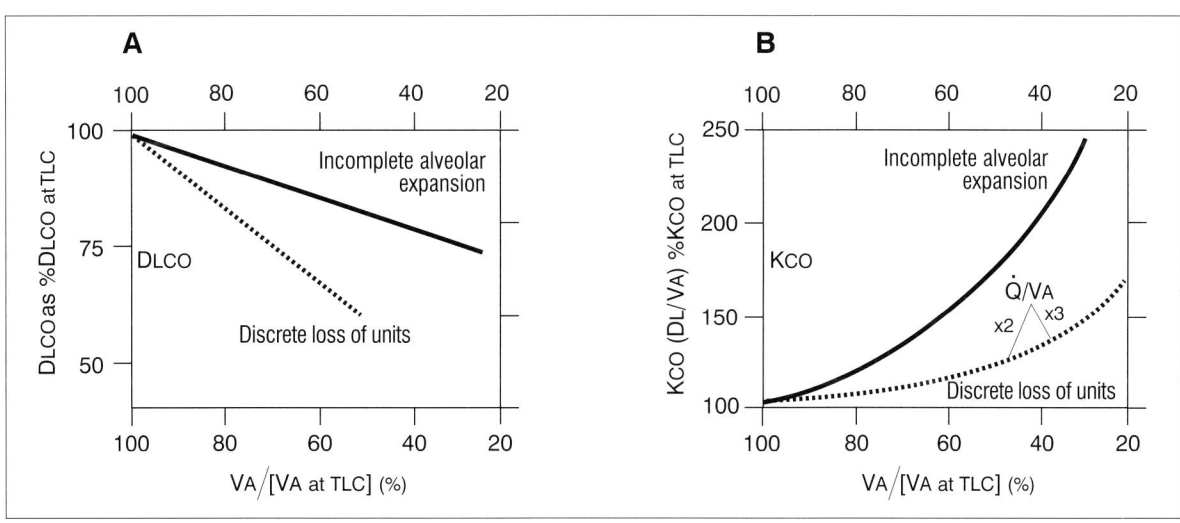

Plots of D_{LCO} and K_{CO} (as percent of D_{LCO} and K_{CO} for V_A at TLC) against V_A (as percent of V_A at TLC), when V_A has been reduced by incomplete alveolar expansion versus 'discrete' loss of units. These plots have been derived from Figure 7 (panels A & B) in Chapter 6.

In B 'discrete loss of units' increases blood flow per unit volume ($\dot{Q}/V_A$) twofold when V_A remaining is 50% and threefold when V_A is 33%.

Table 17.3 Causes of a high Kco

A Loss of units (discrete)	B Incomplete alveolar expansion	C Alveolar hemorrhage	D Increased pulmonary blood volume
See Table 17.1: A.1	See Table 17.1: B	Anti-GBM disease	Left to right shunt (ASD)
Pneumonectomy	Pleural	Pulmonary vasculitis	High cardiac output
Local destruction	Neuromuscular	SLE	
Consolidation/collapse	Chest wall	Wegener's granulomatosis	
Localized infiltrate	Space occupying	Idiopathic hemosiderosis	
	Poor technique		

my, for example) would still increase by 20%, but only to 60% predicted.

Figure 17.1B shows that incomplete expansion of the lungs to a V_A of 70% predicted and a 50% loss of units with a twofold increase in cardiac output have the same effect on K_{CO} (128% versus 125% predicted). A K_{CO} greater than 140% is more likely to be associated with incomplete expansion than loss of units. Of course, other features will help to make the distinction such as (a) respiratory muscle pressures, (b) erect and supine vital capacity, and (c) chest X-ray appearances.

Response of Kco to gain or loss of lung units

After cardiac transplantation, lung volumes increase by 20% on average (because of the reduction in heart volume), but there is no change in the diffusing capacity (64% before versus 67% after) and the K_{CO} declines slightly (65% to 58%).[2] This suggests that the lung units 'regained' as a result of the reduction in central blood volume were involved in the same diffuse pulmonary vascular pathology as the remainder of the lung, and that the original 'loss of units' could be regarded as of the *diffuse* type. Had these regained units been 'normal', i.e. *discrete* loss of units, the D_{LCO} would have increased significantly.

Following bullectomy or lung volume reduction surgery, the well-ventilated compartments contributing to FEV_1, VC, and V_A increase in volume, as previously compressed lung units re-expand. D_{LCO} increases significantly – about as much in percent predicted terms (10–15%) as the vital capacity.[9] K_{CO}, when it has been reported, usually does not change,[10] implying relative homogeneity between the re-expanded and the non-compressed lung units.

On the other side of the coin, pneumonectomy is accompanied by an average 20% fall in D_{LCO} and a 14% increase in K_{CO}.[11] In fact, there was a wide scatter in ΔD_{LCO} (–5% to –42%) and in ΔK_{CO} (–1% to +33%) and, as Corris et al[11] point out, the changes in D_{LCO} and K_{CO} will be influenced by the amount of blood flow and volume which is diverted from the resected lung to the remaining lung. From data in 28 patients, they developed equations to predict the post-pneumonectomy changes:

$$\Delta D_{LCO} (\%predicted) = -0.4x - 8.6$$
$$\Delta K_{CO} (\%predicted) = 0.41x + 2.1$$

where x = percentage flow to resected lung preoperatively, based on a radioisotope lung perfusion scan. For equal flow to both lungs before pneumonectomy (x = 50%) ΔD_{LCO} would be –29% and ΔK_{CO} would be +23 % (from Figure 17.1 a 40% fall in D_{LCO} and a 20% rise in K_{CO} would have been predicted).

Intermittent high Kco

An intermittently high K_{CO} (D_{LCO}) is typical of pulmonary hemorrhage (Figure 17.2).[12,13] Blood which has leaked from immunologically damaged pulmonary capillaries is accessible to inhaled carbon monoxide if the blood is thinly smeared throughout the acini. Local bronchial bleeding does not usually raise the K_{CO} because local hemorrhage blocks or fills acinar units and prevents access to inhaled CO. The

Figure 17.2 Serial measurements in intermittent alveolar hemorrhage

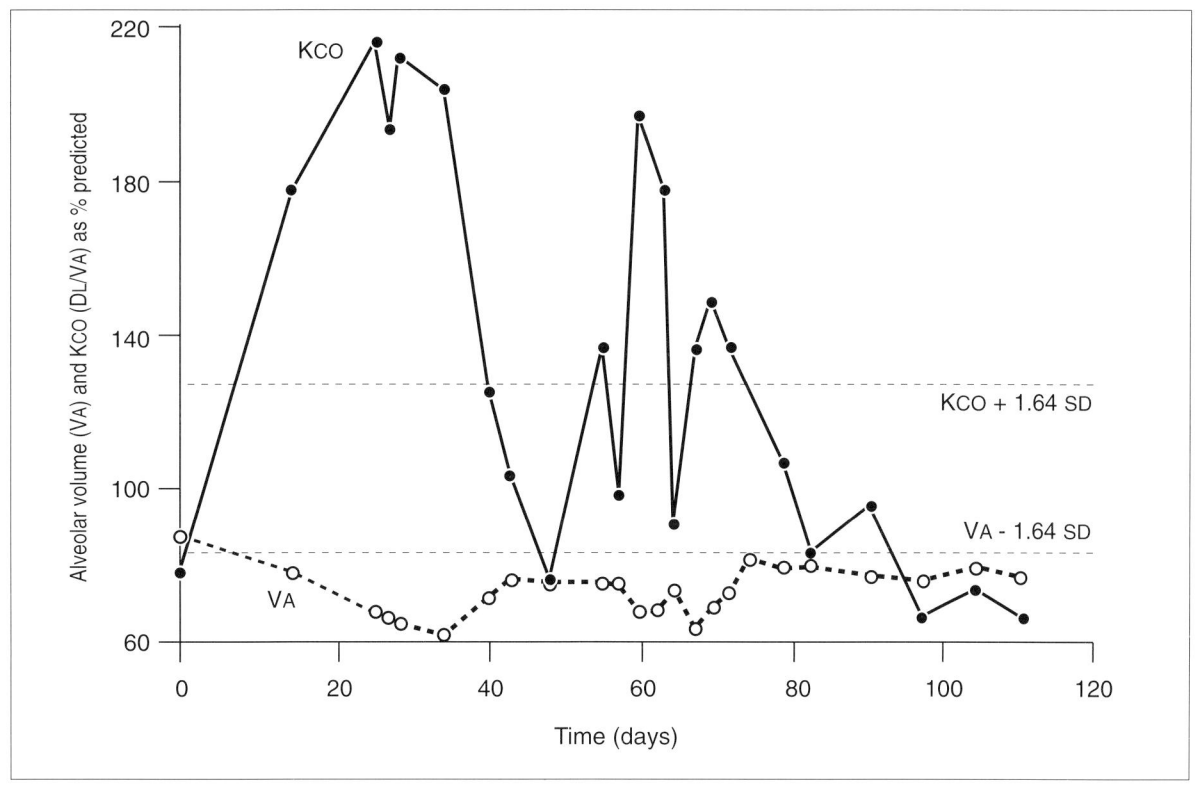

Serial measurements of K_{CO} (corrected for the current [Hb]) and alveolar volume (V_A) in a patient with systemic lupus erythematosus and intermittent pulmonary hemorrhage. K_{CO} peaks reflect excess (shed blood) hemoglobin in alveolar regions accessible to inhaled CO.

Although V_A tends to fall when K_{CO} peaks due to active hemorrhage, the rise in K_{CO} greatly exceeds that expected for the V_A change (see Figure 17.1, panel B).

rise and fall of the K_{CO} is a reflection of the stop/go nature of pulmonary capillary hemorrhage. Once bleeding ceases, macrophages ingest the erythrocytes and the hemoglobin (or hemosiderin) becomes inaccessible to inhaled CO. The half-time of the return of K_{CO} to baseline after bleeding stops is 24 hours.[13] The peaks and troughs in the plot of K_{CO} versus time are amplified if measurements are made frequently (ideally, daily) and if correction is made for the current [Hb] level. See Chapter 16 for further discussion.

INTERSTITIAL LUNG DISEASE

Schwarz et al[14] provide a useful overview of the infiltrative and interstitial diseases. The interstitium, in this context, refers to a potential space between the alveolar epithelium and the capillary endothelium, containing extracellular matrix proteins (collagen, fibronectin, and laminin) and macrophages and fibroblasts. Although the pathology in interstitial lung disease is focused on the alveoli, bronchioles and small pulmonary arteries are sometimes involved in the inflammatory/fibrotic processes. The histological picture is very varied. The principal elements are an 'injury' to the alveolar-capillary basement membranes resulting in migration of neutrophils, eosinophils, or lymphocytes into the interstitium and alveolar air spaces. Proliferation of fibroblasts and collagen deposition follow. Repair and regeneration occur with varying degrees of resolution of the cellular infiltration. The repair process is always accompanied by alveolar wall thickening. The fibrotic reaction may be 'appropriate', e.g. in the resolution of hypersensitivity pneumonitis (also called extrinsic allergic alveolitis [EAA]), or 'excessive' (as in CFA/IPF) where there is

Table 17.4 The more common categories of interstitial lung disease

Histological pattern	Diseases
Diffuse alveolar damage	ARDS, O_2 toxicity, drugs, radiation
	Infections (Legionella, Mycoplasma, viruses)
	SLE
Interstitial pneumonia	CFA/IPF
	Connective tissue diseases
	Hypersensitivity pneumonitis (= EAA)
	Wegener's granulomatosis
	Asbestosis
Lymphocytic pneumonia	Autoimmune disease
	Graft versus host disease
Eosinophilic pneumonia	Drugs, parasites, fungi
	Bronchopulmonary aspergillosis
	Churg-Strauss syndrome
Granulomatous	Sarcoidosis
	Hypersensitivity pneumonitis (= EAA)
	Berylliosis, silicosis
Honeycomb lung	All causes of interstitial pneumonia
	Sarcoidosis
Diffuse alveolar hemorrhage	*with capillaritis:* Wegener's, SLE, systemic vasculitis
	without capillaritis: anti-GBM disease, IPH

Abbreviations: ARDS – adult respiratory distress syndrome; SLE – systemic lupus erythematosus; EAA – extrinsic allergic alveolitis; IPH – idiopathic pulmonary hemosiderosis; anti-GBM disease – anti-glomerular basement membrane disease (syn: Goodpasture's syndrome).

The functional pattern in interstitial lung disease

- Reduction of all lung volumes.
- Increase in P_Lmax and in P_Lmax/TLC (coefficient of retraction).
- Increase in FEV_1/VC ratio.
- Low D_{LCO}.
- Variable K_{CO} (D_L/V_A).
- On exercise
  - reduced exercise capacity and $\dot{V}O_2$peak
  - hyperventilation with increased ventilatory equivalent ($\dot{V}_E/\dot{V}O_2$)
  - low tidal volume and high breathing frequency
  - fall in SaO_2, PaO_2 and widening of A-aPO_2.

disorganization and destruction of the alveoli and the microvasculature until the lung periphery (particularly in the dependent zones) resembles the structure of a 'honeycomb'.

If airflow obstruction is present (likely causes are obliterative bronchiolitis, or COPD in an elderly patient with CFA/IPF who has a history of cigarette smoking) lung volumes may not be much reduced and residual volume may even be increased. The increase in lung elastic recoil at TLC (P_Lmax) is partly caused by the stiffness of the lung from increased deposition of collagen and partly by the loss of lung volume which gives the inspiratory muscles greater mechanical advantage[4] (see Chapter 3, Figure 1). The FEV_1/VC ratio is usually higher than expected (> 0.75) because of a selective loss of alveolar units in relation to the airways which subtend them, and because the increase in P_L above FRC acts as a retractive force to hold open the intrapulmonary airways. The value of K_{CO} (D_L/V_A) depends on whether the loss of lung units is *discrete* or *diffuse*. The worsening of arterial hypoxemia on exercise is caused by diffusion limitation and a fall in the $D_L/\dot{Q}$ ratio (see Chapter 6, Figure 2).

Sarcoidosis and CFA/IPF are the interstitial lung diseases most commonly seen in the pulmonary function laboratory. Sarcoidosis occurs more frequently in the young and middle-aged and CFA/IPF is seen more often in the elderly.

Sarcoidosis

Sarcoidosis is a condition of unknown cause, characterized by tissue infiltration with epithelioid granulomas which are rounded, organized collections of cells (0.1–1.0 mm in diameter). The center of the granuloma consists of macrophages, often fused into giant cells, and amorphous non-necrotic (non-caseous) material; lymphocytes make up the periphery. Granulomas can occur in almost any organ of the body but they are particularly common in the intrathoracic (hilar and mediastinal) lymph nodes and in the lung, generally in a peribronchial location. Bilateral hilar lymphadenopathy (BHL) (in about 80–90% of patients) and lung infiltrates (in about 50%) are the characteristic chest X-ray findings. Pulmonary fibrosis and honeycomb lung (usually in the upper lung zones, as opposed to the lower zones in CFA/IPF) occur in 5–10% of patients with sarcoidosis. The intrapulmonary granulomas replace the normal alveolar architecture, but the structure of non-granulomatous lung nearby is normal (in the absence of fibrosis).

The values shown in Table 17.5 are very similar to those reported by Dunn et al[15] in a smaller series (n = 20) of patients with sarcoidosis (D_{LCO} 80%, D_L/V_A [K_{CO}] 98% predicted).

In Group A, 26% had VC < 85% predicted, and 29% had a D_{LCO} < 80%. In Group B, the figures for VC < 85% pred. were 54% and for D_{LCO} < 80% pred. were 50% (very similar proportions were reported by Winterbauer and Hutchinson[16]). These findings suggest that the vital capacity is as sensitive as the diffusing capacity in detecting lung involvement in sarcoidosis, and supports the concept of a *discrete loss of units* pattern in this condition. If corticosteroids are given, about 45% of patients show an increase in VC and D_{LCO}, irrespective of whether the chest X-ray improves.[16]

Cryptogenic fibrosing alveolitis/ idiopathic pulmonary fibrosis

Patients with diffuse fibrosis and lung parenchymal destruction associated with autoimmune and connective tissue diseases (most commonly systemic sclerosis, polymyositis, and rheumatoid arthritis) or confined to the lung and of unknown cause (CFA/IPF) usually present later in the course of their disease than patients with sarcoidosis. Thus, when pulmonary function is first measured, the disease has progressed to a stage where the loss of lung volume is associated with diffuse lung fibrosis.

The mean values reported by Dunn et al[15] in 21 patients with IPF were similar to those in Table 17.6 (VC 74%, D_{LCO} 43%, D_L/V_A [K_{CO}] 54%). In contrast to sarcoidosis, the measurement of D_{LCO} would appear to be a more sensitive measure of disease than the vital capacity.

Table 17.5 Sarcoidosis (unpublished Hammersmith Hospital series)

Chest X-ray	n		FEV_1/VC ratio	VC % pred	D_{LCO} % pred	K_{CO} % pred
A. Lungs clear	77	Mean	0.8	94	91	112
		Highest	0.95	133	155	170
		Lowest	0.41	55	40	71
B. Lung infiltrates	82	Mean	0.8	83	76	105
		Highest	0.96	120	134	157
		Lowest	0.56	52	32	52

Comment: In Group A, the mean results are within normal limits. Those with the lowest values probably would have had lung infiltrates on a CT scan. Group B had significantly lower values compared to Group A for VC and D_{LCO} (p < 0.001 on unpaired t-test), but not for K_{CO}. Values in the lower range in Group B would be compatible with diffuse lung fibrosis. In Group B the reduction in VC% (VA% pred. was similar) is accompanied by a normal K_{CO}, suggesting a pattern of discrete loss of alveolar units. In both groups, low FEV_1/VC ratios were found in a minority (10%), 13/16 of whom were non-smokers. Granulomatous infiltration of the bronchial mucosa can lead to narrowing of the larger intrapulmonary airways and reduce maximal expiratory flow.

Table 17.6 Cryptogenic fibrosing alveolitis/idiopathic pulmonary fibrosis (unpublished Hammersmith Hospital series)

n = 45	FEV_1/VC ratio	VC % pred	D_{LCO} % pred	K_{CO} % pred	V_A % pred
Mean	0.78	73	54	84	66
Highest	1.0	117	103	139	107
Lowest	0.42	34	25	41	35

Comment: The overall pattern is of volume loss without airflow obstruction, and a low D_{LCO} caused by reductions in both K_{CO} and V_A. If the loss of lung units had been discrete, the K_{CO} at a V_A of 66% should have been 118% predicted (Figure 17.1). Thus K_{CO} of 84% suggests a diffuse destructive process. Nevertheless, the highest values for K_{CO} (139%) would be compatible with discrete loss of alveolar units, either localized fibrosis or alveolar infiltration without fibrosis. Three patients whose K_{CO} was > 120% predicted had VCs in the range 56–68%. The low FEV_1/VC ratio in 20% of the cases was always associated with a history of smoking and with 10–12% higher lung volumes than those without airflow obstruction, similar to the previous report of Hanley et al.[17]

CLINICAL ANALYSIS AND TEACHING

Appendix 17.I presents some examples of pulmonary function test results (spirometry and diffusing capacity only), with the clinical diagnosis, and a *comment* or interpretation in the form of a laboratory report. For teaching (or self teaching) purposes, the data can be written up on a blackboard or on a sheet of paper, *without the clinical diagnosis*, and an interpretation attempted. This *blinded* interpretation should first outline the physiological abnormality, which can then be fitted to a pathological entity. Any set of results can be taken from your laboratory. The minimum requirement is spirometry and diffusing capacity/transfer factor, including V_A and K_{CO} (D_L/V_A). Additional data such as TLC and RV, mouth pressures, PaO_2 and/or SaO_2 at rest and on exercise, and flow-volume curves can be included. When teaching the uninitiated, it is inhibiting to present too much data per patient. Keep it simple. Peak flow values do not help the interpretation. It is surprising how much information can be squeezed out of just spirometry, D_{LCO}, V_A, K_{CO}, and TLC. This exercise is an excellent teaching tool.

CONCLUSIONS

1. The D_{LCO} is best interpreted in terms of its components, alveolar volume (V_A) and alveolar efficiency (K_{CO}).
2. The causes of a low V_A are:
   (a) *discrete* loss of lung units (lung remaining is **normal**)
   (b) *diffuse* loss of lung units (lung remaining is **abnormal**)
   (c) incomplete alveolar expansion
   (d) airflow obstruction.
3. The most common causes of a low K_{CO} are emphysema, pulmonary vascular disease, and diffuse lung fibrosis.
4. Very high K_{CO} (> 140%) occurs with incomplete alveolar expansion, and a moderately high K_{CO} (110–130%) is seen with discrete loss of lung units. The level of elevation of K_{CO} helps to distinguish one from the other.
5. In interstitial lung disease, sarcoidosis is usually an example of discrete loss of alveolar units, and CFA/IPF is more often an example of diffuse loss of units.
6. An intermittently high K_{CO} suggests alveolar hemorrhage.

References

1. Roberts CM, MacRae KD & Seed WA. Multi-breath and single breath helium dilution lung volumes as a test of airway obstruction. *Eur Respir J* 1990; **3**: 515–20.
2. Niset G, Ninane V, Antoine M, Yernault J-C. Respiratory function in congestive heart failure: correction after heart transplantation. *Eur Respir J* 1993; **6**: 1197–1201.
3. Hosenpud JD, Stibolt TA, Atwal K, Shelley D. Abnormal pulmonary function specifically related to congestive heart failure: comparison of patients before and after cardiac transplantation. *Am J Med* 1990; **88**: 493–6.
4. Gibson GJ & Pride NB. Pulmonary mechanics in fibrosing alveolitis; the effects of lung shrinkage. *Am Rev Respir Dis* 1977; **116**: 637–47.
5. McCredie RM, Lovejoy FW & Yu PN. Pulmonary diffusing capacity and pulmonary capillary blood volume in patients with intracardiac shunts. *J Clin Lab Med* 1964; **63**: 914–23.
6. Collard P, Njinou B, Nedjadnik B, Keyeux A, Frans A. Single breath diffusing capacity for carbon monoxide in stable asthma. *Chest* 1994; **105**: 1426–9.
7. Chinn DJ, Cotes JE, Flowers R, Marks A-M, Reed JW. Transfer factor (diffusing capacity) standardized for alveolar volume: validation, reference values and applications of a new linear model to replace K_{CO} (T_L/V_A). *Eur Respir J* 1996; **9**: 1269–77.
8. Hughes JMB, Chinn DJ, Cotes JE, Reed JW. Transfer factor standardized for alveolar volume (correspondence). *Eur Respir J* 1997; **10**: 764–5.
9. Wakabayashi A. Thoracoscopic laser pneumoplasty in the treatment of diffuse bullous emphysema. *Ann Thorac Surg* 1995; **60**: 936–42.
10. Pride NB, Barter CE & Hugh-Jones P. The ventilation of bullae and the effect of their removal on thoracic gas volumes and tests of overall pulmonary function. *Am Rev Respir Dis* 1973; **107**: 83–98.
11. Corris PA, Ellis DA, Hawkins T, Gibson GJ. Use of radionuclide screening in the preoperative estimation of pulmonary function after pneumonectomy. *Thorax* 1987; **42**: 285–91.
12. Ewan PW, Jones HA, Rhodes CG, Hughes JMB. Detection of intrapulmonary haemorrhage with carbon monoxide uptake. Application in Goodpasture's syndrome. *N Engl J Med* 1976; **295**: 1391–6.
13. Greening AP & Hughes JMB. Serial estimations of carbon monoxide diffusing capacity in intrapulmonary haemorrhage. *Clin Sci* 1981; **60**: 507–12.
14. Schwarz MI, King TE & Cherniack RM. General principles and diagnostic approach to the interstitial lung diseases. In: Murray JF & Nadel JA (eds) *Textbook of Respiratory Medicine*, 2nd edn. Philadelphia: WB Saunders 1994: 1803–26.
15. Dunn TL, Walters LC, Hendrix C, Cherniack RM, Schwarz MI, King TE. Gas exchange at a given degree of volume restriction is different in sarcoidosis and idiopathic pulmonary fibrosis. *Am J Med* 1988; **85**: 221–6.

16 Winterbauer RH & Hutchinson JF. Use of pulmonary function tests in the management of sarcoidosis. *Chest* 1980; **78**: 640–7.
17 Hanley ME, King TE, Schwarz MI *et al.* The impact of smoking on the mechanical properties of the lungs in idiopathic pulmonary fibrosis and sarcoidosis. *Am Rev Respir Dis* 1991; **144**: 1102–6.

APPENDIX 17.I
Clinical examples of abnormal D_{LCO}

With airflow obstruction
Case 1

Age/sex	FEV_1/VC ratio	VC % pred	D_{LCO} % pred	K_{CO} % pred	V_A % pred	Diagnosis
69/F	0.23	53	27	46	53	emphysema

Comment: D_{LCO} is reduced by the combination of alveolar destruction and low transfer efficiency (K_{CO}) and the reduced number of contributing units (V_A). TLC was 110%, much greater than VC% or V_A%. Very low FEV_1/VC and K_{CO} is typical of emphysema.

Case 2

Age/sex	FEV_1/VC ratio	VC % pred	D_{LCO} % pred	K_{CO} % pred	V_A % pred	Diagnosis
49/F	0.48	52	64	126	50	bronchiectasis

Comment: K_{CO} is high, but not really high enough at V_A 50% for lack of expansion (Figure 17.1), more in keeping with an increase in cardiac output per alveolus (Figure 17.1) due to 'discrete loss of units' and patchy disease. TLC was reduced at 89% (previous lobectomy). Discrete loss of units and airflow obstruction suggest bronchiectasis. D_{LCO} is not usually as low in asthma.

Case 3

Age/sex	FEV_1/VC ratio	VC % pred	D_{LCO} % pred	K_{CO} % pred	V_A % pred	Diagnosis
49/F	0.6	57	66	105	66	rheumatoid arthritis

Comment: K_{CO} of 105% is low for V_A 66% (Figure 17.1) and suggests inadequate local blood flow compensation for 'discrete loss of units', i.e. alveolar inefficiency, even in the better ventilated lung compartment. Compatible with diffuse interstitial lung disease/fibrosis. Airflow obstruction and low K_{CO} in a non-smoker suggests a pathology of combined alveolitis-obliterative bronchiolitis.

Without airflow obstruction
Case 4

Age/sex	FEV_1/VC ratio	VC % pred	D_{LCO} % pred	K_{CO} % pred	V_A % pred	Diagnosis
58/M	0.93	68	32	63	63	sarcoidosis

Comment: D_{LCO} is reduced because of a combination of loss of volume and alveolar inefficiency. There is no airflow obstruction so TLC is probably in the range 65–75%. High FEV_1/VC suggests fibrosis as does low V_A and K_{CO}. Chest X-ray was in keeping with interstitial fibrosis.

Note: All values are percent predicted normal, except for FEV_1/VC which is the absolute ratio.

Case 5

Age/sex	FEV$_1$/VC ratio	VC % pred	D$_{LCO}$ % pred	K$_{CO}$ % pred	V$_A$ % pred	Diagnosis
64/M	0.76	40	56	155	45	pleural mesothelioma

Comment: Low V$_A$ and high K$_{CO}$ pattern suggests 'discrete loss of units' and/or incomplete alveolar expansion. D$_{LCO}$ and K$_{CO}$ too low at V$_A$ 45% for pure 'incomplete expansion' (Figure 17.1). Chest X-ray shows large tumor extending into lung. Thus, the picture is a mixture of 'extrapulmonary restriction' and 'discrete loss of units'.

Case 6

Age/sex	FEV$_1$/VC ratio	VC % pred	D$_{LCO}$ % pred	K$_{CO}$ % pred	V$_A$ % pred	Diagnosis
27/F	0.9	101	63	66	102	MCTD

Comment: Normal volumes (V$_A$ and VC) but low alveolar efficiency (K$_{CO}$). Suggests a pathological process primarily involving pulmonary vasculature, i.e. a vasculitis in view of clinical diagnosis of mixed connective tissue disease (MCTD).

Case 7

Age/sex	FEV$_1$/VC ratio	VC % pred	D$_{LCO}$ % pred	K$_{CO}$ % pred	V$_A$ % pred	Diagnosis
69/M	0.7	48	57	158	37	collapse of right lung

Comment: Severe volume loss (VC and V$_A$) with compensatory high K$_{CO}$. For pure extrapulmonary restriction, K$_{CO}$ should exceed 200% at V$_A$ 37%. An increase in blood flow per alveolus of 270% (100/37) because of flow diversion from 'lost units' would increase K$_{CO}$ (see Figure 17.1, panel B) to 140%, i.e. compensation for 'discrete loss of units'.

Case 8

Age/sex	FEV$_1$/VC ratio	VC % pred	D$_{LCO}$ % pred	K$_{CO}$ % pred	V$_A$ % pred	Diagnosis
21/F	0.74	29	36	115	31	SLE

Comment: Example of shrinking lung syndrome in systemic lupus erythematosus (SLE), from combination of microatelectasis and extrapulmonary restriction (myopathy with low mouth pressures). K$_{CO}$ should exceed 200% but is low (even if nominally 'normal') because of accompanying vasculitis.

18 Examples of Pulmonary Function in Different Conditions

J M B Hughes

- **INTRODUCTION**
- **CASE REPORTS**

1. Bullous lung disease: effect of bilateral bullectomy
2. Chronic myeloid leukemia: GVHD post bone marrow transplant
3. Extrinsic allergic alveolitis (hypersensitivity pneumonitis)
4. Acromegaly
5. Pulmonary vasculitis
6. Alveolar hemorrhage in systemic lupus erythematosus
7. Poliomyelitis (old): diaphragm weakness
8. Becker's muscular dystrophy and cardiomyopathy
9. Two cases of bronchiectasis
10. Rheumatoid arthritis with fibrosis and bronchiolitis
11. Cryptogenic fibrosing alveolitis (idiopathic pulmonary fibrosis)
12. Dermatomyositis responding to immunosuppressive therapy
13. Bilateral phrenic nerve injury and generalized muscle weakness
14. Sarcoidosis: response to corticosteroids
15. Emphysema and cryptogenic fibrosing alveolitis combined
16. Asthma
17. High K_{CO} without alveolar hemorrhage: variability in reference values
18. Polymyositis with fibrosing alveolitis
19. Sarcoidosis: response to corticosteroids and methotrexate
20. Facio-scapulo-humeral muscular dystrophy
21. Emphysema: heterozygous α_1-antitrypsin deficiency

INTRODUCTION

This chapter presents examples of pulmonary function in different conditions. The emphasis is on the routine tests, but examples of respiratory muscle assessment, simple exercise testing, and flow-volume curves are included. This chapter aims to show:

- pulmonary function patterns in non-respiratory as well as respiratory conditions
- the value of serial testing, both for diagnosis and for monitoring therapeutic response.

These cases can also be used as a teaching resource. They can be presented, without the clinical diagnosis, for discussion in seminars. The presenter can ask the group first to make a physiological/functional diagnosis, and then to suggest some pathological conditions which would be compatible with this functional pattern.

All values of D_{LCO} and K_{CO} have been corrected to a standard hemoglobin level,[1] and the references section gives the source of normal values for spirometry and lung volumes[2] and D_{LCO} and K_{CO}.[3] TLC has been measured by body plethysmography. V_A as % predicted = TLC % predicted − 0.5 L. *In the absence of airflow obstruction*, note there is usually concordance between VC and V_A (and TLC, where given) as percent predicted.

CASE REPORTS

1. Male, aged 53 years. Bilateral apical giant bullae: effect of bilateral bullectomy

Date months	FEV_1/VC ratio	FEV_1 L	VC % pred	TLC L	RV L	D_{LCO} % pred	K_{CO} % pred	V_A L
0	0.42	0.5	24	11.0	9.8	21	69	2.2
19	0.5	1.0	41	5.5	3.5	51	76	4.9

Comment: Bullae occupied at least 60% of thoracic volume at TLC (equivalent to 6.6 L), but K_{CO} was better than would be expected if emphysema were very widespread. Post bullectomy, the increase in FEV_1, VC, V_A, and D_{LCO} is due to re-expansion of previously compressed and atelectatic lung.[4] Note [TLC – V_A] was 8.8 L preoperatively and 0.6 L postoperatively. The patient had an excellent functional result in terms of relief of dyspnea and increase in exercise capacity and quality of life.

2. Male, aged 17 years. Chronic myeloid leukemia

Post-BMT months	FEV_1/VC ratio	FEV_1 % pred	VC % pred	D_{LCO} % pred	K_{CO} % pred	V_A % pred	Comment
0	0.77	72	80	80	98	82	Pre-BMT
7	0.83	74	75	57	72	81	Effect of conditioning
31	0.72	37	43	52	95	56	GVHD (1)
33	0.78	73	80	58	67	88	Response to corticosteroids
69	0.40	20	42	42	87	49	GVHD (2)
74	0.39	32	70	57	78	75	Response to corticosteroid increase

Comment: Pulmonary function not completely normal prior to bone marrow transplantation (BMT) (a leukemia or chemotherapy effect). There is about 25% reduction in D_{LCO} and K_{CO} after BMT because of the toxic effects of total body irradiation[5] and chemotherapy on the microcirculation, but lung volumes do not fall. Onset of rejection of lung by donor marrow (graft versus host disease – GVHD) shown by fall in all lung volumes[5] and further fall in D_{LCO}, but with minimal changes visible on plain chest radiograph. Note rise in K_{CO} with each GVHD episode, implying 'loss of units' with blood flow diversion. Good response to corticosteroids two months later. Continuing GVHD activity over next 3 years leads to airflow obstruction (obliterative bronchiolitis) with severe fall in FEV_1/VC ratio. Some response to increase in the dose of corticosteroids is seen at month 74.
See references[5-7]

3. Male, aged 60 years. Extrinsic allergic alveolitis (hypersensitivity pneumonitis)

Time months	FEV$_1$/VC ratio	FEV$_1$ % pred	VC % pred	D$_{LCO}$ % pred	K$_{CO}$ % pred	V$_A$ % pred	Comment
0	0.88	58	51	23	43	57	
8	0.82	102	99	111	130	90	Post-corticosteroids

Comment: Hypersensitivity to pigeon droppings (pigeon fanciers' lung). Extensive infiltrates on chest X-ray on presentation. Pattern suggests widespread alveolar damage (not fibrosis in view of subsequent response). Remarkable reversibility on corticosteroid therapy.

4. Male, aged 54 years, current smoker. Acromegaly

FEV$_1$/VC ratio	VC % pred	TLC % pred	D$_{LCO}$ % pred	K$_{CO}$ % pred	V$_A$ % pred	MEF$_{50}$/MIF$_{50}$
0.71	128	131	115	106	112	1.4

Comment: Acromegaly is associated with increased secretion of growth hormone from the pituitary gland, resulting in overgrowth of skeletal and soft tissues. The thoracic cavity may enlarge,[8] as in this case, but in two thirds of cases the lung volumes are normal. In those with increased lung volumes, the D$_{LCO}$ and K$_{CO}$ are not raised, suggesting an increase in alveolar size rather than alveolar number. (FEV$_1$/VC ratio is slightly reduced in this case, possibly due to smoking, but lowish ratios are seen in healthy subjects with supernormal FEV$_1$ and VC.) Overgrowth of the soft tissues of the pharynx and larynx is an important respiratory feature of acromegaly, leading to upper airflow obstruction and sometimes to obstructive sleep apnea (OSA). In extrathoracic variable upper airflow obstruction, inspiratory flows on a maximal flow-volume curve are reduced relative to flow on expiration at the same absolute lung volume (Figure 18.1). In addition to inspection of the loop, the ratio of maximal expiratory to inspiratory flow at 50% VC (MEF$_{50}$/MIF$_{50}$) is a useful index. The normal value is about 0.8, and ratios > 1.2 suggest upper airflow obstruction, as here. In a recent series, upper airflow obstruction occurred in 50% of 35 patients,[9] and was a more common abnormality than large lungs (34%).
Note also upper airflow obstruction occurring in thyroid disease.[10]

Figure 18.1

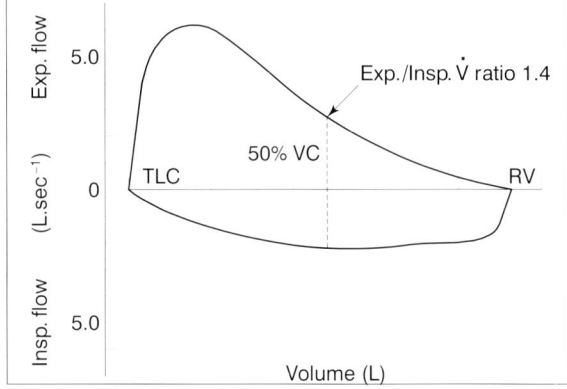

Inspiratory and expiratory flow-volume loops in Case 4, showing extrathoracic variable upper airflow obstruction.

5. Male, aged 66 years. Pulmonary vasculitis

Time months	FEV$_1$/VC ratio	VC % pred	D$_{LCO}$ % pred	K$_{CO}$ % pred	V$_A$ % pred	Hemoglobin g.dL^{-1}
0	0.83	95	105	124	89	6.6 Hemorrhage ?
0.3	0.76	107	81	89	96	8.9
3	0.81	89	38	51	79	9.5
10	0.79	100	82	104	82	11.9

Comment: Presented with renal insufficiency and hemoptysis at −0.2 months; anti-GBM negative. Initial high K$_{CO}$ (0 months) possibly indicates resolving alveolar hemorrhage, though Hb correction factor[1] may 'overcorrect' at Hb < 8.0 g.dL^{-1}. Subsequent pulmonary function pattern is of rapid fall in D$_{LCO}$ and K$_{CO}$ which is later reversed, but with relatively minor reduction in lung volumes. This is compatible with pulmonary vascular involvement.

6. Female, aged 22 years. Alveolar hemorrhage in systemic lupus erythematosus

Time days	FEV$_1$/VC ratio	VC % pred	D$_{LCO}$ % pred	K$_{CO}$ % pred	V$_A$ % pred	Hemoglobin g.dL^{-1}
0	0.93	82	59	80	87	10.3
15	0.91	82	119	180	78	9.5 Hemorrhage
26	0.88	72	123	217	67	7.7 Hemorrhage
29	0.87	69	118	214	65	8.3 Hemorrhage
48	0.86	84	51	77	77	9.2
62	0.84	76	104	180	68	7.4 Hemorrhage
64	0.91	54	57	92	74	9.0

Comment: All values of D$_{LCO}$ and K$_{CO}$ have been corrected for the current hemoglobin level (g.dL^{-1}) using the Cotes equation[1] (D$_{LCO}$ corrected = D$_{LCO}$ observed.[10.2 + Hb]/1.7.Hb). Note that, with alveolar hemorrhage, D$_{LCO}$ and K$_{CO}$ rise. The increase in K$_{CO}$ is greater than expected for the modest decrease in V$_A$. Baseline level of D$_{LCO}$ and K$_{CO}$ is often low because of alveolar damage secondary to capillary hemorrhage. D$_{LCO}$ and K$_{CO}$ return to baseline on day 64, only two days after active hemorrhage (day 62), indicating that the rise in D$_{LCO}$ and K$_{CO}$ reflects active and ongoing bleeding. See Chapters 16 and 17.

7. Male, aged 49 years. Poliomyelitis (old), diaphragm weakness

P₁max cmH₂O	PEmax cmH₂O	FEV₁ % pred	VC % pred	DLco % pred	Kco % pred	VA % pred	VC erect-supine (L)
−41 N < −70	+ 57 N > +90	76	61	74	106	70	3.4 − 2.6 = 0.8 (−24%)

Comment: Reduced respiratory muscle strength; reduction in supine VC suggests weakness of diaphragm. Maximum transdiaphragmatic pressure (Pdi) low at 31 cmH₂O. Lung volumes reduced, but Kco somewhat low (> 150% expected if lack of alveolar expansion was the sole pathology). Patient had nocturnal hypoventilation and morning headaches associated with acute hypercapnia. Treatment with nasal intermittent positive pressure ventilation (NIPPV) has been successful.

8. Male, aged 24 years. Becker's muscular dystrophy and cardiomyopathy

FEV₁/VC ratio	VC % pred	TLC % pred	RV % pred	DLco % pred	Kco % pred	VA % pred	P₁max cmH₂O	PEmax cmH₂O
0.87	77	88	132	50	61	84	−15 N <−70	+ 68 N >+90]

Comment: Respiratory and global muscle strength (P₁max and PEmax) are greatly reduced in keeping with muscular dystrophy, but the Kco should be high (> 150%) if volume reduction is caused by muscle weakness and incomplete alveolar expansion. Becker's dystrophy is associated with cardiomyopathy and cardiac failure, which would explain the low DLco and Kco and the slight increase in RV (see Chapter 16).

9. Two cases of bronchiectasis

Age (yrs) /sex	FEV₁/VC ratio	VC % pred	TLC % pred	DLco % pred	Kco % pred	VA % pred
A. 34/M	0.50	49	49	45	117	47
B. 45/M	0.68	84	84	83	95	91

Comment: Case A has the more typical pattern for bronchiectasis with airflow obstruction and a high normal Kco (discrete loss of units); in his case the left lung has been virtually destroyed and blood flow diverted to the right lung, raising the Kco.
Case B is a non-smoker who has a diffuse bronchitis/bronchiectasis associated with ulcerative colitis.[11] There is minimal lung destruction, and so no diversion of blood flow to increase Kco.

10. Female, aged 31 years, non-smoker. Rheumatoid arthritis with fibrosis and bronchiolitis

Time: years	FEV_1/VC ratio	VC % pred	TLC % pred	RV % pred	D_{LCO} % pred	K_{CO} % pred	V_A % pred
0	0.79	82	78	64	84		
12	0.6	57	80	132	66	105	66

Comment: At year 0, aged 31, the pattern was of mild volume loss and reduction of D_{LCO}; without a measurement of K_{CO}, we cannot determine whether the pathological process is fibrosis and/or vasculitis (K_{CO} < 100%) or localized (discrete) disease (K_{CO} > 100%). At year 12, airflow obstruction has developed with a fall in the FEV_1/VC ratio and a rise in RV, because of obliterative bronchiolitis.[12] The K_{CO} is low for the V_A of 66% and suggests interstitial fibrosis, confirmed by X-ray CT scanning. TLC has remained constant, the restrictive effect of fibrosis being offset by the hyperinflation associated with the bronchiolitis.

11. Male, aged 63, smoker. Cryptogenic fibrosing alveolitis – CFA (idiopathic pulmonary fibrosis – IPF)

FEV_1/VC ratio	VC % pred	D_{LCO} % pred	K_{CO} % pred	V_A % pred	Max. exercise (watts)	SaO_2% rest	SaO_2% exercise
0.72	100	27	34	87	60 [32% pred]	94	87

Comment: Normal volumes and low diffusion might suggest pulmonary vascular disease, possibly hepatopulmonary syndrome with intrapulmonary shunting (see Chapter 16). In fact, D_{LCO} and K_{CO} are too low for most pulmonary vascular pathologies. This is an unusual case of fibrosis without volume loss. Open lung biopsy showed extensive interstitial fibrosis in keeping with CFA, and X-ray and CT scan showed fibrosis and cystic 'honeycomb' change. The FEV_1/VC ratio is low for such extensive fibrosis (> 0.85 would be expected), and the past history of heavy cigarette smoking suggests that fibrosis and hyperinflation coexist.[13] Hyperinflated regions must have supernormal VC, and surrounding fibrosis may help them to empty fully. The fall in SaO_2 on exercise is caused by diffusion limitation and a low D_{LCO} to cardiac output ratio on exercise ($\dot{Q}$ increases normally but D_{LCO} does not).

12. Female, aged 50 years. Dermatomyositis responding to immunosuppressive therapy

	FEV_1/VC ratio	VC % pred	D_{LCO} % pred	K_{CO} % pred	V_A % pred
Before therapy	1.0	51	25	49	51
After therapy	0.95	87	52	78	76

Comment: Typical rash of dermatomyositis, but no evidence of muscle involvement (normal peripheral muscle biopsy and normal mouth pressures). Characteristic pattern before treatment of interstitial lung disease with extensive and diffuse alveolar damage, confirmed by X-ray and CT scanning. Fibrosing alveolitis is often associated with dermatomyositis, and when it is present the response to therapy is usually disappointing. Marked improvement in this instance probably related to the disappearance of an alveolar cellular infiltrate.

13. Male, aged 56 years. Bilateral phrenic nerve injury and generalized muscle weakness

	P₁max cmH₂O	PEmax cmH₂O	Sniff Pes cmH₂O	Sniff Pdi cmH₂O	Cough Pga cmH₂O	VC (L) seated	VC (L) lying
Leaving ICU	−40	+61	−48	34	88	2.5	1.5
after 6 months	−56 N < −70	+120 N > +90	−85 N < −60	65 N > 80	288 N > 120	3.5	2.4

	L twitch Pdi cmH₂O	R twitch Pdi cmH₂O	R + L twitch Pdi cmH₂O	R Quadriceps twitch force kg	R Quadriceps max voluntary contraction (kg)
Leaving ICU	0	6	6	2.5	23.2
after 6 months	3 N > 8	8 N > 7	13 N > 15	7.4 N > 25	42.7 N > 100

Comment: After coronary artery surgery, this patient was difficult to wean from the ventilator and spent 4 weeks in ICU. On leaving the ICU, the low VC (with postural drop of 40%) and reduced P₁max, sniff Pes, and sniff Pdi all suggest diaphragm weakness; this is confirmed by failure to generate any Pdi when the L phrenic nerve is stimulated maximally by cervical magnetic stimulation (twitch Pdi); R twitch Pdi is also low and suggests bilateral injury. In addition, the prolonged stay in ICU has resulted in severe generalized muscle weakness (low PEmax, low Pga, and reduced quadriceps strength); also, the reduction in P₁max is greater than can be explained by diaphragm weakness alone.

6 months later, both hemidiaphragms have improved their function on twitch Pdi, and overall diaphragm strength (sniff Pdi) is ~ 50% of *mean* normal; global inspiratory muscle strength (sniff Pes) is two thirds *mean* normal and adequate. There is still a postural reduction in VC (32%) but absolute values of VC have increased by 1.0L. The expiratory muscles (PEmax and Pga) and quadriceps are substantially stronger.

This case presented by courtesy of J. Moxham, whose chapter (4) should be consulted.

14. Female, aged 35 years. Sarcoidosis – response to corticosteroids

Date months	FEV$_1$/VC ratio	VC % pred	D$_{LCO}$ % pred	K$_{CO}$ % pred	V$_A$ % pred	Comment
0	0.92	60	42	84	54	Corticosteroids started
4	0.9	83	62	85	79	Corticosteroids reduced
14	0.87	86	52	70	80	Corticosteroids increased again
37	0.79	96	73	89	89	Corticosteroids maintained at low dose

Comment: Initial chest X-ray showed widespread infiltration. Pulmonary function pattern consistent with diffuse alveolar damage/interstitial infiltration, rather than the more usual loss of units pattern seen in sarcoidosis. Good response to corticosteroid therapy, radiologically and functionally. Minor relapse seen at 14 months as steroid dose was being reduced, but a further good response occurred. Absence of change in K$_{CO}$ implies a very diffuse and homogeneous infiltrative process. See Chapter 17 for 'typical' patterns in sarcoidosis.

15. Male, aged 47 years. Emphysema and fibrosing alveolitis

Time years	FEV$_1$/VC ratio	VC % pred	D$_{LCO}$ % pred	K$_{CO}$ % pred	V$_A$ L	TLC L	RV L
0	0.15	83	77	78	102	8.4	4.7
8	0.25	114	41	39	110	9.2	4.4

Comment: FEV$_1$ initially 0.6 L, and at year 8 1.2 L. Severe airflow obstruction at the beginning had a reversible element and responded to inhaled bronchodilator and corticosteroid drugs. The predominant diagnosis was emphysema. Over the next 8 years, TLC and VC increased by 1.0 L (V$_A$ by 0.5 L) but, surprisingly, RV decreased by 0.3 L which is unlike progressive emphysema. The CT scan showed a mixture of honeycomb lung on the left side and emphysema on the right side (see Figure 18.2). Severe reduction of D$_{LCO}$ and K$_{CO}$ is caused by a combination of emphysema and fibrosing alveolitis.

Figure 18.2

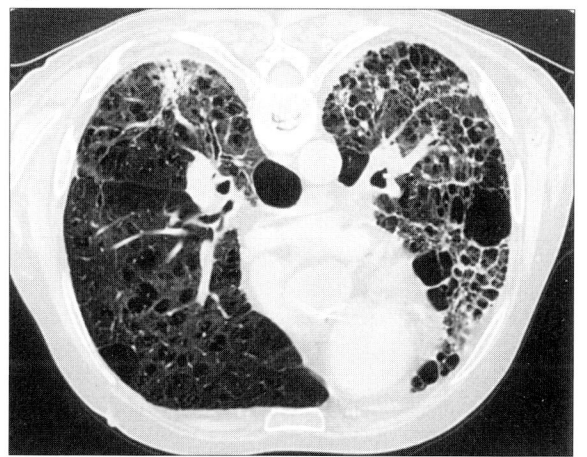

Transaxial CT scan in prone position at cardiac atrial level showing honeycomb change of CFA in left lung (on the right in the figure) and emphysematous changes in the other lung.

16. Female, aged 34 years. Asthma

FEV$_1$/VC ratio	FEV$_1$ % pred	D$_{LCO}$ % pred	K$_{CO}$ % pred	V$_A$ % pred	FEV$_1$ (L) predicted	FEV$_1$ (L) pre-bronch	FEV$_1$ (L) post-bronch	ΔFEV$_1$ (L)
0.7	69	112	132	100	2.3	1.6	2.25	0.65

Comment: Straightforward case of reversible airflow obstruction. Note high normal D$_{LCO}$ and K$_{CO}$, which are often found in asthma and seem to relate to better perfusion of the lung apices in the erect posture,[18] possibly secondary to mild pulmonary hypertension. The bronchodilator challenge is positive with an absolute ΔFEV$_1$ > 0.2 L. ΔFEV$_1$ as percent predicted FEV$_1$ is 28%, and as percent of initial FEV$_1$ 41%.

Figure 18.3

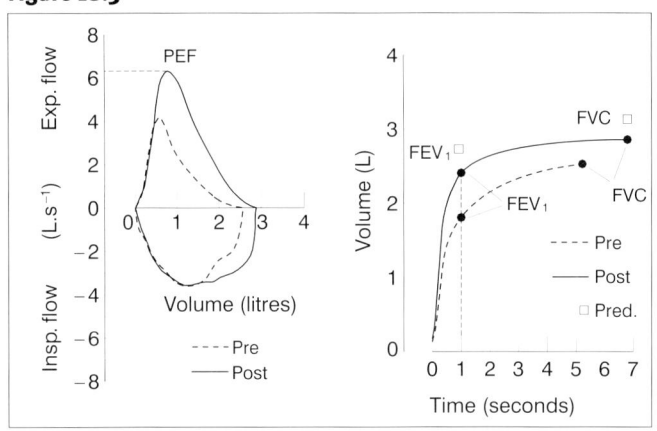

Maximum expiratory flow-volume curve, pre- and postbronchodilator.

Spirogram before and after bronchodilator inhalation (2.5 mg salbutamol [albuterol]) by nebulizer.

17. High K$_{CO}$ without alveolar hemorrhage; variability in reference values

Sex/ht (m)/ age (yrs)	FEV$_1$/VC ratio	VC % pred	D$_{LCO}$ % pred	K$_{CO}$ % pred	V$_A$ % pred	Reference value for D$_{LCO}$ and K$_{CO}$
Case A F/1.5/75	0.7	116	208	175	85	Reference no 3
Repeat calculation	0.7	116	101	128	85	Reference no 14
Case B F/1.7/67	0.76	72	107	173	63	Reference no 3
Repeat calculation	0.76	72	86	139	63	Reference no 14

Comment: An unexplained very high K$_{CO}$ seen in two women > 65 years of age. This is a consequence of a wide range of reference values for D$_{LCO}$ and K$_{CO}$, in some of which[3] women > 60 years are not represented; as a result the age exponent in one regression equation[3] was higher than in other series[14,15] and the predicted D$_{LCO}$ and K$_{CO}$ lower, as can be seen in the table. The possibility of alveolar hemorrhage was raised, but repetition of the tests gave the same result. Another explanation is that true height may be underestimated if there is osteoporosis and curvature of the spine. Arm span can be used as a surrogate for vertical height. The high K$_{CO}$ (even with alternative regression equations[14,15]) may be explained in part by the lowish V$_A$ and failure to inspire to true TLC; incomplete alveolar expansion can increase K$_{CO}$ to 150–200% predicted. Reference equations for K$_{CO}$ are more variable than for other indices; see Chapter 19 for recommendations.

18. Female, aged 42 years. Polymyositis with fibrosing alveolitis

FEV$_1$/VC ratio	VC % pred	D$_{LCO}$ % pred	K$_{CO}$ % pred	V$_A$ L	P$_I$max cmH$_2$O	P$_E$max cmH$_2$O
0.88	40	26	67	41	−29 N < −35	+42 N > +50

Comment: Combination of diffuse alveolar damage (small lung volumes and low D$_{LCO}$ and K$_{CO}$) and inspiratory and expiratory respiratory muscle weakness strongly suggests the polymyositis/dermatomyositis complex of diseases.[16] SLE is a possibility with a combination of inspiratory and expiratory muscle weakness, but the K$_{CO}$ would not generally < 80% predicted.

19. Female, aged 53 years. Sarcoidosis – response to corticosteroids and methotrexate

Time months	FEV$_1$/VC ratio	VC % pred	D$_{LCO}$ % pred	K$_{CO}$ % pred	V$_A$ % pred	SaO$_2$% rest	SaO$_2$% at end of walk test	3 min walking distance (m)
0	0.85	43	16	56	33	94	80	160
16	0.71	67	42	79	58	97	86	240

Comment: 18 year history of untreated active pulmonary sarcoidosis. Chest X-ray and CT scan showed severe bilateral upper zone fibrosis and scattered infiltrates in rest of lung fields. Treatment was started with corticosteroids and weekly methotrexate and a favorable response obtained; patient noticed less subjective dyspnea on exertion. Initial pulmonary function pattern in keeping with diffuse interstitial disease and fibrosis; 25% increase seen in all indices as a result of therapy. K$_{CO}$ increased presumably because the 'regained' lung units were granulomatous (a reversible pathological change) rather than fibrotic, and must have had near normal K$_{CO}$. A simple unpaced walk test provided evidence of improvement – either in exertional dyspnea, or in her degree of motivation.

20. Male, aged 35 years. Facio-scapulo-humeral muscular dystrophy

FEV$_1$/VC ratio	VC % pred	D$_{LCO}$ % pred	K$_{CO}$ % pred	V$_A$ % pred	TLC % pred	RV % pred
0.85	60	75	120	63	63	82

P$_I$max cmH$_2$O	P$_E$max cmH$_2$O	Sniff Pes cmH$_2$O	Sniff Pdi cmH$_2$O	R + L twitch Pdi cmH$_2$O	Cough Pga cmH$_2$O	C$_L$,dyn L.cmH$_2$O^{-1}
−37 N < −70	+39 N > +90	−39 N < −60	53 N > 80	4 N > 15	74 N > 120	0.08 N > 0.06

Comment: Onset of muscle weakness of neck and shoulder muscles at age 19 years. Exertional dyspnea for 10 years. Dyspnea on lying supine with abdominal paradox (inward movement of the abdomen on inspiration in the supine posture). Hypoxemia and hypercapnia at rest (PaO$_2$ 78 mmHg [10.4 kPa]; Paco$_2$ 49 mmHg [6.5 kPa]). All lung volumes are reduced; note concordance between VC, V$_A$, and TLC as % predicted. K$_{CO}$ is raised due to lack of alveolar expansion, but not as much as expected (c. 150%). Inspiratory (P$_I$max, sniff Pes, sniff Pdi) and expiratory (P$_E$max, cough Pga) P$_I$max pressures are greatly reduced. Unpotentiated cervical magnetic stimulation of the diaphragm (R + L twitch Pdi) is also very low. Sleep study is indicated (with SaO$_2$ and PaCO$_2$ monitoring) to assess nocturnal hypoxemia and exclude upper airway collapse (OSA). Nocturnal ventilation with NIPPV may be prescribed.

21. Female, aged 65 years. Emphysema – heterozygous a_1-antitrypsin deficiency

FEV_1/VC ratio	VC % pred	TLC % pred	RV % pred	D_{LCO} % pred	K_{CO} % pred	V_A % pred
0.42	123	132	160	67	67	99

Comment: Heavy cigarette smoker, but also heterozygous α_1-antitrypsin deficiency (MZ phenotype), with serum α_1-antitrypsin level at 0.9 g.L^{-1}, just below the normal range (1.1–2.1). Chest X-ray showed basal bullae, often seen in homozygous α_1-antitrypsin deficiency. Pulmonary function pattern is typical of emphysema with low FEV_1/VC ratio, well-preserved VC and V_A, elevated TLC, and low D_{LCO} and K_{CO}. Low serum α_1-antitrypsin level together with cigarette smoking is probably a risk factor for the development of emphysema. Decreases in lung density measured with CT scanning[17] and in K_{CO}[19] correlate with decreases in airway wall surface area per unit alveolar volume (i.e. microscopic emphysema) and can indicate the severity of emphysema better than a macroscopic assessment of 'holes' in the lung parenchyma from a CT scan or a lung slice in vitro.

References

1. Cotes JE, Dabbs JM, Elwood PC, Hall AM, McDonald A, Saunders MJ. Iron-deficiency anaemia: its effect on transfer factor for the lung (diffusing capacity) and ventilation and cardiac frequency during sub-maximal exercise. *Clin Sci* 1972; **42**: 325–35.
2. Quanjer Ph H. Standardized lung function testing. *Bull Eur Physiopathol Respir* 1983; **19** (suppl 5): 1–95.
3. Bradley J, Bye C, Hayden SP, Hughes DTD. Normal values of transfer factor and transfer coefficient in healthy males and females. *Respiration* 1979; **38**: 221–6.
4. Pride NB, Barter CE & Hugh-Jones P. The ventilation of bullae and the effect of their removal on thoracic gas volumes and tests of overall lung function. *Am Rev Respir Dis* 1973; **107**: 83–98.
5. Schwarer AP, Hughes JMB, Trotman-Dickenson B, Krausz T, Goldman JM. A chronic pulmonary syndrome associated with graft versus host disease after allogeneic marrow transplantation. *Transplantation* 1992; **54**: 1002–8.
6. Roca J, Granena A, Rodriguez-Roisin R, Alvarez P, Agusti-Vidal A, Rozman C. Fatal airway disease in an adult with chronic graft-versus-host-disease. *Thorax* 1982; **37**: 77.
7. Ralph DD, Springmeyer SC, Sullivan KM, Hackman RC, Storb R, Thomas ED. Rapidly progressive airflow obstruction in marrow transplant recipients: possible association between obliterative bronchiolitis and chronic graft versus host disease. *Am Rev Respir Dis* 1984; **129**: 641–44.
8. Brody JS, Fisher AB, Gocmen A, DuBois AB. Acromegalic pneumonomegaly: lung growth in the adult. *J Clin Invest* 1970; **49**: 1051–60.
9. Trotman-Dickenson B, Weetman AP & Hughes JMB. Upper airflow obstruction and pulmonary function in acromegaly: relationship to disease activity. *Quart J Med* 1991; **79**: 527–38.
10. Miller MR, Pincock AC, Oates GD, Wilkinson R, Skene-Smith H. Upper airway obstruction due to goitre: detection, prevalence and results of surgical management. *Quart J Med* 1990; **74**: 177–88.
11. Higenbottam T, Cochrane GM, Clark TJH, Turner D, Millis R, Seymour W. Bronchial disease in ulcerative colitis. *Thorax* 1980; **35**: 581–8.
12. Geddes DM, Corrin B, Brewerton DA, Davies RJ, Turner-Warwick M. Progressive airway obliteration in adults and its association with rheumatoid disease. *Quart J Med* 1977; **46**: 427–44.
13. Hanley ME, King TE, Schwarz MI *et al.* The impact of smoking on the mechanical properties of the lungs in idiopathic pulmonary fibrosis and sarcoidosis. *Am Rev Respir Dis* 1991; **144**: 1102–6.
14. Roberts CM, MacRae KD, Winning AJ, Adams L, Seed WA. Reference values and prediction equations for normal lung function in a non–smoking white urban population. *Thorax* 1991; **46**: 643–50.
15. Salorinne Y. Single breath diffusing capacity: reference values and application in connective tissue diseases and in various lung diseases. *Scand J Respir Dis* 1975; **96** (suppl): 1–86.
16. Marguerie C, Bunn CC, Beynon HLC, Bernstein RM, Hughes JMB, So AK, Walport MJ. Polymyositis, pulmonary fibrosis and autoantibodies to aminoacyl-tRNA synthetase enzymes. *Quart J Med* 1990; **77**: 1019–38.
17. Hayhurst MD, MacNee W, Wright D, McLean A, Lamb D, Flenley DC. The diagnosis of pulmonary emphysema by CT scanning. *Lancet* 1984; **ii**: 320–2.
18. Collard P, Njinou B, Nedjadnik B, Keyeux A, Frans A. Single breath diffusing capacity for carbon monoxide in stable asthma. *Chest* 1994; **105**: 1426–9.
19. McLean A, Warren PM, Gillooly M, MacNee W, Lamb D. Microscopic and macroscopic measurements of emphysema: relation to carbon monoxide gas transfer. *Thorax* 1992; **47**: 144–9.

19 Presentation of Pulmonary Function Test Results to the Clinician

J M B Hughes

- **INTRODUCTION**
- **THE LABORATORY REFERRAL FORM**
  The Pulmonary Function Test request form
- **WHAT IS AN ABNORMAL RESULT?**
  Standardized residuals versus percent predicted
  Presentation of results
- **NORMAL VALUES**
  Which reference values?
  Normal values for K_{CO} (D_L/V_A)
  Normal values for other tests
- **REPORTING ROUTINE PULMONARY FUNCTION TESTS**
  Spirometric and diffusing capacity paradigms of common pathologies
  Obstructive versus restrictive patterns
  Obstructive pattern
  Restrictive pattern
  Do absolute lung volumes always need to be measured?

INTRODUCTION

The routine tests carried out by the Pulmonary Function Laboratory fulfill several functions:

- quantitative assessment of the functional status of the lung parenchyma* (alveoli and capillary bed) and airways
- when appropriate, measurement of bronchodilator response and respiratory muscle strength
- monitoring of disease progress or of response to treatment

- preoperative assessment
- support or lack of support for the clinical diagnosis

What does the clinician expect from the Laboratory? What the clinician would like is:

- clear presentation of the results in relation to 'normal' values
- a brief commentary on the pattern of abnormality, and its diagnostic implications
- for follow-up studies, an indication of significant changes or trends
- where appropriate, comments on the quality of the data and any reservations

* Lung *parenchyma* refers to structures within the acinus – respiratory bronchioles, alveolar ducts, alveoli including the interstitium and intra-acinar blood vessels.

What the clinician may get is an unattractive piece of paper, crammed with figures, many of which (were he/she to understand them) are repetitive or variations on a theme, and therefore redundant; the commentary or 'report' which is attached merely states the obvious, e.g. that test A is normal, test B is high, and test C is low – adding, as if it were a bonus, 'this report has been produced by a computer'!

The theme of this chapter is that there should be better dialogue between the Pulmonary Function Laboratory and the clinician who refers the patient for routine tests. The key to this is:

- the clinician should provide relevant clinical information on the referral form
- the laboratory should provide a clear, concise, and informative report.

THE LABORATORY REFERRAL FORM

This chapter focuses on the standard tests such as spirometry, lung volumes, and diffusion. It is not necessary for the laboratory to do every test on every patient, and the decision on which tests to do must be based on the clinical situation. The clinician who is experienced in Pulmonary Function Testing will specify on the referral form the tests that are needed. But the referral form should always include clinical information relevant to pulmonary function test selection and reporting. Even the most expert clinician should realize that the staff of the Pulmonary Function Laboratory are keen to learn and widen their experience, and this can only be done if they are kept informed.

Clinicians who are not themselves experts in pulmonary function should provide a clinical diagnosis and sufficient information for the laboratory staff to decide which of the routine tests are appropriate. For example, any suspicion of neuromuscular disease or muscle weakness should be mentioned so that measurements of $P_{I}max$ and $P_{E}max$ can be made. The possibility of upper (extrathoracic) airflow obstruction should be considered (enlargement of the thyroid gland or a previous tracheostomy) because measurement of inspiratory as well as expiratory flow-volume loops would be appropriate.

The Pulmonary Function Test request form

Information should be provided on the following items, as a minimum:

- clinical diagnosis (not just 'dyspnea')
- smoking status (current, ex-smoker, or never-smoker)
- current hemoglobin level (for correction of D_{LCO} [T_{LCO}])
- chest X-ray appearance
- requests for additional tests (bronchodilator response, $P_{I}max$ and $P_{E}max$, pulse oximetry or arterial [arterialized] blood gas estimation, exercise testing, walk tests [± additional oxygen], histamine/methacholine challenge etc.)

These recommendations are merely a guide to good practice. The clinical diagnosis could just as well say 'unexplained dyspnea' or 'hemoptysis; cause undetermined' or 'possible asthma'. The clinical diagnosis and chest X-ray appearance may be irrelevant if the test report is generated by a computer. Nevertheless, these details are an important part of the dialogue between the referring clinician and the laboratory staff. For example, unexpected findings on pulmonary function testing in relation to the clinical information should prompt the laboratory staff to suggest additional measurements (such as $P_{I}max$ and $P_{E}max$) or to measure the vital capacity supine as well as erect. Good communication will always lead to a better service.

WHAT IS AN ABNORMAL RESULT?

Standardized residuals versus percent predicted

Normal values are calculated from reference equations (see Which Reference Values?) based on a population of healthy never (not ex-) smoking people. These equations predict a reference value on a continuous scale (a regression line) taking age, sex, and height as the principal determinants. Height measurements are unreliable if there is kyphosis of the spine or vertebral collapse due to osteoporosis; arm span is an group and habitual activity are the other important factors. Every prediction has a confidence limit, and the variability on either side of the regression line is called the *residual standard deviation* (RSD). The predicted range is generally set at ± 1.64 RSD which includes 90% of a population with a 'normal' or Gaussian distribution. The *standardized residual* (SR) is a measure of deviation from predicted in terms of the expected variation within a normal population, adjusted for the age, height, and sex of the subject.

Standardized residual (SR) = [observed–predicted values]/RSD

An SR of −1.644 means a value at the 5th percentile, −1.96 at the 3rd percentile and −2.6 at the first percentile. Conversely, SR +1.96 equals the 95th percentile. Predicted ranges (or RSDs) change little with the age or size in subjects of a given gender, so that a deviation of 1 RSD in a tall person means less in terms of *percent predicted* than a similar deviation in someone of short stature. The constancy of the RSD is unlikely to hold at the extremes of age (the results of almost everyone > 80 years fall within the normal range) and size, or for indices of forced expiratory flow and the FEV_1/VC ratio.

Presentation of results (see Table 19.1)

Several points should be noted:

1. The predicted values for volumes are not quite internally consistent. Predicted [FVC + RV] does not equal predicted TLC, being 0.2–0.3 L less. There are probably two reasons. First, the FVC regression equation was not determined as [TLC − RV], but from a separate ventilatory maneuver. Second, the predictions for VC were derived from the forced maneuver (FVC) rather than the slow vital capacity (the difference between them is small in normal subjects but FVC may be > 0.3 L less than slow VC in airflow obstruction). Similarly, the predicted FEV_1 and VC do not exactly match the predicted ratio (FEV_1/VC).

   These particular reference equations,[1,2] which are in general use throughout the UK and in Europe, are derived from white subjects of European descent who are non-smokers without previous disease which would compromise ventilatory function. The age and height range for the regression line is 18–70 years and 1.5–1.95 m. There is no functional change between the ages of 18 and 25 years for spirometry, lung volumes, or diffusion, so age 25 should be entered for those > 18 < 25 years. Strictly speaking, these predictions should not be extrapolated beyond 70 years (see Table 19.1B), but in practice many patients > 75 years are studied in the Pulmonary Function Laboratory, and good predictions are lacking.

2. For FVC and TLC, the observed values have been set at 80% predicted. For the younger and taller man (A), the observed value is outside the lower limit of 'normal' (−1.64.RSD), but for the older and smaller subject (B) the FVC and TLC of 80% predicted are within the 90% confidence limits. The same pattern is seen in the case of D_{LCO}. Indeed in the older man (B), an FVC of 62% and a D_{LCO} of 60% predicted would be classified as 'normal' (−1.64 RSD).

3. The changes in RV in Table 19.1 are smaller than the 20% expected from the TLC decrease because of internal inconsistencies in the TLC and FVC regression equations, as mentioned earlier. Of course, the same *absolute* change in RV (in L) will have a greater effect on RV (as per cent predicted) than on TLC because RV is only 25–40% of the total lung capacity. The same argument applies to standardized residuals which for the same *absolute* volume change will be 1.5–1.7 times greater for RV than for FVC or TLC. On the other hand, for example A (Table 19.1), an RV of 120% predicted would be within the normal range (±0.925 RSD) unlike the 20% decrease in TLC and FVC in A.

In conclusion, it is a mistake to expect precision in defining 'normal' or 'abnormal' from reference equations. Neither *'percent predicted'* nor *'standardized residuals'* are perfectly accurate. The best indicator of abnormality or 'decrease in function' is by reference to a measurement made on the same subject at an earlier point in time, using the patient as his/her own control. The relationship between *percent predicted* and ± 1.64 RSD is variable. In example A, the cut-off for 'outside the 90% confidence limits' would have been 82% (FVC), 85% (TLC), and 81% (D_{LCO}), but this level in *percent predicted* becomes less as subjects become older and smaller, being 62%, 78%, and 60% respectively in example B. The RSD is a fixed quantity irrespective of age and size and is over-generous in the small and elderly. *Percent predicted* is probably a better index of 'normality' for them, and for children and adolescents in whom the variability around the

Table 19.1 Examples of pulmonary function and indices of 'deviation from normal'
A. White male, aged 25 years, European descent, height 1.85 m*

	Observed	Predicted	% predicted	Predicted range (±1.64 RSD)	Standardized residual
VC (L)	4.43	5.54	80	6.54–4.54	−1.8
TLC (L)	6.16	7.7	80	8.85–6.55	−2.2
RV (L)	1.73	1.85	94	2.51–1.19	−0.3[†]
D_{LCO} (ml.min^{-1} mmHg^{-1})	30	37.6	80	44.4–30.6	−1.8
[D_{LCO} (mmol.min^{-1} kPa^{-1})]	10	12.5	80	14.8–10.2	−1.8

B. White male, aged 75 years, European descent, height 1.55 m

FVC (L)	2.1	2.64	80	3.64–1.64	−0.87[†]
TLC (L)	4.24	5.3	80	6.45–4.15	−1.51[†]
RV (L)	2.14	2.45	87	3.11–1.78	−0.76[†]
D_{LCO} (ml.min^{-1} mmHg^{-1})	13.7	17.1	80	24–10.2	−0.8[†]
[D_{LCO} (mmol.min^{-1} kPa^{-1})]	4.55	5.69	80	8.0–3.39	−0.8][†]

* Predictions taken from references 1,2. H = height in meters; A = age in years. † = between 5th and 95th percentiles.
FVC = 5.76H − 0.026A − 4.34 (1.64.RSD = 1.0)   TLC = 7.99H − 7.08 (1.64.RSD = 1.15)
RV = 1.31H + 0.022A − 1.23 (1.64.RSD = 0.67) D_{LCO} = 11.11H − 0.066A − 6.03 (1.64.RSD = 2.32) [traditional units: times 0.33 for SI]

regression line increases as the absolute value increases. Subjects from ethnic groups other than those of European descent have smaller lung volumes for their height – the conversion factors varying from 0.87–0.9[1] – but there is no conversion needed for the D_{LCO} (T_{LCO}).[2] Conversion factors are available for black Americans.[3]

On the actual Pulmonary Function Test report itself, there are good reasons for quoting, in addition to the observed value, the percent predicted value and the standardized residual (SR). One more number can be accommodated without the report becoming cluttered, and a choice should be made between the predicted value itself or the range (± 1.64 RSD).

If standardized residuals are used, their definition and a severity scale should be appended at the foot of the Pulmonary Function Test report, e.g.:

Standardized residuals (SRs): ± 1 SR contain 90% of the reference population		
Severity scale for SRs:	mild	1.64–3.0
	moderate	3.0–4.0
	severe	> 4.0

The standardized residual is a useful way of quantifying the observed result in terms of the normal range. Most authorities recommend this approach, but it has not yet been taken up by many pulmonary function laboratories. The SR is not completely independent of the extremes of age and size, and for some indices of forced expiratory flow (e.g. MEF_{25} [syn: $\dot{V}max_{25}$], ATS nomenclature: FEF_{75}) the normal range is so wide that SRs are insensitive at detecting abnormality.

NORMAL VALUES

Which reference values?

There is an extensive literature concerning reference values,[1–6] and there are some useful commentaries on them.[7–9] The variation in reference equations between studies is quite considerable. For a given age (45 years), height (1.75 m), and sex, the predicted value for FEV_1 and FVC in nine studies, summarized by the ATS,[3] varies around the mean of all values by 7.4–13.3%, and in five studies of TLC by 5–7.5%. In 10 studies of D_{LCO} in men, at the same age and height, the variation around the mean value (after excluding the highest and lowest predictions) was 24% (in women 17%). For K_{CO} (D_L/V_A) the range around the mean value was 10% in men and 14% in women.

These differences in reference values which remain once age, sex, and height have been eliminated are not well understood. Ethnic differences and factors relating to equipment, technique, and calculation account for 25% and 7.5% of the residual variability between groups, and the remainder (67.5%)[8] is thought to be related to respiratory disease in childhood, genetic variation, passive smoking, air pollution, and the level of physical activity; the importance of each factor is unknown. All studies in the last 20 years have excluded current or ex-smokers. Cohort effects are emerging in that healthy individuals today tend to have FEV_1 values >100% based on the predictions of 20 years ago.

The Working Party in Europe on 'Standardization of Lung Function Tests' under the auspices of the European Community for Steel and Coal reviewed all the available studies of normal values in healthy non-smokers and developed 'summary equations' based on the pooled data from these reports. These regression equations were published in a lengthy report in 1983.[5] The validity of pooling data from disparate sources with ill-understood differences and the validity of the statistical analysis was seriously challenged.[9] Whether valid or not, these regression equations for spirometry, lung volumes, and diffusing capacity have been widely used and publicized throughout Europe, including the United Kingdom. The Working Party updated their recommendations 10 years later,[1,2] but saw no reason to alter the regression equations for routine lung function (except in the case of K_{CO} [see later]) since more recently published reference data from several European centers were broadly in agreement with the existing summary equations.

The American Thoracic Society's Working Party (which included several members of the European Working Party!) adopted a different stance.[3,4] They felt that data from various studies with unexplained differences should not be pooled – particularly not data from different continents. They proposed that each laboratory should choose equations from the literature, ideally drawn from sources close to home, which best suited a group of healthy subjects (10–15 of each sex) studied in that particular laboratory.

Normal values for K_{CO} (D_L/V_A)

The difficulties in establishing standard reference values are highlighted in the case of K_{CO}. The K_{CO}, as pointed out in Chapter 6, contains no volume information, being derived from the rate of disappearance of CO from alveolar gas during breath-holding. As a measure of efficiency, it should be independent of lung volume and body height, like the FEV_1/VC ratio. Nevertheless, height was a parameter in 10/18 studies quoted in the ATS summary document.[3] The present consensus is that only age and sex are important. Even the role of gender is questionable, since as a measurement of gas exchanging efficiency under resting conditions K_{CO} should be the same in men and women, like PaO_2 ($PaCO_2$ is slightly lower in women, probably due to sex hormone influences on the level of ventilation); however, only one[10] out of many studies has shown that K_{CO} is independent of gender.

In the studies referenced by the ATS,[3] the mean value for K_{CO} (age 45 years) in men from 10 studies was 5.08 ml.min^{-1} mmHg^{-1} L^{-1} (traditional units) (1.69 mmol.min^{-1} kPa^{-1} L^{-1} [SI units]) and in 8 studies in women K_{CO} was 5.3 (1.77). But the European reference value[5] is 5.8 (1.93) for men, and 6.18 (2.06) for women, which is considerably above any of the ATS quoted values. This discrepancy was noted by Love and Seaton,[11] who found in epidemiological studies that K_{CO} in healthy subjects was consistently 24% less than the European standard reference value. They showed that if the predicted value for D_{LCO} was divided by the predicted value for TLC (using EEC equations), i.e. $D_{LCO}\,pred/TLCpred$, a K_{CO} reference value was obtained which was in accord with their own normal population. Surprisingly, the Working Party agreed and the use of $D_{LCO}\,pred/TLCpred$ to predict K_{CO} is now recommended in Europe.[2] No RSD accompanies this reference value for K_{CO}. This solution is quite illogical because K_{CO} is not a size dependent measurement.

If one wishes to choose reference values for K_{CO} which are around the mean of published values in various studies, the reference equations of Roberts et al from London[22] would seem a reasonable choice. For a North American source of data of a similar nature, the data of Miller et al[13] would be suitable. All 'position papers' on normal values agree that D_{LCO} and K_{CO}[2] are more of a problem for selecting reference equations than spirometry and lung volumes, where there is reasonable conformity on both sides of the Atlantic (FEV_1 and TLC in women from European regressions exceed the average of the three most commonly used North American reference values[14–16] by 13% and 11% respectively, but other differences in spirometry and lung volumes are trivial). We have labored the point concerning K_{CO} because there is misunderstanding of the essential nature of the measurement, and because we have stressed its key role in the interpretation of routine pulmonary function tests in Chapter 17.

The ideal study of normal values as a function of age would be longitudinal rather than cross-sectional. Watson et al[17] studied 42 never-smokers (all men, average age 37.2 years) over a 10 year period. The decline in D_{LCO} and K_{CO} was 0.1 and 0.01 in SI units (0.3 and 0.03, in traditional units) per year. In the published cross-sectional studies the 'age' exponent (per year) [in SI units] for D_{LCO} varies from 0.043–0.1 (mean for 12 studies 0.073) and for K_{CO} from 0.007–0.017 (mean for 10 studies 0.011). Thus there is reasonable agreement between the cross-sectional studies and the longitudinal survey.

Normal values for other tests

A joint North American and European Working Party has reported on infant lung function testing,[18] and reference values are available for children and adolescents.[19–21] For other tests, the European recommendations on reference values for lung elasticity should be consulted.[5] For respiratory muscle strength and mouth pressures, consult Chapter 4, and for PaO_2 and $A\text{-}aPO_2$ see Chapter 5. For the single-breath nitrogen test of uneven ventilation (phase III) and for closing volume and closing capacity, consult Roberts et al.[12] As Gibson[7] has pointed out, there are still some neglected areas, such as measurements of airway resistance using the forced oscillation technique, and measurements made during sleep.

REPORTING ROUTINE PULMONARY FUNCTION TESTS

Should the routine tests of spirometry, flow-volume curves, lung volumes, and diffusing capacity (transfer factor) be reported at all? Clearly, the results should be scrutinized for internal consistency and errors before being sent out. The reporting of routine tests by medical staff is now a rare event. Test reports are prepared by the Laboratory staff, or produced automatically by a computer program. Computers can be instructed to recognize 'patterns' and a very simple example is given below, but a computer-generated report cannot use the information provided by the clinician on the request form and tailor the report to the individual patient. A compromise would be for the laboratory to generate a 'Computer Report' *and* a 'Personalized Report'.

Spirometric and diffusing capacity paradigms of common pathologies

The patterns illustrated in Table 19.2, which all differ from one another, should not be taken too literally. They are 'typical' examples of well-established disease. A Pulmonary Function Report might say 'compatible with ...' or 'supports (or does not support) the clinical diagnosis of ...'. But many patients with these pathologies, for various reasons, will not fit these paradigms. For a given pulmonary pathology, there is a wide spectrum of functional values (and the patterns themselves may differ from those in Table 19.2) as the disease progresses from the early to the end stage. In addition, two pathologies may coexist, such as smoking-related COPD and fibrosing alveolitis (CFA/IPF). This makes computer interpretation 'difficult' (and it tends towards the 'trivial'), and the Pulmonary Function Laboratory staff, with knowledge of the clinical problem, should be able to provide the clinician with an interpretation of the results which is more relevant to that particular patient.

The *diagnostic information* provided by routine pulmonary function testing is usually underplayed. The tests are considered to be sensitive in the detection of abnormality, but non-specific concerning the cause. In general terms this is true, but pulmonary function patterns can suggest, confirm, or refute a clinical diagnosis quite persuasively, even if not with absolute authority. Nevertheless, the detection of alveolar hemorrhage from intermittent rises of K_{CO} (Chapter 17) is highly specific. The D_{LCO} is an important and entirely non-invasive 'window' on the pulmonary circulation. A low D_{LCO} accompanied by normal lung volumes is suggestive of a pulmonary vascular pathology (Chapter 16). *But*, occasionally emphysema and fibrosing alveolitis (especially with pre-existing COPD) can present with a low D_{LCO} and virtually normal lung volumes. Pulmonary function tests within the normal range do not definitively rule

Table 19.2 Spirometric and diffusion patterns of common conditions

FEV$_1$/VC ratio	VC % predicted [SR]	D$_{LCO}$ (T$_{LCO}$) % predicted [SR]	K$_{CO}$ (D$_L$/V$_A$) % predicted [SR]	Disease process
< 0.5	< 100% [< −1.0]	< 60% [< 3.0]	< 80% [< −1.64]	Emphysema
< 0.7	< 100% [< −1.0]	> 100% < 125% [> 1.0 < 1.64]	> 100% < 80% [> 1.0 < 1.64]	Asthma
< 0.7	< 80% [< −1.64]	< 80% [< −1.64]	> 100% < 125% [> 1.0 < 1.64]	Bronchiectasis
< 0.7	< 80% [< −1.64]	< 80% [< −1.64]	< 100 < 1.0	Bronchiolitis
> 0.7	< 80% [< −1.64]	< 100% [< 1.0]	> 125% [< 1.64]	Incomplete alveolar expansion
> 0.7	< 80% [< −1.64]	< 80% [< −1.64]	> 100% < 125% [> 1.0 < 1.64]	Discrete loss of units e.g. pneumonectomy
> 0.8	< 80% [< −1.64]	< 60% [< −3.0]	< 80% [< −1.64]	Diffuse loss of units e.g. generalized fibrosis
> 0.7	> 80% [> −1.64]	< 60% [< −3.0]	< 80% [< −1.64]	Pulmonary vascular pathology
> 0.7	< 100% [< −1.0]	> 80% [> −1.64]	> 150% [> 3.0]	Alveolar hemorrhage (if intermittent)

SR = standardized residual (no of RSDs by which the observed value deviates from 'normal')
Concordance between levels of *percent* predicted and *SR values* is only approximate, and is affected by the RSD of the regression equation and the absolute predicted value.
See Chapter 17 for interpretation of D$_{LCO}$ and K$_{CO}$ (D$_L$/V$_A$) in incomplete expansion and discrete and diffuse loss of units, and Chapter 16 for pulmonary vascular pathology and alveolar hemorrhage.

out any pulmonary involvement in a disease process, because of the variability of function within so-called 'normal' populations around the mean reference value, i.e. ± 1.64 RSD ~ 80–120% predicted. The best reference is the subject himself, and the tests should be repeated six or twelve months later to check stability of function.

Obstructive versus restrictive patterns

Interpretation should go beyond the recognition of these two patterns of pulmonary function, but they are so basic to any understanding that a few remarks will be made, based on the discussion in the ATS document *Lung Function Testing: Selection of Reference Values and Interpretative Strategies*.[3]

Obstructive pattern

- A low FEV$_1$/VC ratio is the gold standard among routine tests for the detection of airflow obstruction, although a few normal subjects with supernormal FEV$_1$ and VC values may have a low ratio.
- In doubtful cases (FEV$_1$/VC borderline normal), inspection of the shape of the flow-volume curve is better than relying on indices from the curve such as MEF$_{25}$ (syn: V̇max$_{25}$), ATS nomenclature: FEF$_{75}$) or MEF$_{50}$ (FEF$_{50}$) where the normal variation is very wide.

- The slow VC will generally give a larger vital capacity than the FVC, especially in airflow obstruction, and is the preferred measurement.
- The severity of airflow obstruction is gauged better from the FEV_1 than from the FEV_1/VC ratio.

Restrictive pattern

- Restrictive is not a good term, since it refers to all causes of small lung volumes (a small TLC is necessary for the diagnosis) and should not be thought to indicate restrictive *lung* disease (e.g. fibrosis). 'Small lungs' is a better term, but it is unlikely to replace the more familiar 'restrictive'.
- Diagnosis is based on a reduced TLC, but in the presence of a normal FEV_1/VC ratio, a reduction in VC is 'suggestive' of the diagnosis.

Do absolute lung volumes always need to be measured?

This question sounds like heresy. Nevertheless, if the FEV_1/VC ratio is absolutely normal, the extra information generated by the measurement of TLC and RV is small. This is particularly so in the case of follow-up measurements. In addition, the helium dilution single-breath alveolar volume (V_A), obtained as part of the D_{LCO} measurement, acts as a 'surrogate' for TLC, *in the absence of airflow obstruction*. The single-breath V_A [+V_{Danat}] as percent predicted TLC is 93.6% ± 7.56 in normal subjects,[22] so a V_A < 80% predicted TLC suggests strongly a restrictive pattern ('small lungs') when associated with a reduced VC and a normal FEV_1/VC ratio. In fact, as percent predicted, all lung volumes (FEV_1, VC, TLC, V_A) tend to be concordant in the absence of airflow obstruction.

For many years, at Hammersmith, we have *not* measured TLC and RV in cases where the FEV_1/VC ratio is normal, relying on VC and V_A for information on lung volumes. This has greatly increased the number of patients coming through the laboratory each day, without significant loss of diagnostic or functional information. There is no point in doing tests where the information gain is slight. If greater efficiency is to be asked from Pulmonary Function Laboratories in the future, the value of each test should be questioned. There is always a tendency to do 'what we have always done'.

References

1. Quanjer Ph H, Tammeling GJ, Cotes JE, Pedersen OF, Peslin R, Yernault J-C. Lung volumes and forced ventilatory flows. *Report of Working Party "Standardization of Lung Function Tests"*. *Eur Respir J* 1993; **6**(suppl 16): 5–40.
2. Cotes JE, Chinn DJ, Quanjer PH, Roca J, Yernault J-C. Standardization of the measurement of transfer factor (diffusing capacity). *Report of Working Party "Standardization of Lung Function Tests"*. *Eur Respir J* 1993; **6**(suppl 16): 41–52.
3. American Thoracic Society. Lung function testing: selection of reference values and interpretative strategies. *Am Rev Respir Dis* 1991; **144**: 1202–18.
4. Crapo RO & Gardner RM. Single breath carbon monoxide diffusing capacity (transfer factor), recommendations for a standard technique. *Am Rev Respir Dis* 1987; **136**: 1299–307.
5. Quanjer Ph H. Standardized lung function testing. *Bull Eur Physiopathol Respir* 1983; **19**(suppl 5): 1–95.
6. Cotes JE. Lung Function; Assessment and Application in Medicine, 5th edn. Oxford: Blackwell Scientific 1993: 17.
7. Gibson GJ. Standardized lung function testing. *Eur Respir J* 1993; **6**: 155–7.
8. Becklake MR. Concepts of normality applied to the measurement of pulmonary function. *Am J Med* 1986; **80**: 1158–64.
9. Thornton JC & Miller A. Standardized lung function testing. *Bull Eur Physiopathol Respir* 1984; **20**: 571–2.
10. Bradley J, Bye C, Hayden SP, Hughes DTD. Normal values of transfer factor and transfer coefficient in healthy males and females. *Respiration* 1979; **38**: 221–6.
11. Love RG & Seaton A. About the ECCS summary equations (letter). *Eur Respir* 1990; **3**: 489.
12. Roberts CM, MacRae KD & Seed WA. Multi-breath and single breath helium dilution lung volumes as a test of airway obstruction. *Eur Respir J* 1990; **3**: 515–20.
13. Miller A, Thornton JC, Warshaw R, Anderson H, Tierstein AS, Selikoff IJ. Single breath diffusing capacity in a representative sample of the population of Michigan, a large industrial state. *Am Rev Respir Dis* 1983; **127**: 270-7.
14. Morris JF, Koski A & Johnson LC. Spirometric standards for healthy nonsmoking adults. *Am Rev Respir Dis* 1971; **103**: 57–67.
15. Crapo RO, Morris AH & Gardner RM. Reference spirometric values using techniques and equipment that meet ATS specifications. *Am Rev Respir Dis* 1981; **123**: 659–64.
16. Knudson RJ, Lebowitz MD, Holberg CJ, Burrows B. Changes in the normal expiratory flow-volume curve with growth and aging. *Am Rev Respir Dis* 1983; **127**: 725–34.
17. Watson A, Joyce H, Hopper L, Pride NB. Influence of smoking habits on change in carbon monoxide transfer factor over 10 years in middle aged men. *Thorax* 1993; **48**: 119–24.
18. Quanjer PhH, Stocks J, Polgar G, Wise M, Karberg K, Borsboom G. Compilation of reference values for lung function measurements in children. *Eur Respir J* 1989; **2**(suppl 4): 184s-261s.
19. Stocks J & Quanjer Ph H. Reference values for residual volume, functional residual capacity and total lung capacity. ATS workshop on lung volume measurements. Official Statement of the European Respiratory Society. *Eur Respir J* 1995; **8**: 492–506.

20 Rosenthal M, Bain SH, Cramer D, Helms P, Denison D, Bush A, Warner JO. Lung function in white children aged 4 to 19 years. I. Spirometry. *Thorax* 1993; **48**: 794-802.

21 Rosenthal M, Cramer D, Bain SH, Denison D, Bush A, Warner JO. Lung function in white children aged 4 to 19 years. II. Single breath analysis and plethysmography. *Thorax* 1993; **48**: 803–8.

22 Roberts CM, MacRae KD, Winning AJ, Adams L, Seed WA. Reference values and prediction equations for normal lung function in a non-smoking white urban population. *Thorax* 1991; **46**: 643–50.

Glossary of Abbreviations

Lung volumes

CV		closing volume (volume change from initiation of airway closure to RV)
CC		closing capacity (CV + RV)
EELV	(syn: FRC)	end-expired lung volume during resting breathing
EEV	(syn: Vr)	elastic equilibrium volume (*used in pediatric literature*)
ERV		expiratory reserve volume (FRC – RV)
FEV_1		forced expiratory volume in one second
FIV_1		forced inspiratory volume in one second
FRC	(syn: EELV or Vr*)	functional residual capacity (*not necessarily equal to EELV or Vr)
FVC		forced vital capacity
IC		inspiratory capacity (TLC – FRC)
IVC		inspiratory vital capacity
RV		residual volume
TGV	(syn: FRCpleth)	thoracic gas volume (measured by body plethysmography, usually close to FRC)
TLC		total lung capacity
V_A		alveolar volume (measured by gas dilution, generally in single inspiration to TLC)
VC		slow vital capacity
V_L		volume of the lungs at which a measurement is made
Vr	(syn: EEV)	relaxation volume of the respiratory system (P_L = Pcw)

Gas flow ($\dot{V}$)

FV		flow-volume curve
MEF_{vol}	(syn: $\dot{V}vol$)	maximum expiratory flow at a specific volume
MEF_{25}	(syn: $\dot{V}max_{25}$) etc.	maximum expiratory flow with 25% of VC remaining in the lung, etc.
		ATS nomenclature: FEF_{75} [forced expiratory flow after 75% of VC expired]
MMEF	(syn: FEF_{25-75} or $\dot{V}max_{75-25}$)	maximum mid-expiratory flow
MEFV		maximum expiratory flow-volume curve started from TLC
MIFV		maximum inspiratory flow-volume started from RV
MIF_{vol}	(syn: FIF_{vol})	maximum inspiratory flow at a specific volume
MIF_{50}	(syn: FIF_{50})	maximum inspiratory flow with 50% of VC remaining in the lung
MEF_{FRC}	(syn: $\dot{V}_{FRC}$)	maximum expiratory flow at FRC during PEFV in infants
M-P ratio		ratio of flow at same absolute lung volume for MEFV ($\dot{V}m$) and PEFV ($\dot{V}p$) curves
PEF	($\dot{V}max$)	peak expiratory flow

PEFV		partial expiratory flow-volume started below TLC (partial MEFV curve)
PIF		peak inspiratory flow
V̇insp, V̇exp		flow on inspiration or expiration (for airway resistance or measurements, or on exercise)

Pressures

CPAP		continuous positive airway pressure
$P_{0.1}$	(*syn:* $Pm_{0.1}$)	mouth occlusion pressure 0.1 s after onset of inspiration
Pab		abdominal pressure (usually estimated from Pga)
Palv	(*syn:* P_A)	alveolar pressure
Pao		pressure at airway opening (mouth, nose, tracheostomy)
Pb	(*syn:* Patm)	barometric pressure
Pbox		plethysmographic pressure
Pcw	(*syn:* Pw)	chest wall recoil pressure (Pbody surface – Ppl)
Pdi		transdiaphragmatic pressure (Pab – Ppl)
Pes	(*syn:* Poes)	esophageal pressure
PEEPe		externally applied positive end-expiratory pressure
PEEPi		intrinsic positive end-expiratory pressure
Pga		gastric pressure
PImax	(*syn:* MIP)	lowest mouth pressure during a maximum inspiratory effort
PEmax	(*syn:* MEP)	highest mouth pressure during a maximum expiratory effort
P_L	(*syn:* Pst(L))	lung recoil pressure (static) (Palv – Ppl)
P_L, dyn		lung recoil pressure (dynamic) during tidal breathing
$P_L$max		maximum lung recoil pressure (static) at TLC
Pmo		mouth pressure
Pmus		net pressure generated by respiratory muscles
Pna		nasal pressure
Ppl		pleural pressure (usually measured from Pes)
Pres		pressure to overcome resistive properties of lungs
Prs		recoil pressure of respiratory system (lungs + chest wall)
Ptm		transmural pressure (intraluminal – extraluminal)
Ptn		transnasal pressure (Pnasopharynx – Pnasal opening)
Ptp		transpulmonary pressure (Pao – Ppl, dynamically; P_L or (Palv – Ppl) under static conditions)

Resistance and compliance

C_L		static compliance of the lung
C_L,dyn		dynamic compliance of the lung
Ccw	(*syn:* Cw)	compliance of chest wall
Crs		compliance of respiratory system (C_L + Ccw)
E		elastance (1/compliance)
Gaw		airway conductance (1/resistance)
k		shape factor of PV curve
PV		static pressure-volume curve of the lungs
Raw		airways resistance (1/conductance)
Rcw		resistance of chest wall

Rint		airway resistance measured by the airflow interruption technique
R_L		resistance of airways and lung tissue
Rna		nasal resistance
Rrs		resistance of respiratory system (airways, lung tissue, chest wall)
Rti		lung tissue resistance
s		seconds
sGaw	(syn: Gaw/V_L)	specific airway conductance (corrected for lung volume [V_L] at which measurement is made)
τ		tau (Greek): time constant of the respiratory system (Crs × Rrs)
TT_{di}		tension time index of diaphragm (T_I/T_{TOT} × Pdi/Pdimax)
W		work of breathing (change in pressure × change in volume)
Xrs		reactance (sum of compliance and inertance) of the respiratory system
Zrs		impedance (sum of reactance and resistance) of the respiratory system

Ventilation

f	(syn: RR)	breathing frequency (respiratory rate)
F_IO_2		fractional concentration of inspired oxygen (often as percentage)
MVV	(syn: MBC)	maximum voluntary ventilation (maximum breathing capacity)
T_I		inspiratory time
T_E		expiratory time
T_{TOT}		total respiratory cycle duration
T_I/T_{TOT}		inspiratory duty cycle
V_T/T_I		mean inspiratory flow
$\dot{V}_E, \dot{V}_I$		minute ventilation measured in expiration or inspiration
$\dot{V}_Emax$		maximum ventilation during a progressive exercise test
$\dot{V}_A$		alveolar ventilation
V_T		tidal volume
V_D		dead space (anatomic [anat] or physiological [physiol])
V_D/V_T		proportion of tidal volume ventilating dead space
$\dot{V}_E$ reserve		$\dot{V}_Emax$ predicted – $\dot{V}_Epeak$ (on exercise)

Gas exchange and blood flow

$A-aPO_2$	(syn: $P(A-a) O_2$, $A-aDO_2$, PAO_2-PaO_2)	alveolar-arterial oxygen tension difference
AT		anaerobic threshold on exercise
β		capacitance coefficient (effective solubility): $mmHg^{-1}$
βO_2		oxygen capacitance coefficient (tangent to ODC)
CaO_2		arterial blood oxygen concentration
$C(A-a)O_2$		arteriovenous oxygen content difference
$Cc'O_2$		end-capillary blood oxygen concentration
CvO_2		mixed venous blood oxygen concentration
CO		carbon monoxide
COHb%		percentage saturation of Hb with CO
CI		cardiac index ($\dot{Q}$ corrected for body surface area)
DO_2		oxygen delivery ($CaO_2 \times \dot{Q}$)

HR	*(syn:* fC*)*	heart rate
HR reserve (HRR)		HR max predicted – HR peak (on exercise)
Hb		hemoglobin concentration
Hct	*(syn:* PCV*)*	hematocrit (PCV = packed cell volume)
NO		nitric oxide
ODC		oxygen dissociation curve
P (in gas exchange)		partial pressure ~ gas tension
P_{50}		PO_2 at which Hb is 50% saturated with oxygen
PaO_2, $PaCO_2$		arterial gas tension
P_AO_2, P_ACO_2		alveolar gas tension
$Pc'O_2$, $Pc'CO_2$		end-capillary gas tension
$P\bar{e}tO_2$, $PetCO_2$		end-tidal gas tension
P_EO_2, P_ECO_2		mixed expired gas tension
PvO_2, $PvCO_2$		mixed venous gas tension
$PtcO_2$, $PtcCO_2$		transcutaneous gas tension
P_IO_2		inspired oxygen tension
P_{H_2O}		pressure of water vapor
Ppa		pulmonary arterial pressure
Ppw		pulmonary wedge pressure
Ppv		pulmonary venous pressure
Qp		pulmonary blood volume
$\dot{Q}$	*(syn:* C.O.*)*	cardiac output
$\dot{Q}s$		shunt flow
$\dot{Q}_T$		total pulmonary blood flow (~ cardiac output)
$\dot{Q}s/\dot{Q}_T$		shunt fraction
R	*(syn:* RER*)*	respiratory exchange ratio
RQ		respiratory quotient
$SaO_2\%$		percentage saturation of hemoglobin with oxygen in arterial blood
$SpO_2\%$		percent saturation of Hb with oxygen using pulse oximetry
$\dot{V}O_2$	*(syn:* $\dot{M}O_2$*)*	oxygen consumption
$\dot{V}O_2max$		maximal oxygen consumption
$\dot{V}O_2peak$		peak (highest achieved) oxygen consumption
$\dot{V}CO_2$	*(syn:* $\dot{M}CO_2$*)*	carbon dioxide production
$\dot{V}_A/\dot{Q}$		ventilation-perfusion ratio
WR	*(syn:* $\dot{W}$*)*	work rate [watts(SI): kg.m.min^{-1} (trad)] ~ power output

Diffusion

D_{LO_2}		diffusing capacity for oxygen
D_{LCO}	*(syn:* T_{LCO}*)*	diffusing capacity for carbon monoxide
D_M		membrane conductance for gas diffusion
K_{CO}	*(syn:* D_L/V_A*)*	rate of uptake of carbon monoxide (~ transfer coefficient)
	(syn: T_L/V_A*)*	*(syn:* diffusing capacity per unit alveolar volume*)*
kCO		slope of alveolar CO concentration-time curve (time^{-1}) (equivalent, except in units, to K_{CO})
Qc		microvascular (capillary) blood volume
T_{LCO}	*(syn:* D_{LCO}*)*	transfer factor for carbon monoxide
θ		rate of reaction of gas with hemoglobin: min^{-1} mmHg^{-1}

Miscellaneous

ATPD		ambient temperature and pressure, dry
ATPS		ambient temperature and pressure, saturated with water vapor
ATS		American Thoracic Society
bd		bronchodilator
BHR	(syn: AHR)	bronchial (airway) hyper-responsiveness
BMI		body mass index (weight/body surface area)
BTPS		body temperature and pressure, saturated with water vapor
BTS		British Thoracic Society
ERS		European Respiratory Society
EVLW		extravascular lung water content
LTOT		long term (domiciliary) oxygen therapy
MMD		mass median diameter (for aerosol sizing)
NIPPV	(syn: nPPV)	nasal intermittent positive pressure ventilation
NCPAP		nasal continuous positive airway pressure
PD_{20}	(syn: PC_{20})	provocative dose (concentration) for 20% decrease in function
PFT		pulmonary function test(s)
pred	(syn: reference value)	predicted normal
RC/AB		ratio of rib cage to abdominal movement or displacement
RFT		respiratory function test(s)
RIP	(syn: Respitrace™)	respiratory inductance pneumograph
RSD		residual standard deviation
SBN_2		single-breath expired nitrogen slope
SR		standardized residual (observed-predicted/RSD)
STPD		standard temperature and pressure, dry
VAS		visual analogue scale

Clinical terms

$\alpha_1 PI$	(syn: $a_1 AT$)	α_1-proteinase inhibitor (α_1-antitrypsin)
ARDS		adult respiratory distress syndrome
BLT		bilateral (double) lung transplantation
CABG		coronary artery bypass graft operation
CPR		cardiopulmonary resuscitation
COPD	(syn: COLD)	chronic obstructive pulmonary (lung) disease
CFA	(syn: IPF)	cryptogenic fibrosing alveolitis
CXR		chest radiograph
CT	(syn: X-ray CT)	computerized tomography (3D X-ray imaging)
EEG		electroencephalogram (electrical activity of the brain)
EKG	(syn: ECG)	electrocardiograph
EMG		electromyograph (electrical activity of skeletal muscle)
HLT		heart-lung transplantation
IPF	(syn: CFA)	idiopathic pulmonary fibrosis
IHD		ischemic heart disease (syn: myocardial infarction, angina pectoris)
ICU	(syn: ITU)	intensive care (therapy) unit
LVRS		lung volume reduction surgery
MRI		magnetic resonance imaging
OSA		obstructive sleep apnea

PE	pulmonary embolism
QoL	quality of life
REM	rapid eye movement in sleep
SLT	single lung transplantation
SOB(OE)	shortness of breath (on exertion)

Index

Page numbers in *italic* print refer to figures and tables.

abdominal movements, 156, 157–8
acetylene, 77, 95
acidosis
   hypoxemic response, 86
   metabolic, 88
   oxygen therapy, 202
acoustic reflection, 42
acromegaly, 54, 153, 276
adenosine triphosphate, 134
adult respiratory distress syndrome (ARDS), 86–7
   hypoxemia, 187
   intensive care, 186, 190
   nitric oxide therapy, 92
   posture, 188
airflow interruption technique, 36–8
airflow resistance, 27–43
   airflow interruption technique, 36–8
   anesthesia, 37
   chest wall, 41
   comparison of different methods, 38–9
   components, 27–8
   dependence on breathing phase/flow, 28–9
   dependence on lung volume, 28–9, 31
   distribution, 38–41
   expiratory, *8*, 28
   inspiratory, *8*, 28
      infants, 171
   intensive care, 37, 193
   localization of site, 17–18
   low alveolar volume, 262
   lung tissue, 41
   measuring, 29–38, 39–41
   nasal (R_{na}), 39–41
   nasopharyngeal, 41
   oropharyngeal, 41
   physiology, 27–9
   reference values, 38
   serial distribution, *28*
airway response, 220
   bronchoconstrictors *see* bronchoconstrictor
      responses
   bronchodilators *see* bronchodilator responses
airways

   developmental physiology, 164–6
   dimensions, assessing, 42
   variations in tone, 29
allergens, 224
albuterol *see* salbutamol
alpha$_1$-antitrypsin deficiency, 284
alveolar-capillary gas transfer, 94–5
alveolar dead space, 82–3
alveolar hemorrhage, 251, *252*, 264, 265, 277
alveolar hypoventilation, 81, 87
alveolar volume (V_A), 52, 98, 260
   calculation, 104
   low, 260–62
alveoli
   loss of alveolar units, 260–61, 263–4
   pressure (P_{alv}), 7
   transmural pressure (P_{tm}), *8*
anatomic dead space, 82–3
anatomic shunt, 85–6
anesthesia, 37
anticholinergic drugs, 222
apnea *see* obstructive sleep apnea
arterial blood gases
   carriage, 77–8
   exercise testing, 138
   infants, 176–8
   intensive care units, 186–7
   non-invasive determination, 176–8
   pre-operative evaluation, 237
   respiratory muscle weakness, 61
arterial oxygen saturation (SaO_2), 76–8, 157
arterial oxygen tension (PaO_2), 76–8
   age changes, 83–4
   arterialized capillary blood, 79
   normal values, 83
   PaO_2/FiO_2 ratio, 84–5
   transcutaneous measurements ($tcPO_2$), 79
aspirin, 223, 224
asthma, 283
   airflow resistance, 31, 39
   airway tone, 29
   bronchoconstrictor responses, 220–22, 226
   bronchodilator responses, 228–9

asthma (cont.)
cough, 232
dyspnea, 122
exercise testing, 145
FEV_1, 228
functional residual capacity, 52–3
impaired gas mixing, 115
lung function tests, 164, 166
maximum effort flow-volume curves, 13
maximum expiratory flow, 17
Maximum-partial (M-P) ratios, 18
occupational, 224
$PaCO_2$, 88
peak expiratory flow, 24
pulmonary function, 283
respiratory muscle function, 70
response to carbon dioxide, 117
schoolchildren, 181
total lung capacity, 55
total respiratory resistance, 35, 39
ventilatory control, 117
atropine, 29

baseline dyspnea index (BDI), 123–4
Becker's muscular dystrophy, 278
Behçet's disease, 249
$beta_2$-adrenoceptor agonists
airway tone, 29
bronchoconstrictor responses, 224
bronchodilator responses, 227
bilateral hilar lymphadenopathy, 267
blood gases *see* arterial blood gases
blood pressure
arousal-induced changes, 158
exercise testing, 138
intrathoracic effects, 156–7
blue bloater syndrome, 87, 117, *119*
body plethysmograph, 10
airway resistance, 29–31
applications, 31
constant volume, *31*
infants, 169, 176
lung volumes, 29, 52
method, 30
pre-school children, 179–80
pressure-volume curve/compliance, 47
technical problems, 29–30
body surface measurements, 174–5

Bohr effect, 77
Borg scale, 125–7
exercise testing, 138
Boyle's law, 47, 52
breath-actuated dosimeters, 223
breath-holding time (BHT), 109
breathing pattern analysis, 110
breathlessness *see* dyspnea
bronchial hyper-responsiveness (BHR), 220–22
non-specific, 226
bronchiectasis, 226, 278
D_{LCO}, 270
total lung capacity, 54
bronchiolitis, 14, 243, 279
bronchoconstrictor responses, 220–27
agents, 222–4
airflow resistance, 41
dose-response curves, 225–6
exercise, 222, 223
mechanisms, 220–22
pharmacological blockade, 224
plateau of maximum response, 225
provocation tests, 222–5
bronchodilator responses, 227–30
airflow resistance, 41
in asthma, 282
dose/choice of bronchodilator, 227
expressing the response, 228
interpretation, 228–30
timing of measurements, 227
bronchography, 41
bronchomalacia, 181
bronchomotor tone, 29
bronchospirometry, 237
bullectomy, 238–9, 275
bullous lung disease, 52, 238–9, 275

capillary blood oxygen, 79
capnographs, 176
capsaicin, 231
carbon dioxide
arterial (PCO_2), 87–8
and hypoxia, 112
interaction with oxygen dissociation curve (Bohr effect), 77
retention, 117
ventilatory control, 111–12
carbon monoxide

alveolar-capillary transfer, 94
diffusing capacity *see* diffusing capacity: carbon monoxide
rate of uptake (Kco), 260, 262–5
reference values, 282, 291–2
carboxyhemoglobin (COHb), 80
cardiac disease
congestive heart failure, 86, 246
dyspnea, 122
left ventricular dysfunction, 245–6
versus lung disease (exercise testing), 144–5
cardiac output
DLCO, 103
intensive care, 188
cardiomyopathy, 278
cardiorespiratory polygraphic monitoring, 178
chemoreceptors, peripheral, 108, 113
chest wall
airflow resistance, 41
compliance (Ccw), 49, 190–92
disease
school children, 181
ventilatory control, 118–19
elasticity, 45–6
infants, 176, *177*
resting volume, 46
Cheyne-Stokes respiration, 116, 157
choke points, 7–8, 12, 18
chloral hydrate, 168
chronic hyperventilation syndrome, 88
chronic myeloid leukaemia, 275
chronic obstructive pulmonary disease (COPD)
abnormal gas exchange, 116
airflow resistance, 31, 39
bronchoconstrictor responses, 226
bronchodilator responses, 227, 229–30
carbon dioxide retention, 117
constant volume body plethysmography, *31*
distribution of resistance, 39–46
domiciliary oxygen therapy, 202
dyspnea, 122
exercise testing, 142, 144
expiratory flow limitation, 8, 21–2
expired nitric oxide, 92
FEV$_1$, 4, 229
FiO$_2$, 86
forced vital capacity, 229
and hypercapnia, 71, 87–8, 117, *118*

hypoxemia, 117
impaired gas mixing, 115
inspiratory muscle weakness, 117
long-term oxygen therapy, 203
lung volume, 52–6
maximum expiratory flow, 17
maximum voluntary ventilation, 6, 69
mechanical load, 117
nasal intermittent positive pressure ventilation, 210–11, 214–15
nocturnal oxygen therapy, 206
peak expiratory flow, *14*, 24
post-transplant, 242
respiratory muscle function, 77, 71–2, 116
response to carbon dioxide, 117
tidal flow-volume curves, 22, *23*
total lung capacity, 55
total respiratory resistance (oscillation method), 34–5, 39
ventilatory control, 117
during sleep, 119
Churg-Strauss syndrome, 244, 249
closing volume, 89–90
compliance, 47–9
chest wall (Ccw), 45–6, 49, 190–92
dynamic, 32–4, 49
infants, 171–3
intensive care, 190–92
lungs (CL), 45–6, 47–9
pre-school children, 180
total respiratory (Crs), 45, *46*, 49
congestive heart failure, 86, 246
connective tissue diseases, 249
constant exhalation DLCO measurement, 98–9
continuous mandatory ventilation (CMV), 186
continuous positive airway pressure (CPAP), 160–61
intensive care, 186
obstructive sleep apnea, 61
cor pulmonale, 202
corticosteroids, 281, 283
cough
decreased effectiveness, 232
frequency, 230, 231–2
gastric pressure, 65
laboratory evaluation, 230–32
MEFV, 17, 20
sensitivity, 230–32

cromoglycate, 224
cryoglobulinemia, *252*
cryptogenic fibrosing alveolitis (idiopathic pulmonary fibrosis), 265–6, 267, 279, 281, 282
   arterial oxygen tension (PaO_2), 86
   long-term oxygen therapy, 203
   lung transplantation, 241
   peak expiratory flow, 24
   total lung capacity, 54–5
cycle ergometers, 137
cystic fibrosis, 181, 226
   long-term oxygen therapy, 203
   lung transplantation, 241

dead space compartment, 82–3
deep inflation (DI), 18, 220
dermatomyositis, 279
diaphragm, 58
   assessment of strength, 65–8
   electromyogram, 65
   endurance, 69
   pacing, 210
   weakness, 59, *60*, 278
diethylenetriamine pentacetate (DTPA), 197–8
diffusing capacity (transfer factor)
   oxygen (D_{LO_2}), 81, 95
   carbon monoxide (D_{LCO}), 93–106
      abnormal, clinical examples, 270–71
      alveolar oxygen concentration, 102
      carbon monoxide back pressure, 103
      cardiac output, 103
      chronic smoking, 103–4
      clinical analysis, 260–65
      components (D_M, Q_C), 100–102
      healthy subjects, 102–4
      hemoglobin concentration, 102
      intensive care, 189
      interpretation, 259–68
      K_{CO} *see* carbon monoxide: rate of uptake
      low alveolar volume (V_A), 260–62
      lung expansion, 102
      measurement, 96–100
      pulmonary vascular disease, 246
normal values, 104
   mitral stenosis, 246
   nitric oxide (D_{LNO}), 101–2
   post-transplantation, 242
   respiratory muscles, 60–61
   Roughton–Forster equation, 102–4

diffusion, 76–7
   limitation, 81, 94–5
disability, 135–6
dosimeters, 223
Down's syndrome, 182
drug sensitivities, 224
dynamic compliance (C_{Ldyn}), 32–4, 49
dynamic lung resistance (R_L), 169–71
dyspnea
   analysis, 129–30
   definition, 121–2
   intensity versus distress 129, *130*
   measurement, 122–9
   and oxygen consumption ($\dot{V}O_2$), 129
   rating scales, 126–9
   reference variables, 127–8
   scaling and experience, 129–30
   versus fatigue, 130
   visual analogue scale, 125, *126*, 127

elastic equilibrium volume (EEV), 45, 52
elasticity, 45–50
electrocardiogram (EKG)
   exercise testing, 138
   pulse transit time, 156
   sleep fragmentation, 156–7
electroencephalogram (EEG)
   arousals, 158
   sleep studies, 155
electromyography (EMG), 159
   diaphragm, 65
   muscle fatigue, 70
emphysema, 281, 284
   airflow resistance, 31
   arterial oxygen tension (PaO_2), 86
   compliance, 49
   diffusing capacity, 270
   functional residual capacity, 52–3
   lung transplantation, 241–2
   lung volume reduction surgery, 239–40
   maximum effort flow-volume curves, 13
end-expiratory lung volume (EELV), 52
   cystic fibrosis, 181
   infants, *165*
endothelial permeability, 196–7
epithelial barrier integrity, 197
Epworth Sleepiness score, 154
equal pressure points (EPP), *8*, 17
esophageal balloon catheter technique, 32–4

infants, 169–71
exercise testing, 133–47
    anaerobic (lactate) threshold, 142–3
    athletic subjects, 141
    cardiac disease, 144–5
    clinical situations, 144–5
    contrainidications, 140–41
    cooperation/motivation, 146
    data presentation, 137–9
    disability assessment, 135–6
    endurance tests, 134–6
    field tests, 136–7
    heart rate, 138
    interpretation, 145–7
    laboratory testing, 137–44
    lung disease, 144–5
    maximal aerobic capacity ($\dot{V}O_2$max), 142
    maximal capacity tests, 134–6
    normal values, 141–2
    physiological response, *146*, 147
    post-transplantation, 243
    preoperative evaluation, 145, 237
    protocols, 141
    quality control, 140
    rationale, 134–6
    reporting, 145–7
    safety, 140–41
    submaximal testing, 144
    tidal-flow volume curves, 21
    ventilatory limit, 143–4
    work capacity, 146
    expiratory flow limitation, *8*, 17, 21–2, *23*, 28
expiratory muscle strength, 64–5
expiratory reserve volume (ERV), 6
    obesity, 55
extrathoracic airway obstruction
    fixed, 15
    functional, 15–16
    maximum effort flow-volume curves, 14–16
    peak expiratory flow, 24
extravascular lung water (EVLW), 195–6
extrinsic allergic alveolitis, 265–6, 276

face masks, 207
facio-scapulo-humeral muscular dystrophy, 283
fibrosing alveolitis *see* cryptogenic fibrosing alveolitis
Fick Equation, 79
Finapres, 156–7
flow-limiting segments (FLS; choke points), 7–8, 12, 18

flow-volume analysis, 7
flow-volume curves, *see* maximum expiratory and inspiratory flow-volume curves
forced expiratory flow indices, 174
forced expiratory maneuvers
    infants, 174
    pre-school children, 180
    vital capacity, 9–10
forced expiratory volume in one second (FEV_1), 4, 9
    best tests/repeatability, 11
    bronchodilator responses, 228–9
    cystic fibrosis, 241
    emphysema, 241
    extrathoracic airway obstruction, 15
    intensive care, 189
    post-bullectomy, 239
    post-pneumonectomy, 235–6, 237
    pre-school children, 180
    reference values, 12
    smokers, 12
    transplant rejection, 243
forced inspiratory vital capacity maneuver, 12–13
forced inspiratory volume in one second (FIV_1), 6
forced oscillation techniques, 34–6
    infants, 171–3
    pre-school children, 180
forced vital capacity (FVC), 4–6, 9
    best tests/repeatability, 11
formoterol, 227
fractional concentration of inspired oxygen (FiO_2), 84–7
functional residual capacity (FRC), 45, 50, 52–3
    airflow obstruction, 28
    infants, 176
    intensive care, 188, 189–90
    obesity, 53, 55
furosemide (frusemide), 224
gas exchange, 76–92
    alveolar-capillary, 94–5
    diseased lungs, 82–8
    inefficiency, quantitating, 83–6
    intensive care, 186–9
    three-compartment model, 82–3

gastro-esophageal reflux, 232
Goodpasture's syndrome, 250–51
graft-versus-host disease, 275
Guillain-Barré syndrome, 24, 60, 186

helium and MEFV curves, 17–18, 99

hemoglobin
  carbon monoxide diffusion, 94, 95
  and D_{LCO}, 101, 102
  oxygen transport, 76–8
  sickle-cell disease, 247
hepatopulmonary syndrome (HPS), 255–6
hereditary hemorrhagic telangiectasia (HHT), 252–4
Hering-Breuer inflation reflex, 173, 179
histamine
  administration, 223
  bronchoconstrictor responses, 164, 222–6
hypercapnia, 86
  and COPD, 72, 87–8, 117, *118*
  rebreathing response, *113*
  respiratory muscle weakness, 61, *62*
hypersensitivity pneumonitis (extrinsic allergic alveolitis [EAA]), 265–6, 276
hyperventilation
  chronic, 88
  exercise, 134
  gas exchange, 86, 87
  sustained, 69
  syndrome, 116–17
hypocapnia
  hyperventilation syndrome, 117
  hypoxemia, 86
hypothyroidism, 153
hypoventilation, 59, 80–81, 116
  alveolar, 81, 88
  hypercapnia, 61
  primary alveolar (Ondine's curse), 116
hypoxemia
  breathing pattern, *119*
  causes, *80*
  compensatory mechanisms, 86
  exercise-induced, 134
  inspired oxygen fraction (FiO_2), 186–7
  respiratory muscle weakness, 61
  responses, 86–7
  see also arterial oxygen tension
hypoxia
  carbon dioxide, 112
  oxygen therapy, 202
  rebreathing response, *113*

idiopathic pulmonary fibrosis *see* cryptogenic fibrosing alveolitis
impairment, 135
impedance
  pneumography in infants, 176
inert gas dilution technique, 50–51
infants
  expiratory flow limitation, 22
  respiratory function, 168–80
inspiratory airway resistance (Raw), *8*, 28
  infants, 171
inspiratory capacity (IC), 6
inspiratory effort, measuring, 155–6
inspiratory flow, *8*, 28
  limitation, 17, 22, 155–6
inspiratory resistive loading, 69–70
inspiratory work, 33
inspired oxygen fraction (FiO_2), 186–7
intensive care unit, 186–98
  airway resistance measurement, 37, 193
interstitial lung disease, 265–7
  hypercapnia, 117
  hypoxemia, 117
  respiratory muscle changes, 116
  ventilatory control, 117–18
intrapulmonary shunting, 251–2
intrathoracic airway dimensions, 28
intrathoracic airways obstruction
  maximum effort flow-volume curves, 13–14
  peak expiratory flow, 24
  tidal flow-volume curves, 21–2
  see also COPD, emphysema and asthma
intrinsic positive end-expiratory pressure (PEEPi), 53, 192–3
ipratropium, 29, 227
iso-volume pressure-flow curve, 42

K_{CO} *see* carbon monoxide, rate of uptake
kyphoscoliosis, 52, 118, 181

lactic acidemia, 142–3
lactic acidosis, 136
larynx
  obstruction, 16
  paralysis, 15
left ventricular dysfunction, 245–6
leukotrienes, 224
liver transplantation, 256
lobectomy, 236
long-term oxygen therapy (LTOT), 203–6
lung cancer, surgery, 234–8
lung disease, maximal exercise, 134–5
lung function

tests *see* pulmonary function tests
typical values, *164*
lung recoil pressure (P$_L$), 7, *8*, 16–17
    maximum (P$_L$max), 47, *49*
    role in reducing maximum expiratory flow, 16–17
lung transplantation, 241–3
lung volume reduction surgery, 239–40
lung volumes, 50–55
    airflow resistance, 28–9, 31
    calculation, *50*
    determinants, 52–3
    in disease, 54–5
    infants, 176
    intensive care, 189–90
    measurement, 50–52
    postural effects, 54
    pre-school children, 180
    respiratory muscles, 60–61
lungs
    airflow resistance, 41
    bullae, 238–9, 275
    collapse, 271
    compliance (C$_L$), 45–6, 47–9, 190–92
    denervated, physiology, 243
    dynamic resistance (R$_L$), 169–71
    elasticity, 45–6
        infants, 176, *177*
    parenchyma, 195–7
    pressures, 27–8
    two compartment filling/emptying, 14

magnetic stimulation, 66–7
magnetometry, 176
mandibular advancement devices, 161
maximal aerobic capacity (VO$_2$max), 134–6, 141–2
maximum effort flow-volume curves, 13–22
maximum expiratory flow (MEF), 7–8
    infants, 174
    lung recoil pressure, 16–17
    pre-school children, 180
    reference values, 12
    tests, 42–3
    variation in normal population, 11–12
maximum expiratory flow-volume (MEFV) curve, *7*, *9*, 13–22
    best tests/reliability, 11
    common errors, *10*
    cough, 16, 20
    instruments, 10
    intrathoracic airways obstruction, 13–14
    nasal, 19–20
    partial, 18–19
    quality control, 10
    sarcoidosis, *16*
    variation in normal population, 11–12
maximum inspiratory flow (MIF), 8–9, 12–13
    instruments, 10
maximum inspiratory flow-volume (MIFV) curves, 13–22
    bronchodilation, 229
    intrathoracic airways obstruction, 13–14
    nasal, 19–20
maximum lung recoil pressure (P$_L$max), 47, *49*
maximum mid-expired flow (MMEF), *5*, *6*, *9*
maximum mouth pressures, 61–2
maximum relaxation rate (MRR), 69, 70–71
maximum voluntary ventilation (MVV), *5*, *6*–*7*, 69
mean transit time (MTT), *5*
mechanical loading, 114–15, *116*
mechanoreceptors, 108
Medical Research Council (MRC)
    Dyspnoea Scale, 126, *127*
    long-term oxygen therapy trial, 203, 204
mesothelioma, 271
metabisulfite, 222
methacholine, 42, 164
    bronchoconstrictor responses, 224–6
    dose-response curve, *226*
methane, 99
methemoglobin, 80
methotrexate, 283
microvascular injury, 250–51
minute ventilation, 109–10
mitral valve disease, 245–6
    residual volume, 55
mixed connective tissue disease (MCTD), 249, 271
mouth breathing, expiratory flow limitation, 21–2
mouth occlusion pressure, 110–11
multiple inert gas elimination technique (MIGET), 88, *89*
multiple occlusion technique, 173
muscles *see* respiratory muscles
muscular dystrophy
    Becker's, 278
    facio-scapulo-humeral, 283
    ventilatory control, 118–19
    vital capacity, 62
myasthenia gravis, 24

myopathy, *62*

nasal cavity
    airflow resistance (R_{na}), 39–41
    obstruction, peak inspiratory/expiratory flow, 24–5
    patency, 42–3
    polyps, 181
    volume measurement, 40
nasal continuous positive airway pressure (NCPAP), 155, 156, 160–61
nasal intermittent positive pressure ventilation (NIPPV), 209–10
nasal prongs, 207–8
nasal valve, 19, 41
nebulizers, 223
nedocromil, 224
negative effort dependence, 9–10, 22
negative expiratory pressure (NEP), 22
negative pressure ventilation (nPV), 210
neuromuscular disease, 59
    expiratory muscle strength, 64
    hypercapnia, 71, 119
    hypoxemia, 119
    obstructive sleep apnea, 182
    respiratory muscle changes, 116
    ventilatory control, 118–19
    vital capacity measurement, 189
nitric oxide, 77, 91
    diffusing capacity (D_{LNO}), 101–2
    exhaled, measurement, 91–2
    inhaled, therapeutic use, 92
Nocturnal Oxygen Therapy Trial (NOTT), 203, 204

obesity
    closing volume, 90
    lung volumes, 53, 54, 55
    obstructive sleep apnea, 153
obstructive sleep apnea (OSA), 152–4
    acoustic reflection, 42
    age changes, 153
    airway resistance, 41–2
    daytime sleepiness, 154
    definition, 154
    extrathoracic airway obstruction, 15–16
    hypoxemia, 153–4
    infants, 178
    inspiratory flow limitation, 22
    obesity, 153
    pharyngeal narrowing, 152
    predisposing factors, 153
    respiratory muscle weakness, 61
    school children, 181–2
    syndrome, 154
    treatment, 160–61
    treatment rationale, 153–4
    ventilatory control, 119
Ondine's curse, 116
oronasal airflow, 157
oxygen
    arterial blood, 77–82
    alveolar to arterial gradient (A-aPO_2), 84, *85*
    fetal, 77
    measurement, 78–80
    typical values, 78
    capillary blood, 79
        concentrators, 206
        delivery
        intensive care, 187, 188
    nebulizers, 201
    systems, 206–9
        liquid, 207
        therapy
            acute, 202–3
            air travel, 208–9
            ambulatory, 206–9
            cylinders, 207
            domiciliary, 202–8
            equipment, 206–7
            hypercapnic COPD, 88
            long-term (LTOT), 203–6
            night-time, 205–6
    transport, 76–7
    transtracheal, 208
oxygen consumption (VO_2)
    dyspnea, 129
    exercise, 136
    maximal aerobic capacity (VO_2max), 134–6, 141–2
oxygen cost diagram (OCD), 123
oxygen dissociation curve (ODC), 77–8
    oxygen-carbon dioxide diagram, *81*

palliative surgery, 238
panting, 29–31
partial pressure, 76
peak expiratory flow (PEF), 7, 8, 9, 22–5
    applications, 24–5
    best tests/repeatability, 11
    infants, 174, *175*

nasal, *19*, 20, 24
physiological basis, 22–3
reference values, 12, 22–4
technical aspects, 23–4
peak inspiratory flow (PIF), 12–13
nasal, *19*, 20, 24
perfusion limitation, 95
periodic breathing, 116
persistent pulmonary hypertension of the newborn, 92
pharynx, narrowing/collapse, 152, *156*
phase lag, 175
phrenic nerve
injury, 59, 280
stimulation, 65–7, 71
physiological dead space, 83
physiological shunt, 84, 85
compartment, 83, 188
pink puffers, 117, *119*
plethysmography *see* body plethysmography
pleural pressure (Ppl), 7, *8*, 111
esophageal balloon catheter measurement, 31–2
infants, 171
pneumonectomy, 235–6
pneumonia, 86
pneumotachograph, 9–10, 137
infants, 173
inspiratory flow limitation, 155–6
Poiseuille flow, 28
poliomyelitis, 278
polycythemia
long-term oxygen therapy, 203
secondary, 86, 253
polygraphic monitoring, 178, 180
polymyositis with fibrosing alveolitis, 267, 282
polysomnography, 159
positive end-expiratory pressure (PEEP), 189, 190
compliance, 190–2
instrinsic (PEEP$_1$), 53, 192–3
positive pressure during expiration (EPAP), 209
posture
intensive care, 188–9
lung volumes, 53
pregnancy
PaO$_2$, 83
pulmonary arteriovenous malformations, 254
smoking, 166
preoperative assessment, 234–44
exercise testing, 145, 237
pressure at airway opening (P$_{ao}$), 190–2

pressure-flow curves (neonatal), *172*
pressure-volume (PV) curve, 46, *47*
analysis, 47
changes in disease, 49
measurement, 47, *48*
primary pulmonary hypertension (PPH), 247–8
propranalol, 224
protein accumulation index (PAI), 196–7
provocation tests, 222–5
post-transplantation, 242
provocative concentration (PC), 225–6
provocation dose (PD), 225–6
pulmonary arteriovenous malformations (PAVMs), 86, 252–5
idiopathic, 255
pulmonary artery pressure, 203
pulmonary edema, 195–6
pulmonary embolic disease, 246–7
PaCO$_2$, 88
pulmonary fibrosis
compliance, 49
total lung capacity, 53, 54
pulmonary function *see* respiratory function
Pulmonary Function Status Scale, 125
pulmonary function tests
abnormal results, 288–9
intensive care unit, 186
normal values, 290–2
obstructive pattern, 293–4
pediatric, 164–80
presentation, 287–94
reference values, 290–2
referral forms, 288
reporting, 292–4
request forms, 288
restrictive pattern, 294
Pulmonary Functional Status and Dyspnea Questionnaire, 125
pulmonary hemorrhage, 264–5
pulmonary hypertension, 245–50
lung transplantation, 242
persistent of the newborn, 92
primary, 247–8
pulmonary hypotension, 251–6
pulmonary vasculitis, 248–50, 277
pulmonary venous hypertension, 245–6
pulse oximetry (SpO$_2$), 78, 79–81
exercise testing, 138
infants, 176–8

pulse oximetry (SpO$_2$) (cont.)
    obstructive sleep apnea, *159*
pulse transit time (PTT), 157, 158
pulsus paradoxus, 156

quality of life, 204

radioactive gas measurements, 90–91
radiography
    diaphragm, 61
    lung volumes, 52
rapid thoraco-abdominal compression technique
        (RTC), 174, *175*
    rebreathing D$_{LCO}$ measurement, 99–100
rebreathing techniques, 112–14
reference values, 11–12
relaxation volume (V$_r$), 45, 52
residual volume (RV), 53
respiratory drive, 194
respiratory function
    case reports, 275–84
    pediatric, 164–82
        airway function, 169–75
        assessment, 168–79
        clinical physiology, 166–8
        common conditions, *167*
        developmental physiology, 164–6
        epidemiological studies, 166
        infants, 168–80
        interpretation of results, 182
        long-term oxygen therapy, 203
        pre-school children, 179–80
        reference ranges, 180
        school children, 180–82
        typical values, *164*
    preoperative assessment *see* preoperative assessment
        pulmonary vascular disease, 245
    tests *see* pulmonary function tests
respiratory inductance plethysmography, 110, 175
respiratory muscles, 58–72
    assessment, 58–9
        endurance, 68–70
        fatigue, 69, 70–72
        intensive care, 193–4
        sequential, 68
        strength, 59–68
    disease, 58–9, 116
    endurance, 68–70
    fatigue

assessment, 70–72
load/capacity balance, 58
normal function, 58
strength, 59–68
weakness, 280
    arterial blood gases, 61
    maximum effort flow-volume curves, 16
    peak expiratory flow, 24
    symptoms, 59
respiratory paradox, 156
respiratory pattern generator, 108
respiratory quotient (RQ), 80
Respitrace™, 110
restrictive lung disease
    maximum effort flow-volume curves, 16
    peak expiratory flow, 24
    post-transplant, 242
rheumatoid arthritis, 267, 279
    diffusing capacity, 270
rhinomanometry, 39–41
rib cage movements, 156, 157–8
Roughton-Forster equation, 100–102

salbutamol
    administration, 223
    bronchoconstrictor responses, 220
    bronchodilator responses, 227
salmeterol, 227
sarcoidosis, 266–7, 281, 283
    diffusing capacity, 270
    MEFV curve, *16*
shuttle walk test (SWT), 136–7
sickle-cell disease, 247
    single-breath D$_{LCO}$ measurement, 96–8, *99*, 106, 260–62
single-breath nitrogen expiration test, 89–90
six minute walk test (6MWT), 136–7
sleep, 151–61
    fragmentation, measurement, 157–8
    inspiratory flow limitation, 152
    long-term oxygen therapy, 204
    quality, 155
    rapid eye movement, 61
    respiratory sleep studies, 154–61
    study equipment, 159
    ventilatory control, 108–9, 119
smokers
    D$_{LCO}$, 103–4
    effects in pregnancy, 166

FEV$_1$, 12
PaO$_2$, 83
sniff, 20
sniff esophageal pressure (sniff P$_{es}$), 63–4
sniff nasal pressure (sniff P$_{na}$), 62–3
sniff transdiaphragmatic pressure (sniff P$_{di}$), 64
snoring, 155
    ventilatory control, 119
spirogram, *5*
spirometry, 4–7
    asthma, 181
    instruments, 10–11
    post-transplantation, 242
    pressure-volume curve/compliance, 47, *48*
    reference values, 12, 292–3
sulfur dioxide, 222
sulfur hexafluoride (SF$_6$), 18, 99
sustained pressure development, 69–70
systemic lupus erythematosus (SLE), 249–50, 271, 277
systemic sclerosis, 267

terbutaline
    administration, 223
    bronchoconstrictor responses, 220
    bronchodilator responses, 227
theophylline, 227
thermal dye technique, 195
thoracic gas volume (TGV), 10, 29, 52
thoracic surgery, 234–44
thoraco-abdominal compression technique, 174, *175*
three-compartment gas exchange model, 82–3
threshold loaded breathing, 71–2
tidal breathing
    infants, 174
    measurement, 109–10
    of nebulized agents, 223
tidal flow-volume curves, 20–22
    bronchodilation, 230
    infants, *172*
tonsillar hypertrophy, 181
total lung capacity (TLC), 4, 9, 50, 53
    and airflow resistance, 29, 31
    asthma, 55
    infants, 174
    post-pneumonectomy, 235
    reduction, 4
total lung resistance (R$_L$), 28, 39
    distribution, *39*
    esophageal balloon catheter measurement, 32–4

total respiratory compliance (C$_{rs}$), 45, *46*, 49
total respiratory resistance (R$_{rs}$), 28
    forced oscillation measurement, 34–6
    infants, 171
trachea
    auscultation, 180
    stenosis, 15
tracheostomy-intermittent positive pressure ventilation (T-IPPV), 210
transcutaneous electrical stimulation, 65
transdiaphragmatic pressure, 66, 111
transfer factor *see* diffusing capacity
transitional dyspnea index (TDI), 123–4
transpulmonary pressure, 47, 49
treadmills, 137
tussigens, 230
twitch mouth pressure, 67

UCSD (University of California, San Diego) Shortness of Breath Questionnaire, 124
upper airway
    narrowing, 152–3
    obstruction (nasal polyps), 181
    resistance, 39–41
    shunt, 35
upstream conductance, 17
uvulopalatopharyngoplasty (UPPP), 155

venous admixture (physiological shunt) compartment, 83, 187–8
ventilation
    assisted, 209–12
    continuous mandatory, 186
    control *see* ventilatory control
    demands of exercise, 134
    distribution, infants, 178
    domiciliary, 210–11
    failure, 186
    maldistribution, 89–90
    maximum voluntary, 5, 6–7, 69
    measurement during exercise, 137–40
    minute, 109–10
    mouthpiece, 210
    nasal intermittent positive pressure, 209–10
    negative pressure, 210
    weaning, 194
ventilation/perfusion mismatching, 81–2
    measuring, 88–91
    respiratory muscle weakness, 61

ventilation/perfusion (V_A/Q) ratio, 81–2
    posture, 188–9
ventilation/perfusion scans, 90–91
ventilatory control, 107–20
    assessing, 109–15
    breathing patterns, 115
    carbon dioxide, 111–12
    chemosensitivity, 111–13
    in disease, 105–9
    exercise, 109
    feedback, 108–9
    in health, 108–9
    infants, 178–9
    mechanical loading, 113–15, 116
    response to CO_2, 111–12
    response to hypercapnia, 111–13
    response to hypoxia, 111–13
    sleep, 108–9, 119
    tests, 112–13

Venturi masks, 207
visual analogue scale
    dyspnea, 125, *126*, 127
    exercise testing, 138–40
vital capacity (slow [relaxed] vital capacity), 4–6, *5*
    best tests/repeatability, 11
    chest wall disease, 181
    in disease, 54–5
    forced (FVC), 4–6, 9, 11
    intensive care, 189
    post-pneumonectomy, 234–5
    postural effects, 53
    reference values, 12
    respiratory muscles, 60–61

Wegener's granulomatosis, 248–9

Yan method, 223

RC
734
.P84
H84
1999

DATE DUE

RC
734
.P84
H84
1999

SOUTH UNIVERSITY
709 MALL BLVD.
SAVANNAH, GA 31406

SOUTH UNIVERSITY
709 MALL BLVD.
SAVANNAH, GA 31406